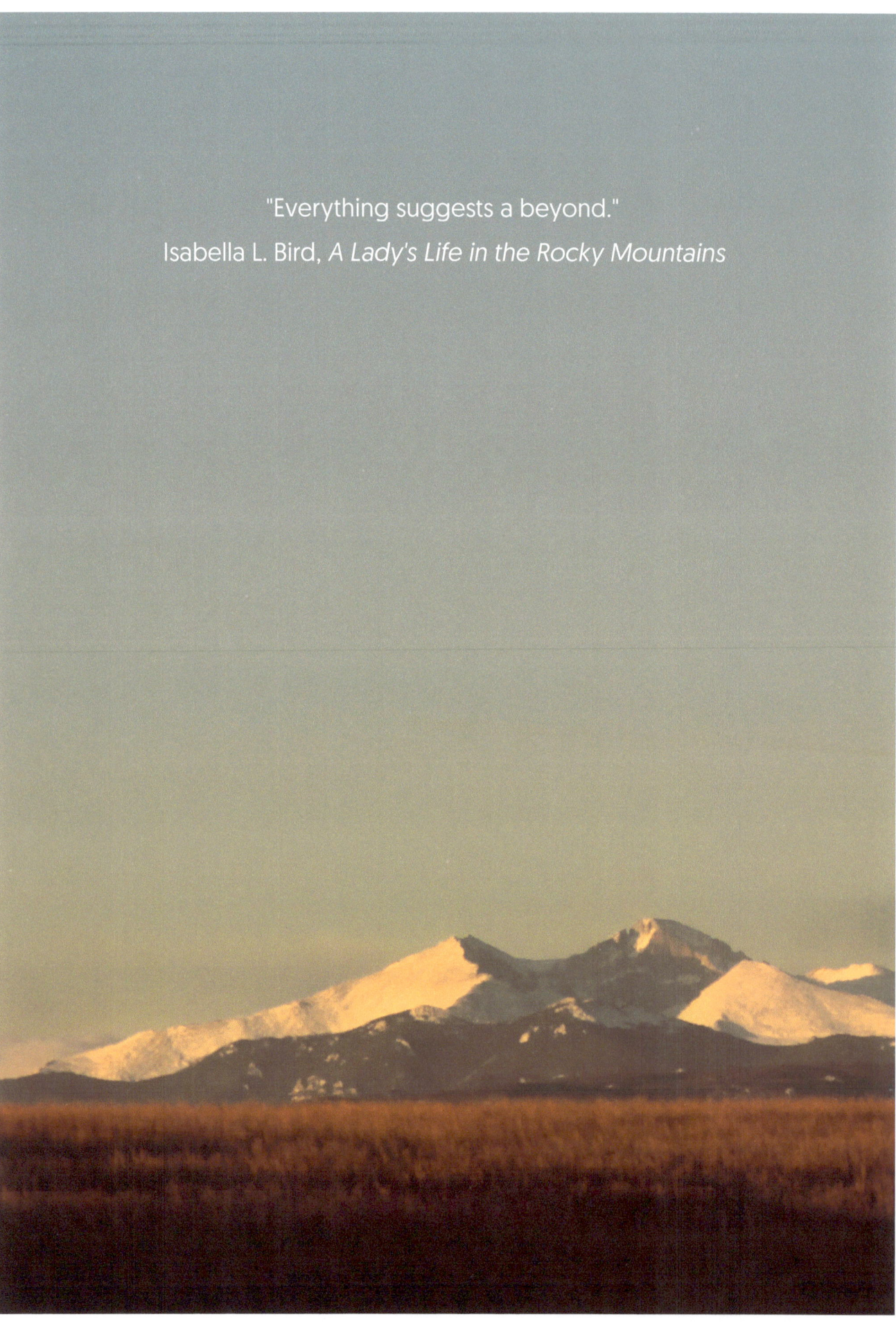

"Everything suggests a beyond."
Isabella L. Bird, *A Lady's Life in the Rocky Mountains*

Food ELEVATED

100 Recipes for Colorful Cooking from the Colorado Front Range

Lisa Boesen

Designed by Erin Dyer

ELEVATED PUBLICATIONS
© 2021 by Lisa A. Boesen
All rights reserved
Published in the United States by
Elevated Publishing
Fort Collins, CO
www.itsyourseason.life

Jacket Design and Layout by Lisa A. Boesen and Erin M. Dyer
Photography by Lisa A. Boesen and Susan M. Dyer

LIBRARY OF CONGRESS
CATALOGING-IN-PUBLICATION DATA.
Boesen, Lisa. A.
Food ELEVATED
100 Colorful Recipes from the Colorado Front Range
Lisa A. Boesen – 1st ed.
p.cm.
ISBN (Hardcover): ISBN 978-0-578-83430-6
PRINTED IN THE UNITED STATES OF AMERICA
First Edition

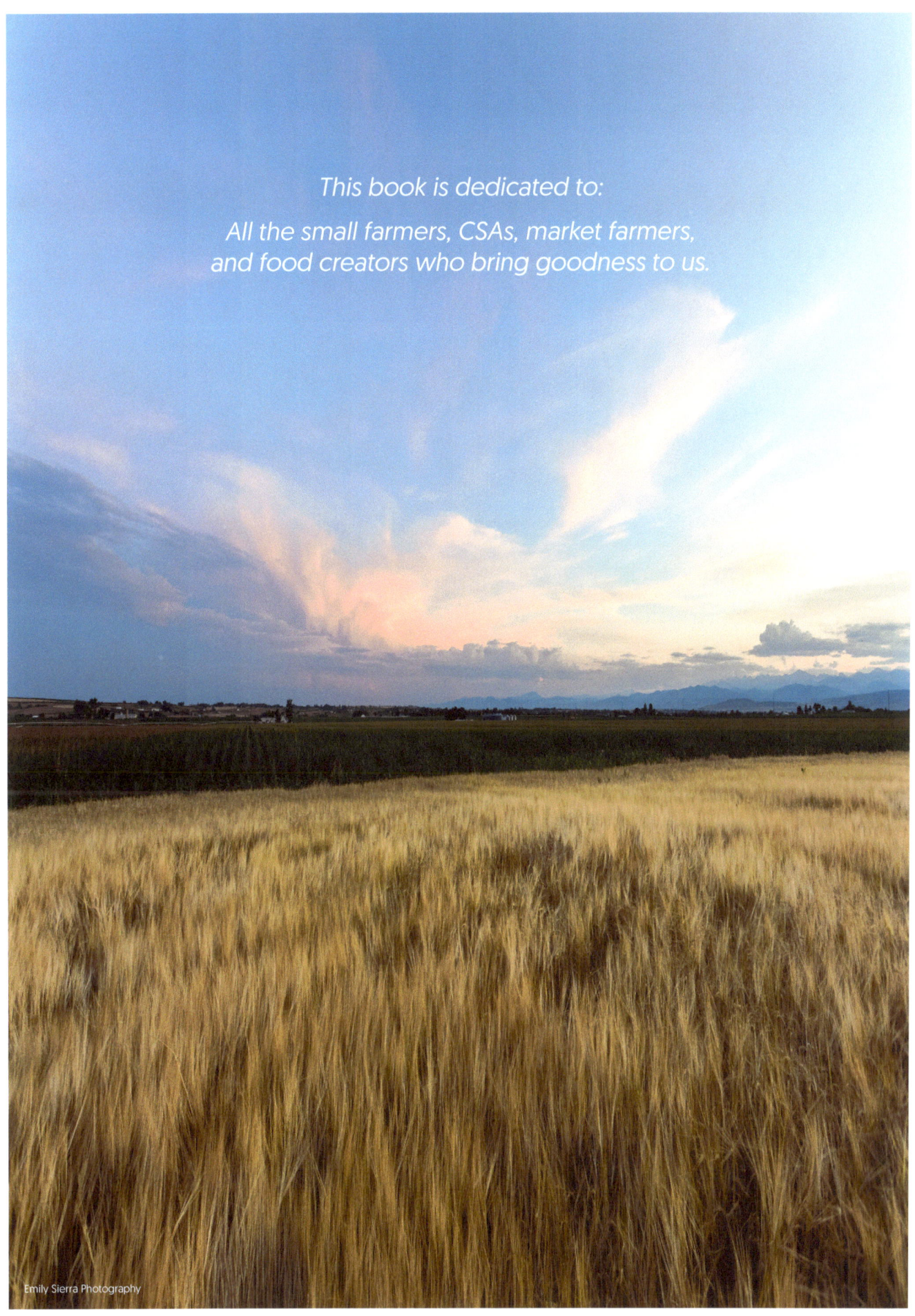

This book is dedicated to:

All the small farmers, CSAs, market farmers, and food creators who bring goodness to us.

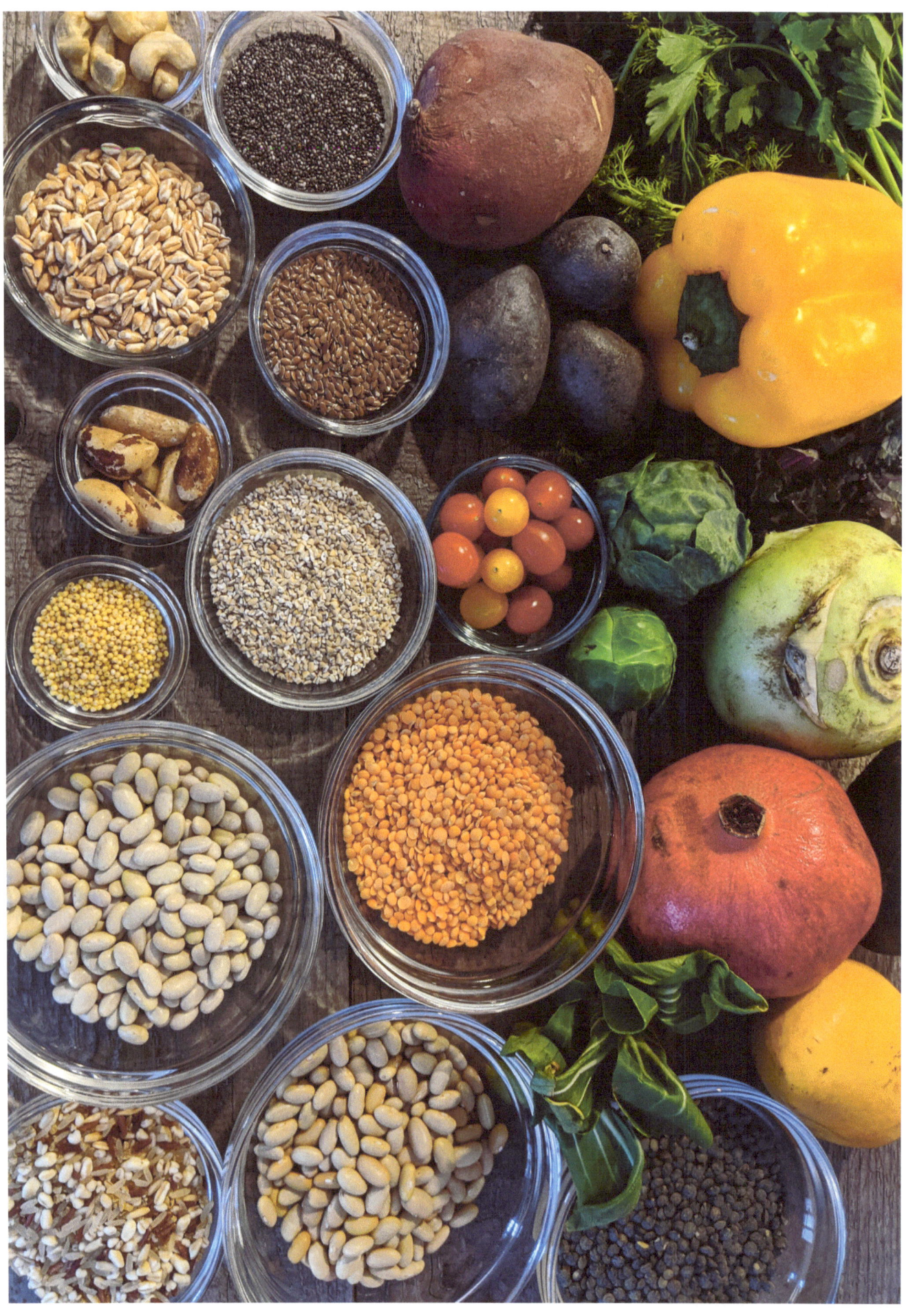

Table of Contents

Recipe List 9
About the Author 10
The Team 11
Acknowledgments 12
Introduction 13
How to Use This Cookbook 14
Measurements/Abbreviations & Serving Sizes 14
Resources 15
SPRING 17
SUMMER 47
AUTUMN 91
WINTER 127
Cuisine-Related Herb, Aromatic, Spice, Nut & Seed Pairings 167
ELEVATIONS: Simple Tips for Brightening Any Dish 168
Beer Pairings 170
Wine Pairings 171

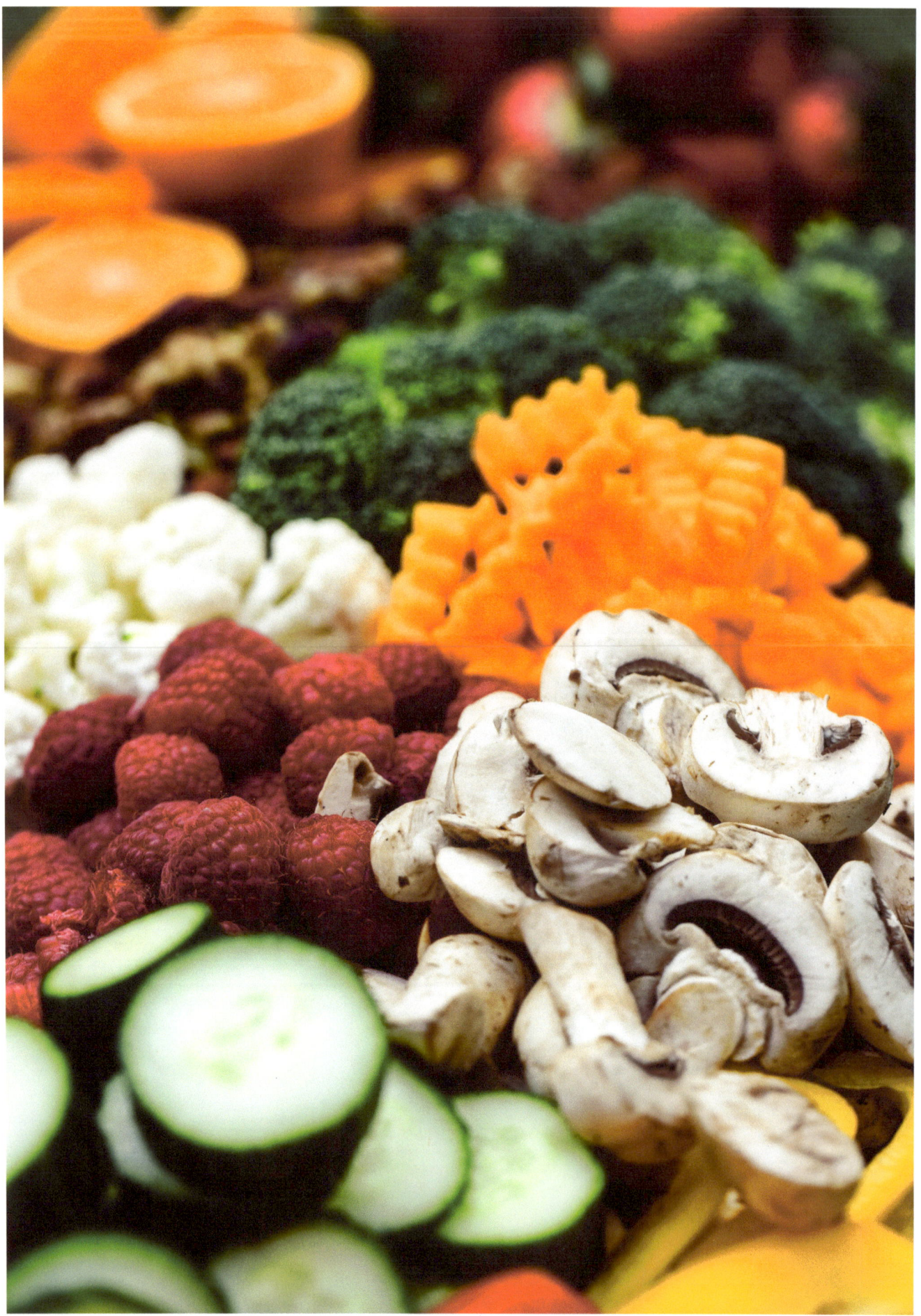

Recipe List

SPRING

Earth Day Three Pea Salad 19
Radish Pea Potsticker Salad 20
Cilantro Green Dip 21
Avocado Pea Mash w/ Plantain Chips 22
Quinoa Millet Pea Bowl 23
Cauliflower Chickpea Green Bean Salad 24
Front Range Niçoise Salad 25
Israeli Couscous Mushroom Bean Soup 27
Mushroom Stem Vegetable Broth 28
Skillet Asparagus w/ Panko Almond Crumbs 31
Roasted Carrots w/ Furikake 32
Perfect Green Beans 33
Fresh Fava Beans w/ Garlic, Mint & Cumin 34
Cinnamon Cap Mushroom Vegetable Medley 35
Italian Grilled Oyster Mushrooms w/ Garlic Chive Pappardelle 36
Conical Morels in White Wine Cream Sauce 37
Buckwheat Crêpes w/ Mushroom Asparagus Cream Sauce 38
Brussels Sprout Asparagus Sugar Pea Stir Fry 40
Creamy Sage Orzo w/ Asparagus & Peas 41
Picnic on the Poudre 42
Rhubarb Two Ways 44

SUMMER

Ramen Noodle Revival 49
Simple Salad with Grated Garlic Dressing 50
Black-eyed Pea Salad w/ Cabbage 52
Heirloom Tomato Salad 56
Grilled Squash w/ Miso & Sesame Glaze 58
Chupe de Elote y Papas 59
Sardinian Saffron Fregola w/ Potatoes & Peas 60
Tri-Color Peppers Three Ways 62
Three Herbs & Sumac Potatoes 65
Potatoes w/ Fennel & Onion 66
Miso Pepper Potatoes 67
Succotash w/ a Twist 68
Smoked Cauliflower & Chickpea Spinach Wrap 70
Basil Pesto w/ Your Choice of Pasta 72
Saffron Pasta w/ Fresh Tomato Sauce 74
Baby Gnocchi Three Ways 75
Award-Winning Red Chili Sauce 76
Eggplant Parmesan 78
Roasted Tomatoes & Mushrooms in Brandy Cream Sauce 81
Albaloo Polo 83
Rustic Peach Crumble 85

AUTUMN

A Tasting of Beets Three Ways 93
Kale, Pear, Candied Garlic, Almond & Honey Salad 95
Apple Parsnip Salad 99
Pumpkin Peanut Soup 102
Kohlrabi Bean Barley Soup 103
Purple Carrot Soup Two Ways 104
Cream of Cauliflower & Carrot Soup 106
Pumpkin Flatbreads 107
Traditional German Rotkohl 108
Super Simple Sauerkraut 110
Sweet Dumpling Squash w/ Ras Al Hanout, Candied Ginger & Dried Fruit 111
Parsnips & Pears 112
Smoked Garlic 113
Patatas y Garbanzos en Pimentón 113
Lentils w/ Celeriac Truffle Purée 114
Indian Cabbage w/ Turmeric and Peas 115
Aspen Moon Farm Polenta w/ Roasted Grape Tomatoes 117
Butternut Squash Potato Tofu Curry 118
Pasta with Pumpkin Cream Sauce 119
French Apple Pie 120
Chocolate Beet Cupcakes 123
Honey Lavender Roasted Italian Plums 124
Cast Iron Skillet Honey Roasted Apples 125

WINTER

Microgreen Gremolata, Pistou & Pesto 129
Toum 130
Roasted Shiitakes Two Ways 131
Greens, Grains & Veg Goodness 132
Vegetable Barley Soup 134
Kale, Bean, Potato & Marjoram Soup 136
Porcini White Bean Rosemary Soup 138
Parsnip Carrot Latkes 139
Smoky Acorn Squash w/ Pomegranate & Feta 140
Kurbis Stumfus 141
French Style Lettuce & Peas 142
Indian Saffron Potatoes in Coconut Milk 143
Delicata Squash w/ Apricots, Poms & Pecans 144
Sage Roasted Shiitakes 145
Roasted Brussels Sprouts w/ Amaretto Cherries 146
Golden Pumpkin Chips 147
Pumpkin Ravioli 148
Espinacas con Garbanzos 150
Butternut Squash, Toasted Lentils & Poms 151
Colorado Smoked Green Chili 154
Mushroom Parmentier 156
Foul Mudammas 159
Kolaches 162
Kolache Fillings Two Ways and Pocepka Topping 164

LEARNING PAGES

The Elusive Morel & More 26
Age of Asparagus 30
Strawberries 101 54
Cherries, Zen & Now 82
Peach Perfect 84
Tomatoes, Corn & Melons, Oh My! 86
Honey Bee FAQs 88
It's About Garlic 94
Apple Me This 96
Keep Squash & Carry On 100
The Beet Goes On 122
Beans – They're What's For Dinner 152
Health for the Holidays 160

About the Author

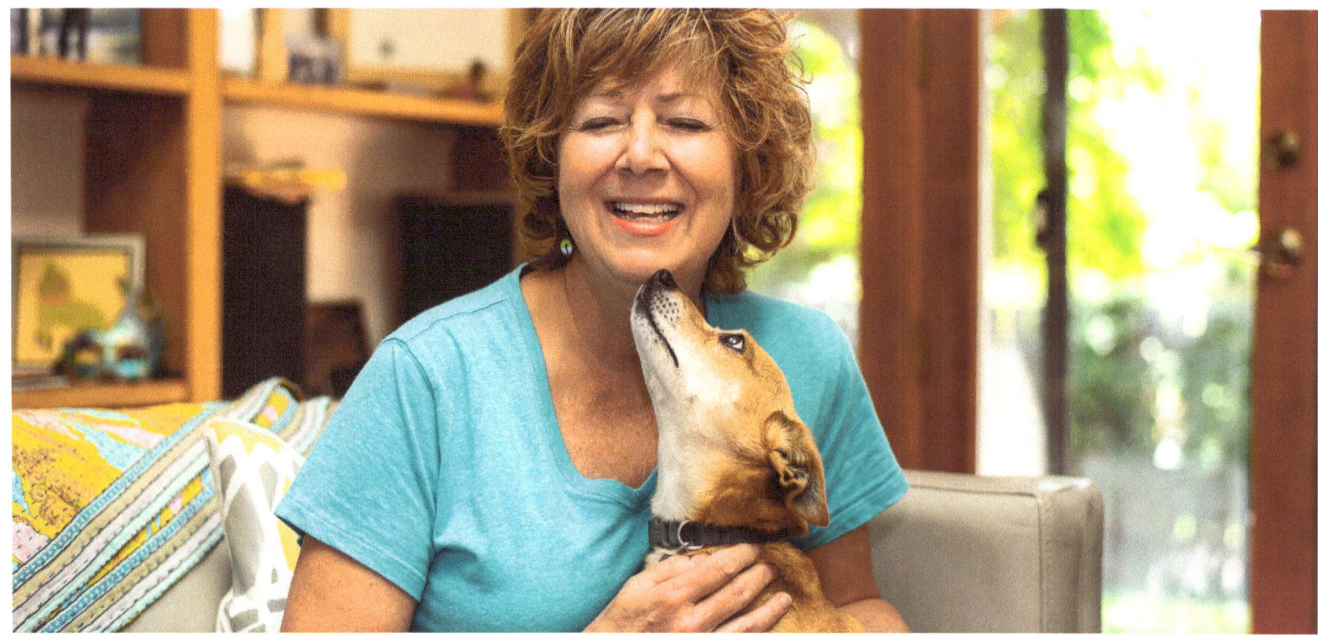

Lisa is a professional speaker, writer, home chef, podcaster, and beekeeper based in Fort Collins, Colorado. Weaving musings about beekeeping, she presents workshops, videos, and chats centered around a healthful lifestyle, self-care, and simple living.

Lisa has been writing since the age of 12, and has studied the art of cooking for over 50 years and counting. She aims for each dish to offer an original taste and unique learning experience. She attended pasta making classes in Italy, completed the Forks Over Knives® plant-based cooking course, and has poured over hundreds of cookbooks and lessons in research of the science of cooking and presentation for the home cook. She flexes her creativity by peering inside the pantry and refrigerator of a relative's house, and transforming their current selection of ingredients into a delicious and nutritious meal.

From marrying pears and parsnips and revisiting the sugar beet industry, to experimenting with herbs, wild and cultivated mushrooms, and purple carrots, Lisa invites you to discover the culinary magic of the Northern Colorado region. You will learn easily accessible, primarily plant-based recipes and techniques as you take pause to enjoy the visual beauty of the fruits and goodness of the Earth.

Lisa has over 40 years of experience in the healthcare industry, including cardiac and pulmonary rehabilitation program management, Human Resources, and Performance Improvement. She holds a Master's Degree in Organizational Management and is a Certified Master Coach. She can be found at *www.ItsYourSeason.Life*, and on Facebook, Twitter, YouTube, Podbean, Instagram, Pinterest, and LinkedIn.

Follow along in *Food ELEVATED* as Lisa shares a visual exploration of Northern Colorado and guides the taste of the region from her kitchen to yours.

◉ @itsyourseason.life	▶ Lisa Boesen	◉ @itsyourseason.life	in linkedin.com/in/lisaboesen
🐦 @lboesen2	🎙 itsyourseason.podbean.com	📌 pinterest.com/lisaboesen	🔗 itsyourseason.life

The Team

This book would not have come to fruition without the team. Erin, in particular, gave many, many—hundreds of—hours and a personal commitment to this project. The cookbook received substance and character through her design, editing, and careful placing of photos. She is my Imagineer!

I am also fortunate to have friends who are wine and beer connoisseurs, who gave their time and talent to this project!

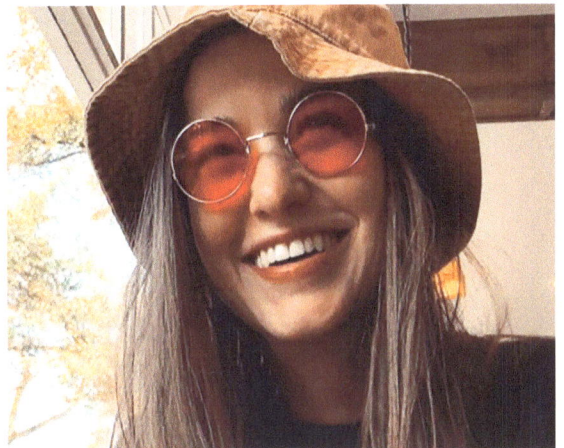

Erin Dyer, BFA

Erin is a graphic designer, illustrator, and photographer from Houston, Texas. She received a BFA in Communications and a minor in Psychology from Texas State University, and a degree in Digital Communication/Graphic Design from Houston Community College. Erin currently resides in Sacramento, California – America's Farm-to-Fork Capital. Her interests include music, thrift shopping, eco-consciousness, the human brain, mental health, and all creative arts. Erin was vegetarian for many years and is vegan since 2016. She loves to support local plant-based restaurants, and is always experimenting with nourishing nosh in her kitchen. Follow her work at *erin-dyer.com*

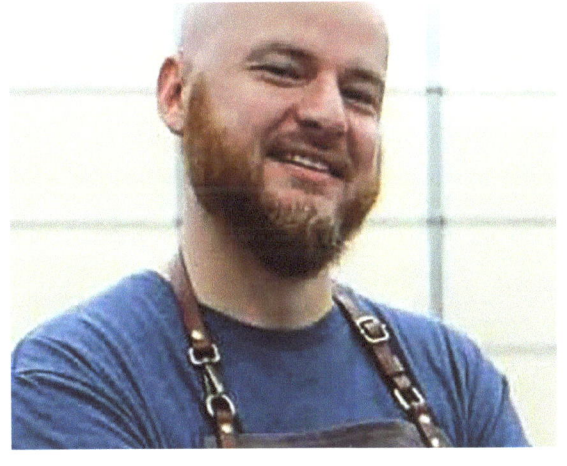

Justin Kruger

Justin is a classically trained chef originally from the Northwest, working at various restaurants including under Chef Tyler Florence in California. His passion and food focus is sustainable local products, as well as contributing the important community work of giving at-risk youth a chance at learning culinary skills. He is an expert homebrewer and loves sharing craft beer with anyone who has the time to spare. He is one half of Two Fat Justins Catering Company (*twofatjustins.com*).

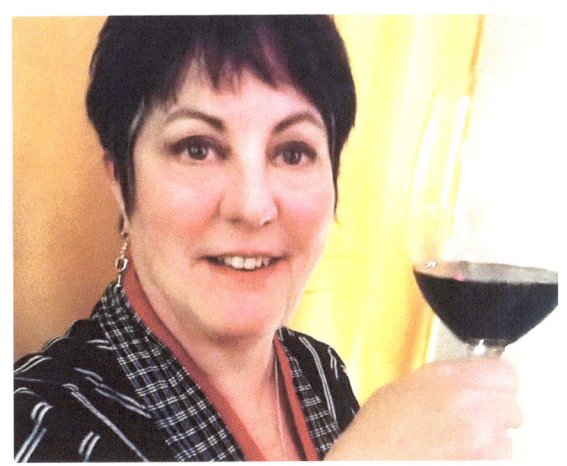

Ann Rawlinson, Sommelier, CMS

Ann is a good cook, a good skier, and knows something about wine. She is a certified Sommelier through the Court of Master Sommeliers, and formerly the sommelier at Wisconsin's premier 5 Diamond, 5 Star resort – The American Club Resort. Ms. Rawlinson now lives in Fort Collins, Colorado, in order to be closer to her son, who is a restaurateur in Summit County. With 300 sunny days annually in Colorado, her favorite quaff in the summer, spring, and fall? Rosé! It goes with everything, especially vegetarian dishes.

Acknowledgements

As with many creative projects, there is a backstage crew. I am most thankful to my husband, Mike, for supporting me, and being my editor and balancing act. And strangely, I am giving a weird, brief nod to cancer that put us on this journey of eating and living healthier.

To my friend Judith Sevel, who helped me with the editing (multiple times).

To my friend Susan Dyer – editor, photographer, motivator, confidant, and 20-year supporter extraodinaire. A friend who makes life beautiful with her camera and heart.

To my social tribe, who joined me for food chats, shared their garden glories, and provided challenges and inspiration as I worked on this cookbook. This group of women is always up for a Northern Colorado experience, which has provided me with adventures whenever and wherever we go.

To the following folks who gave me hours of their time – sharing stories, photographing their produce, gardens and farms and assistance with editing. Over the last two years, I have learned so much from the following contributors:

- *The Spice and Tea Exchange® Fort Collins* – The owners took a chance and collaborated with me on my first launch at tastings! The project worked and I am forever grateful.

- *On the Vine at Richmond Farms* – Just a lovely couple! They tolerated my impromptu visits to take photos and to enjoy a pause amidst their strawberry fields.

- *Gardens on Spring Creek* – For partnering with me on workshops. The Gardens are a wonderful place to learn about Northern Colorado gardening – they offer fantastic events, and provide a beautiful environment in which to enjoy your surroundings and renew your mind.

- *The Fort Collins Senior Center* – For partnering with me on live and virtual engagements, to share our experiences and promote a primarily plant-based lifestyle. The staff has been superb!

- *FarmFresh CSA* – For providing me with fresh produce for recipes, and many of the photographs presented in this cookbook.

- *Clint Johnson* – For his time in sharing stories about his family's farming history.

- *Walt Rosenbery* – For the personal tour of his Masonville Apple Orchards, and for sharing his love for all things apple!

- *Nathan Meyer, The Colorado Peach Company* – For his willingness to review and edit the Peach Perfect learning page.

Food unites us. May it continue to do so!

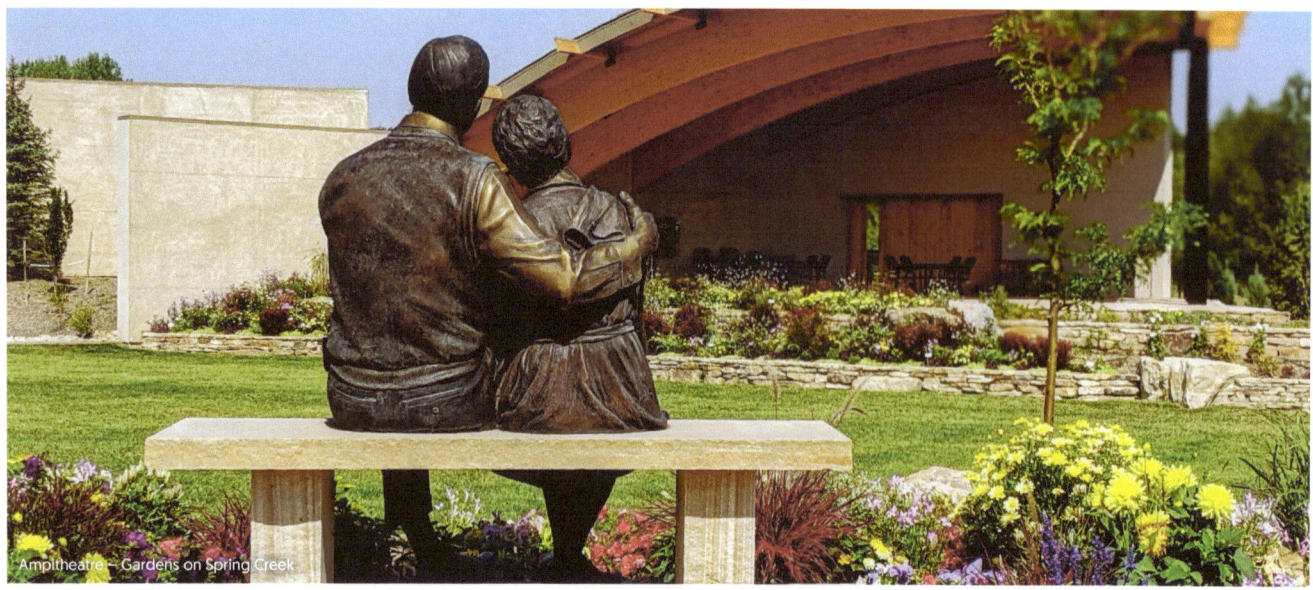

Ampitheatre – Gardens on Spring Creek

Introduction

As I wrote this cookbook, I realized I had been cooking for over 50 years. Over half a century! I started with Julia Child in the 1960s, The Galloping Gourmet *in the 1970s, witnessed the advent of* The Food Network, *and of course, I always had my mom in the kitchen. As a household with both parents working outside the home, my family progressed from the excitement of Banquet TV dinners and Swanson pot pies to—gasp—frozen pizza and the microwave. Prepared and packaged foods were always at our beck and call. My mother was a home economics teacher, and we learned all sorts of ways to assemble food for a dish, but not necessarily how to check a broccoli floret for doneness. Fast forward to 2021 – here we are with purple carrots, orange cauliflower, and learning to prepare and enjoy the goodness of the earth.*

How This Started

My husband and I live in Fort Collins, Colorado – about 60 miles north of Denver. It is nestled along the Poudre River and butts up against the first line of foothills, a.k.a. Front Range, where the Poudre River flows out of the Rockies. On a clear day, you can see the layers of hills and eventually Longs Peak, Mount Meeker, the Mummy Range, and others. For over a century this area has been an agricultural goldmine, brought to fruition in a mostly arid climate through a maze of irrigation ditches that still crisscross many planned neighborhoods, and an ingenuity that brought water to the area by tunneling under the Continental Divide. One can still envision the many farms, and imagine how fertile and active this area of Colorado was generations ago. Small farms still abound, showing the desire of others to till the land, pasture animals, and raise crops in a sustainable manner. Northern Colorado manifests itself in many CSAs (Community Supported Agriculture), market farms, and raised beds that dot the front and backyards of many a home.

What This Book Is

- *Part Recipe and Technique Book* – What do I do with that sweet dumpling squash, parsnip, or purple carrot? How do I tell when green beans are done?
- *Part History Book* – Let's appreciate the agricultural history of the area, and everyone who is currently working hard to create a sustainable and regenerative food environment.
- *Part Photo Album* – Preparing and eating plants is colorful. Adding more plants to a lifestyle may be a mindbender. Let's embed those colors into our memory banks!
- *Part Visual Visit to Northern Colorado* – Walk with me through our gardens, markets, and unique vendors.
- *A Movement to Support Our Local Farmers* – How about the dozens of varieties of apples, local asparagus, and 10 varieties of garlic?

I do not want this book to be the definitive answer to questions about Northern Colorado cuisine or recipes. It is to be a touchstone so visitors reading this book can get a feel for the beauty of the area, and the difficulties of raising vegetables in soil that looks like caliche – in an area that has a very short growing season, droughts, fires and—yes—perhaps even a flood.

This book is written within the context of the four seasons, and includes a bit about what is occurring in Northern Colorado. You will receive a colorful brushing of history in each season, annual events highlighted and of course, recipes that you can adjust for your area, your shopping, and your taste.

What is Front Range Cuisine?

In my opinion, Colorado does not have a "cuisine," per se. The food of Colorado is an amalgamation of Hispanic, Native American, and cuisine mixes from early settlers and immigrants—such as the English, Swedish, Italians, and Germans from Russia—as well as the inclusion of other new international culinary cuisines brought to this area. We are known for our cattle, lamb, and dairy industries. Colorado is also privy to some of the most beautiful farmers markets and Community Supported Agriculture (CSA) bounties that are sustaining themselves at different elevations and terroir.

This book focuses primarily on Colorado fruits, grains, and vegetables. You may choose to add some wonderful responsibly-raised local meat or fish as a side to anything in this cookbook. What else should you focus on? Freshness. And seasonal items, if possible. Sharing history and new cuisines. Simple techniques. Interesting, accessible tastes. Herbs and spices as culinary friends. Ideally in this order. Enjoy!

How to Use This Cookbook

Let's talk about the elephant in the room... plants are good for you. There is always room at the table for anyone who wants to eat more plants. Although my husband and I are primarily plant-based, I am not recommending any one lifestyle or eating pattern except – let's just eat more veg! My hope is that you discover ways to eat more fruits, grains, and veg—and along the way—figure out what works for you. My goal as a home chef and writer is to introduce you to different ways to add, cook, and elevate the fruits of the earth.

By the time you have completed all of the dishes in this cookbook, you may have learned a thing or two, such as the following:

Cooking Techniques
- Experiment with several new veggies and grains
- Mash, purée, sauté, steam, pan sear, grill, roast, smoke, parboil, grate, and ferment
- Bake kolaches – why not celebrate occasionally?

Cuisines
Learn how spices, nuts, seeds, and herbs elevate a dish. Test out new ideas and techniques you may have never tried before. I use a lot of saffron – it's worth it. I also reference The Spice and Tea Exchange® spices quite a bit – although they have online ordering, feel free to use mixes from your favorite spice store, or mixes that match what we are doing in the recipe, no pressure.

Usage and Storage Tips
Learn batch prepping techniques and how to keep produce fresh for longer.

Marriage Tips
Nothing personal of course! We can marry a veg with a fruit and have a new dish.

History
Learn about Colorado's agricultural successes and challenges, and appreciate what farmers do to bring goodness to us.

Measurements/Abbreviations
- lb = pound
- oz = ounce
- tbsp = tablespoon
- tsp = teaspoon
- dash = a few sprinkles, no specific measurement

(err on the side of caution – dash to your taste level)

Serving Sizes
Most dishes amount to 2 servings. These can all easily be doubled for 4 servings or more.

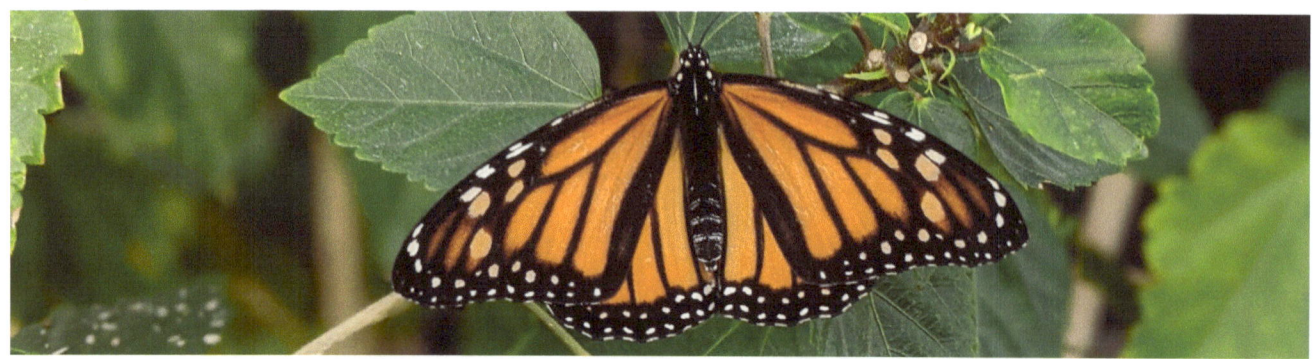

Resources

A very special thanks to the Northern Colorado farmers, vendors and businesses below. Although I may not have been able to include them all in my 100 recipes, I have had the pleasure of using their products and appreciate their efforts to bring goodness to Northern Colorado. This is not an exhaustive list, as monthly we seem to gain more creative options!

- FarmFresh CSA
- Colorado Fresh
- On the Vine at Richmond Farms
- Long Shot Farm
- Hazel Dell Mushrooms
- Hope Mushrooms
- Willow Creek Mushroom Farm
- Sunray Natural
- Sunrise Ranch Farms
- Miller Farms
- Hope Farms
- Pope Farms and Produce and Garden Center
- Raisin' Roots Farm
- Native Hill Farm
- Garden Sweet
- Happy Heart Farm
- Aspen Moon Farm
- Sunspot Urban Farms
- Hoffman Farms
- Masonville Orchards
- EP Greens
- Healthy Harvest Olives
- The Oil Barn
- Rocky Mountain Olive Oil
- Shak Shouka LLC
- Pastamore Gourmet Foods
- Pappardelles Pasta
- Pastificio Boulder
- Mountain Avenue Market
- Turmeric Indian Grocery
- Olive Tree Market
- Root Shoot Malting
- The Spice and Tea Exchange®
- Old Town Spice Shop
- Savory Spice Shop®
- The Cupboard
- Larimer County Farmers Market
- Fort Collins Farmers Market
- Boulder County Farmers Market
- Longmont Farmers Market

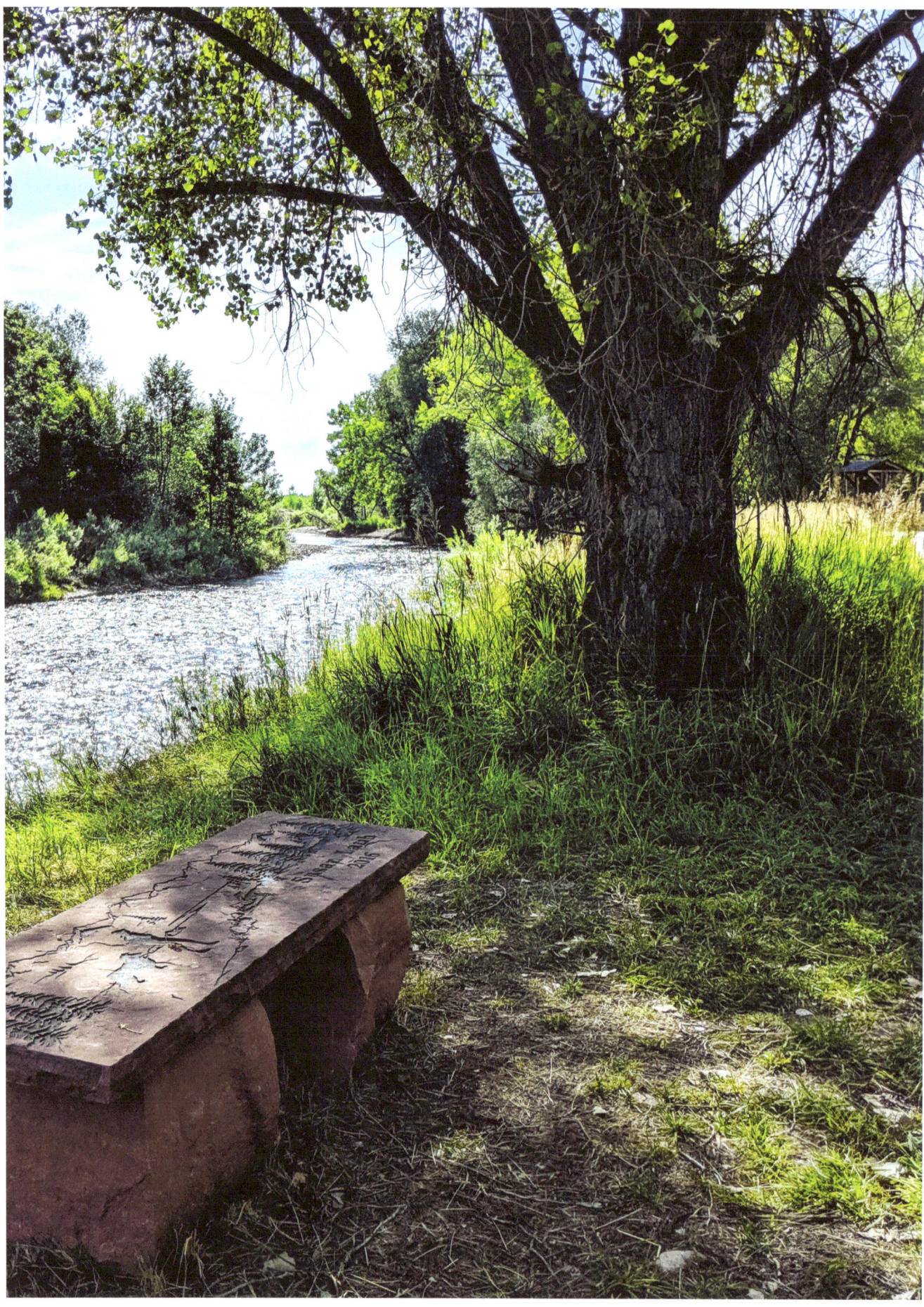

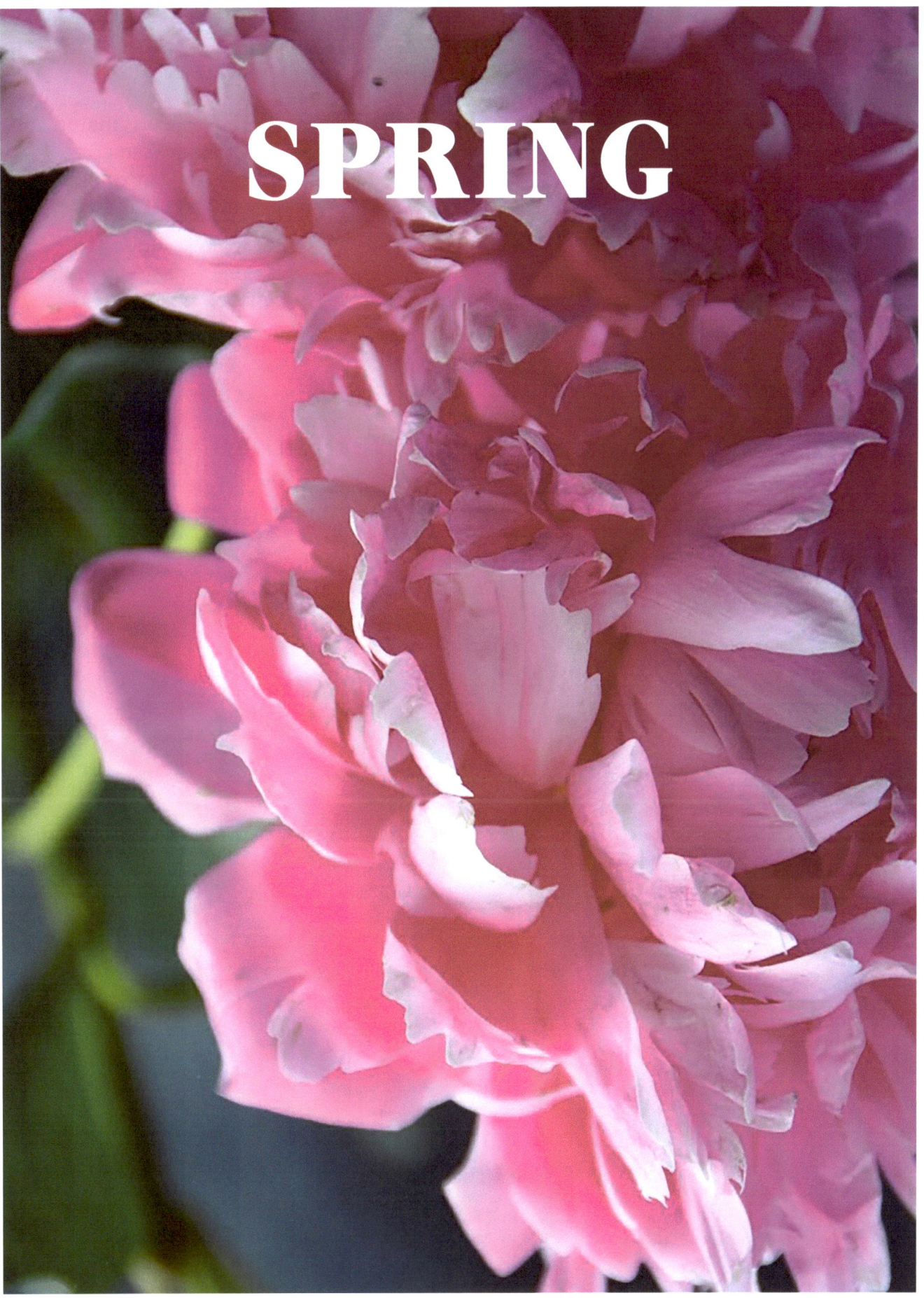

SPRING

The earth awakens. Crocuses are peeking through the snow, and the bees are beginning their early foraging flights. Crimson and pink peonies are popping, garnet irises are standing tall, and the fragrance of lilacs is filling the air. Cyclists on the Poudre River trail are listening to the high mountain snow spring runoff and the gentle hum of Ranch-Way Feed near downtown Fort Collins. Walkers pause and gaze across Cattail Chorus Natural Area looking towards the snow-capped peaks of Mount Meeker and Longs Peak. Others are prepping for rafting and kayaking day trips in late June, or picnics at the river or county open spaces. During the spring season, there are 50 shades of green against a blue sky, snowy mountains, and garden delights.

Home gardening may begin in March with indoor seed-starts. April still brings snow, and the ground is barely manageable. Backyard gardeners here know to hold off planting directly into the ground until after Mother's Day. There is still a danger of frost—or, good heavens—an early June snow storm. Beekeepers are managing nature's ritual of swarming, and the spring farmers markets are open for business.

We are privy to an average of 300 sunny days per year. By June, it is just a few short weeks until the longest day of the year. At this elevation, and as the Spring months dry out and heat up, growth will be quick and there will be something fresh and delicious to eat every week.

What is in store for Spring? Rhubarb, asparagus, lettuce, sugar peas, kale, garlic scapes, carrots, early cauliflower, flowers and herb starts, lettuce, lavender, and later in the season – strawberries.

Ready? Let's greet Spring!

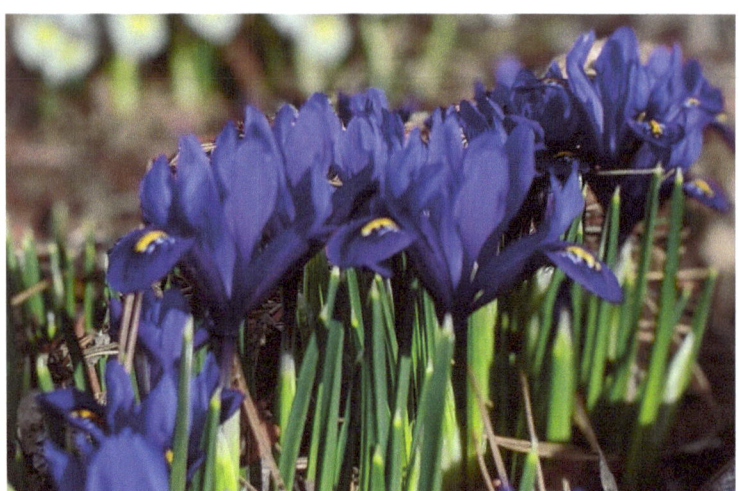
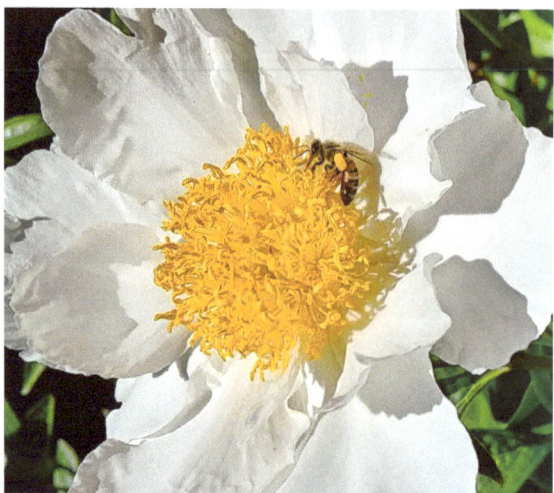
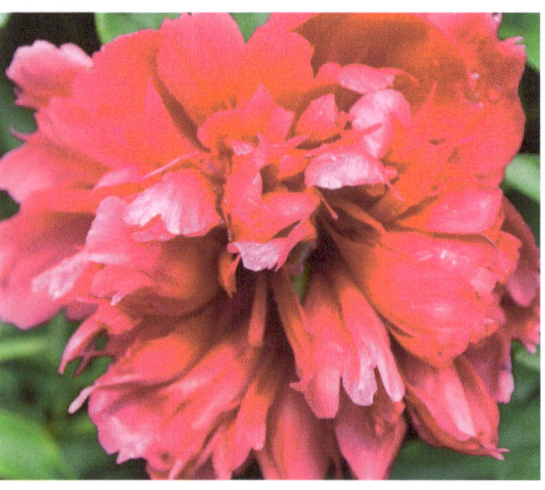
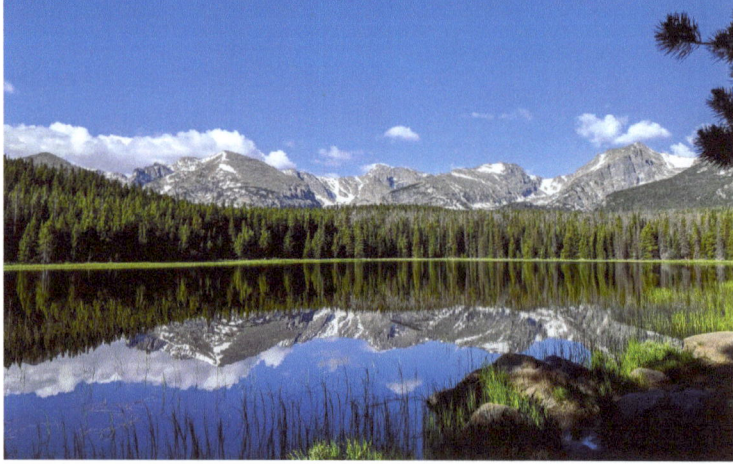

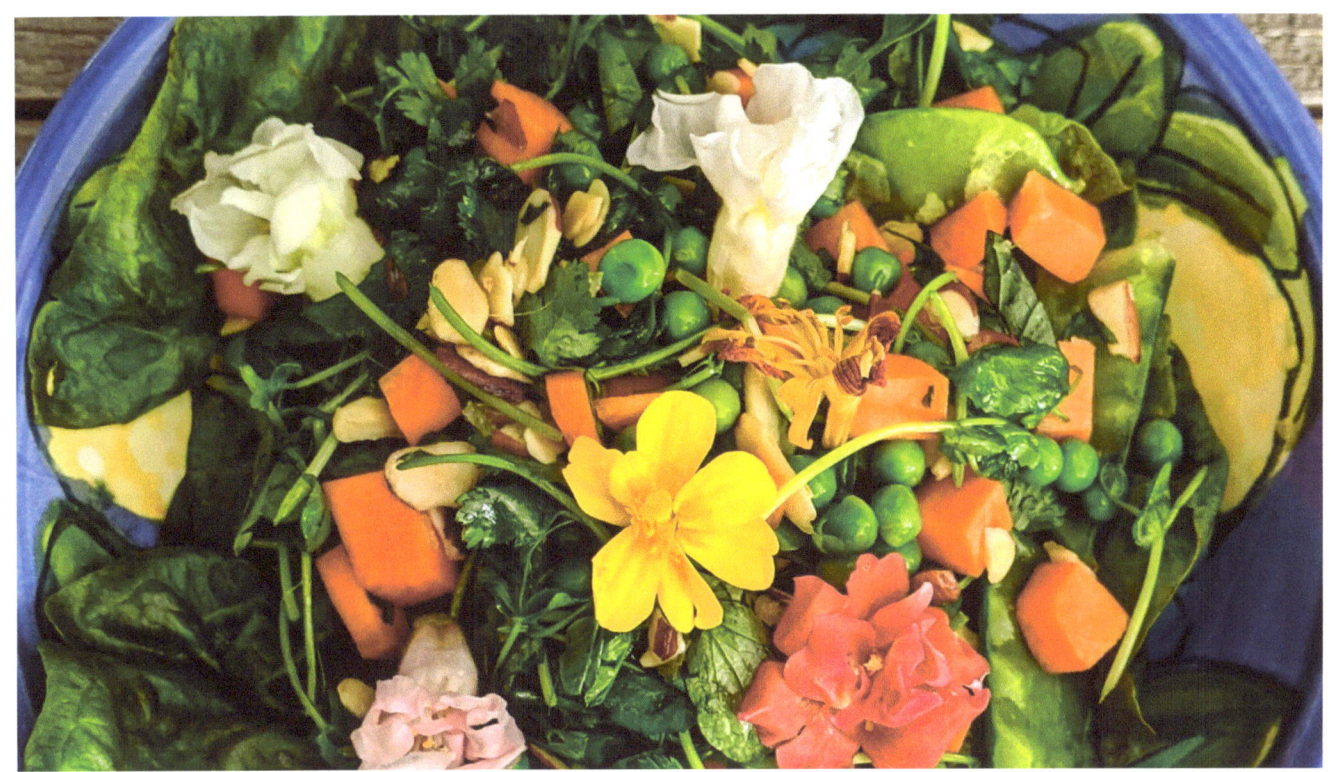

EARTH DAY THREE PEA SALAD

Let's start with an easy but interesting dish – flowers, peas, carrots, and lettuce. Here in Colorado, we may still get one more snow after Earth Day or Mother's Day. A bit later at the market in May, there are fresh peas and gorgeous lettuce heralding in mid-Spring! This lovely lemon design serving dish from the Stark Pottery collection in Longmont compliments the scene.

Ingredients
- 1 medium head of beautiful lettuce
- 1 cup fresh sugar peas
- ½ cup frozen peas, thawed
- 1 handful of pea shoots
- ½ cup diced carrots
- 1 tsp lemongrass mint balsamic vinegar, or your flavored white balsamic vinegar of choice
- 1 tbsp olive oil
- Salt and pepper to taste

For the Garnish
- Chopped mint and/or cilantro
- Fresh edible flowers
- Sliced almonds, toasted or caramelized

Instructions
Assemble vegetables in a bowl.
Whisk the olive oil and balsamic vinegar in another bowl until emulsified. Allow to sit for 5 minutes.
Toss the salad with dressing.
Place in a pretty serving bowl and garnish with chopped mint and/or cilantro, fresh edible flowers, and sliced almonds.
Salt and pepper to taste.

Elevate This: Add some spinach or some locally grown nasturtiums for a bit of bite. And add a spring fruit such as a few sliced, fresh, local strawberries. Less is more.

Serves 2-3 as a salad dish

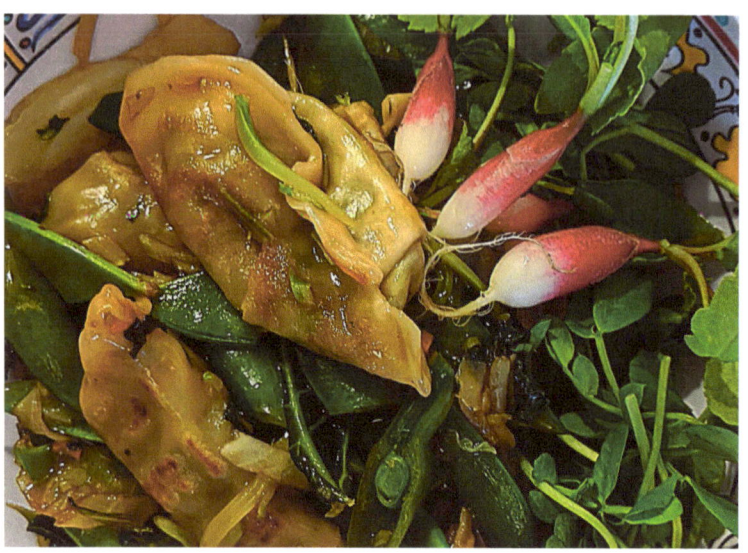
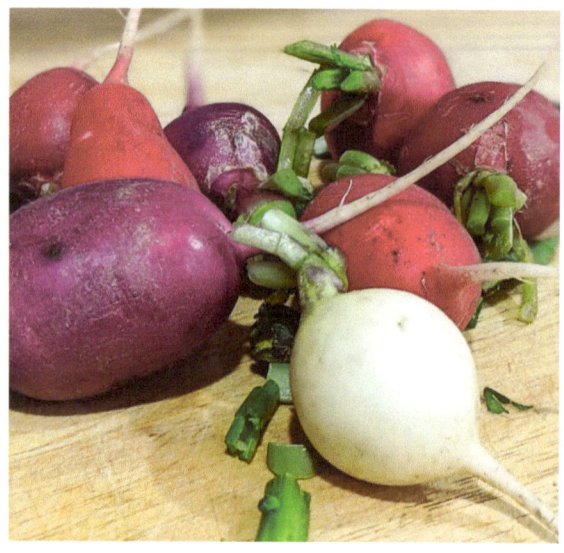

RADISH PEA POTSTICKER SALAD

I love keeping vegetable or vegan potstickers in the freezer. They bring a salad together and are a super easy, quick appetizer. This dish pulls together all the yumminess of the first CSAs and farmers markets in Northern Colorado. Peas, asparagus, kale, bok choy, and other cruciferous spring greens. A vendor gave me a small bag of baby radishes to try, and I'm glad she did.

Ingredients

For the Potsticker Dipping Sauce
- 1 tsp soy sauce
- 1 tsp rice wine vinegar
- 1 tbsp peanut oil
- 1 tsp sugar
- ½ tsp chile oil, sriracha, or Chinese ginger garlic sauce
- 1 tsp cornstarch
- 1 small shake of toasted sesame seed oil (optional)

For the Salad
- 1 tbsp oil
- 6-8 vegetable or vegan potstickers
- 2 cups mix of chopped kale, bok choy, or other cruciferous greens
- ¼ cup water
- 4 asparagus stalks, trimmed and cut into thirds on the diagonal
- 1 handful sugar snap peas
- 1 handful snow peas (optional)
- 6-8 baby radishes, greens intact

Instructions

Mix potsticker dipping sauce ingredients in a small bowl and heat in the microwave for 60 seconds, or until slightly thickened, and set aside.

In a wok or large skillet, heat oil over medium heat. Add potstickers and allow to brown on one side.

Turn over the potstickers. Add the greens and water. Cover and steam for 2-3 minutes.

Uncover the skillet or wok, push the mixture to the side, and place the asparagus and peas in the middle of the pan. Cover and steam for another 2 minutes. Add a tablespoon more of water if necessary.

Uncover. Add the dipping sauce to the middle of the pan. Increase the heat and allow the sauce to thicken. Toss well.

Divide the mixture into two bowls, and artfully place the potstickers and radishes on top.

Elevate This: Top with toasted almond slices, chopped cashews, or peanuts. Sprinkle with toasted white and black sesame seeds. Crispy seasoned shiitake mushrooms or wonton strips will add some crunch. Serve over rice to serve 3-4.

Serves 2 as a salad dish

CILANTRO GREEN DIP

Cilantro grows very well here in the cooler months of spring and summer, except in my garden, of course. But fortunately the CSAs and market vendors bring bunches of beautiful cilantro to their stalls. Cilantro crosses quite a few cuisine boundaries, including: Mexican, Southwest or TexMex, Asian, Indian, Thai, Chinese, Caribbean, Mediterranean, North African, and Eastern European. This dip elevates any dish – it is hard not to put on everything. It is so good I gave it its own page. If it gets you eating more veg, then, yeah!

Ingredients
- 1 bunch of cilantro, stems and all
- ½ cup mayonnaise (regular or vegan)
- ½ cup milk (dairy or non-dairy, almond milk or cashew almond milk work best)
- 3 tbsp Hidden Valley Ranch dressing; or 1 tsp garlic powder, 1 tsp onion powder, and 1 tbsp dried parsley
- Juice of ½ lime, or 1 tbsp bottled lime juice
- ¼ cup jarred jalapeño slices
- 1 tbsp jalapeño brine from the jar, or white vinegar

Instructions
Place all ingredients in a blender and blend until creamy. Adjust seasonings to your taste – you may want less or more. Some like it spicier, and others not so much.

Serve with anything, but I recommend vegetables. My favorites are steamed baby potatoes and sugar snap peas.

Helpful Tip: For vegetable trays, some vegetables taste better parboiled rather than raw. Broccoli florets can be steamed in the microwave for two minutes to brighten the color. Rinse in cool water to stop the cooking process, drain to dry, or wrap in dish towel. Wrap asparagus in wet paper towels and microwave for one minute. Rinse, drain, let dry. The same goes for sugar snap peas – 30 seconds or so will do the trick to brighten their color, while keeping their sweetness and texture.

Elevate This: Try a touch of fresh Thai basil and/or a dash of locally made fermented hot sauce.

Makes 1 cup

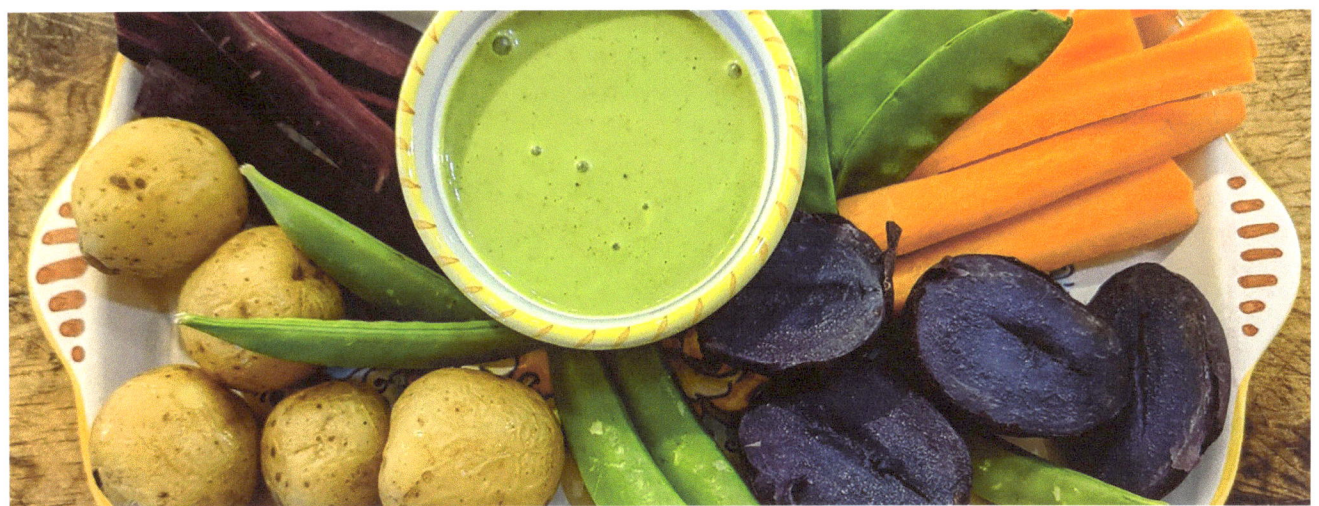

AVOCADO PEA MASH WITH PLANTAIN CHIPS

This mash was the Palate Pleaser course at my first primarily plant-based tasting event at The Spice and Tea Exchange® Fort Collins. I love this recipe because it takes a familiar food that we all know and love—guacamole—and creates a new face for the dish. It's green and refreshing to look at – and the frozen peas give a luscious sweetness, balance, and a bit of "fluff."

Ingredients
- 1 ripe avocado, halved and scooped
- ½ cup frozen green peas; thawed, or microwaved on low for 30 seconds
- ½ tsp lemon juice
- 1 tsp The Spice and Tea Exchange® adobo mix
- 2 tsp olive oil
- 10-12 multi-colored grape tomatoes, quartered

Instructions
Blend the first three ingredients until smooth in a food processor or mash well with a fork for a rustic look. Mix the adobo mix and olive oil in a bowl. Add the tomatoes and allow to marinate for 30 minutes. Serve tomatoes alongside the avocado pea mash. (Alternatively, create a well in the middle of the mash and place the tomatoes in the indention.) Serve in a bowl with plantain chips.

Elevate This: Serve with more fresh vegetables – there can never be enough fresh veg on a table. Experiment with blending different beans such as frozen soybeans or lima beans. Create a new cuisine using Italian or French spice mixes.

Makes 1 cup

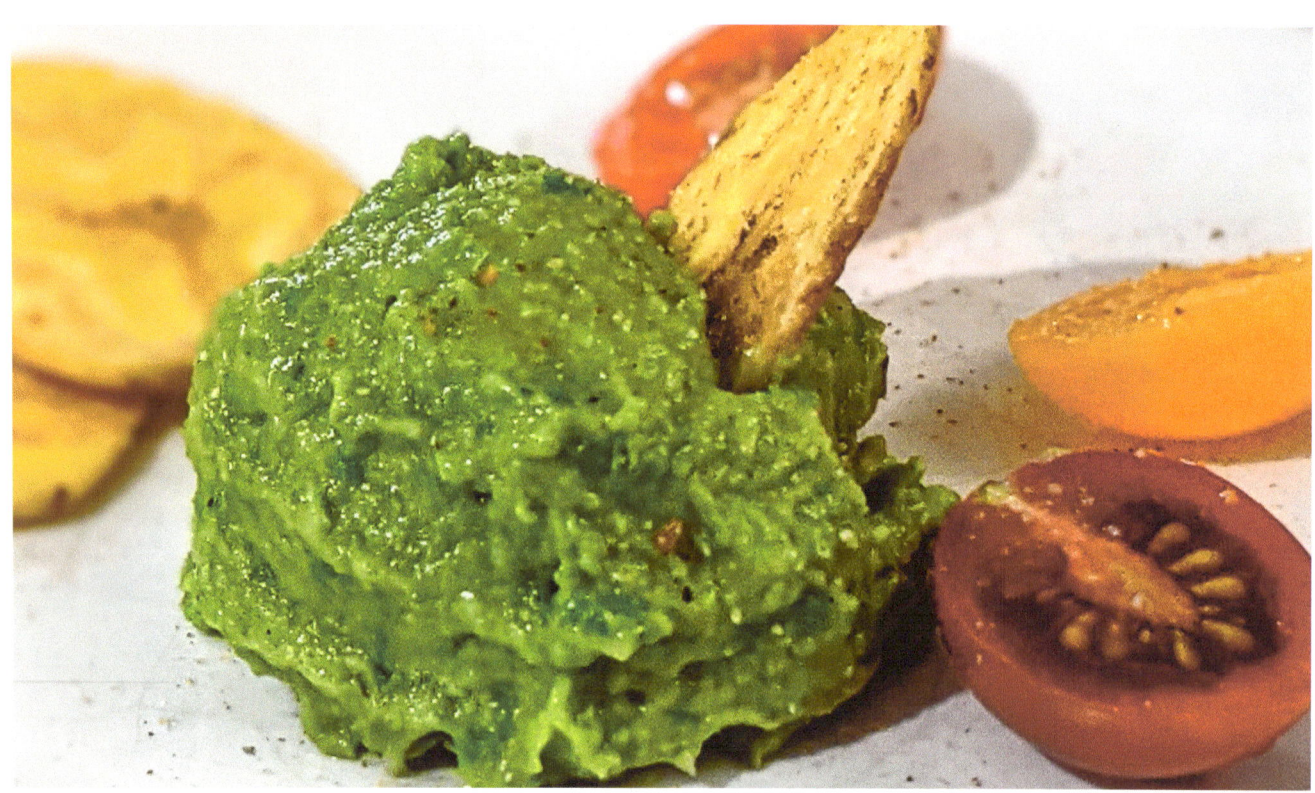

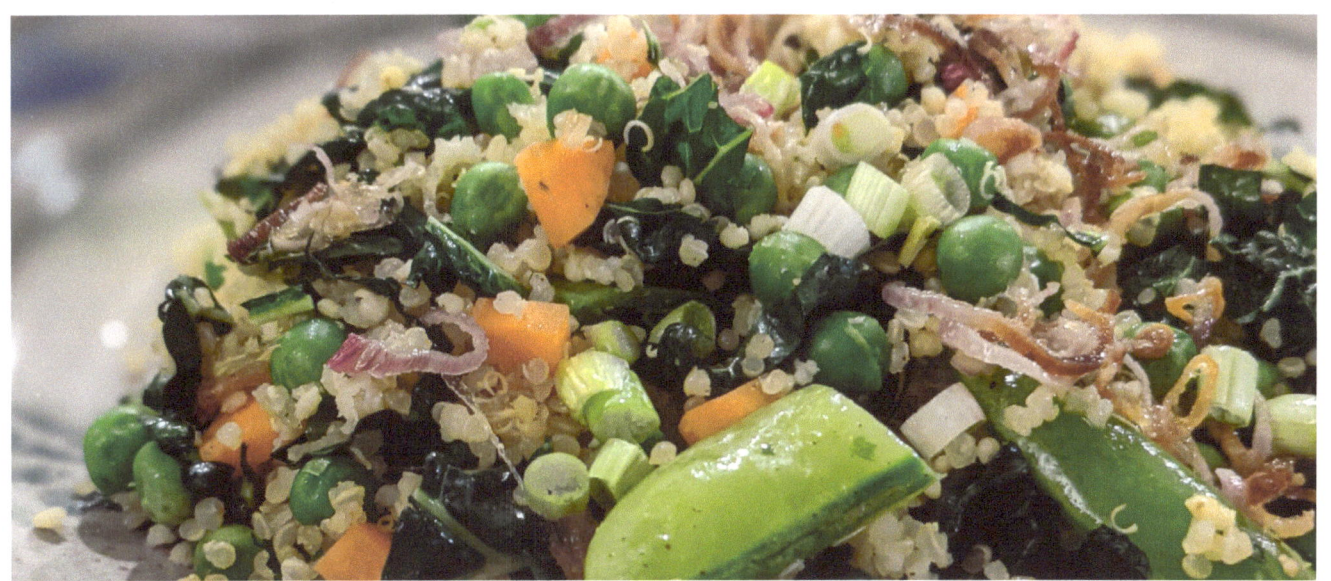

QUINOA MILLET PEA BOWL

Colorado is the number one producer of millet in the country, growing about 6.4 million bushels annually, and earning about $23 million from the crop. A pseudo-grain, millet originated more than 4,000 years ago from a wild West African grass. It makes a perfect crop for Colorado's arid climate. I paired the millet with another power-house seed—quinoa—and some bits and pieces of leftover veg from the farmers market. Enjoy a bit of Colorado. This is a gluten-free dish.

To cook millet or quinoa, rinse the seeds under running water. Place the seeds in a saucepan of 2:1 ratio of water to seed. Bring to a boil, then reduce to medium heat and cook 15-20 minutes, until the quinoa gently pops open or the millet softens. Drain and cool.

Ingredients
- 1 tsp oil
- 1 garlic clove, minced
- 1 cup chopped kale
- 1 carrot, diced
- 1 tsp of your spice mixture of choice – Italian, Provence, Greek, etc.
- 1 cup cooked millet
- 1 cup cooked quinoa
- ½ cup green peas
- ½ cup sugar peas, cut in half on diagonal
- 2 green onions, chopped
- 1 shallot, thinly sliced
- 1 tbsp oil
- ½ tsp sea salt

Instructions
In a skillet, heat the oil over medium heat.
Add the garlic and cook for 30 seconds.
Add the kale and sauté until slightly wilted.
Add the next 7 ingredients and cook until warm.
Combine the shallot, oil, and sea salt in a bowl, and microwave at 1-minute increments until the shallot rings become golden and crunchy.
Add half the shallots to the millet mixture, stir gently, and place in a serving bowl.
Top the bowl with the rest of the caramelized shallot.

Elevate This: Add more protein, such as soy beans or fresh fava beans. Review the *Cuisine-Related Pairings* chart (p. 167). Consider adding a toasted nut such as pistachios, or a dollop of Microgreen Pistou (p. 129). Serve with grape tomatoes and Niçoise olives. Add dried fruit for sweetness. Sautéed shiitakes bring umami.

Serves 2 as a side dish

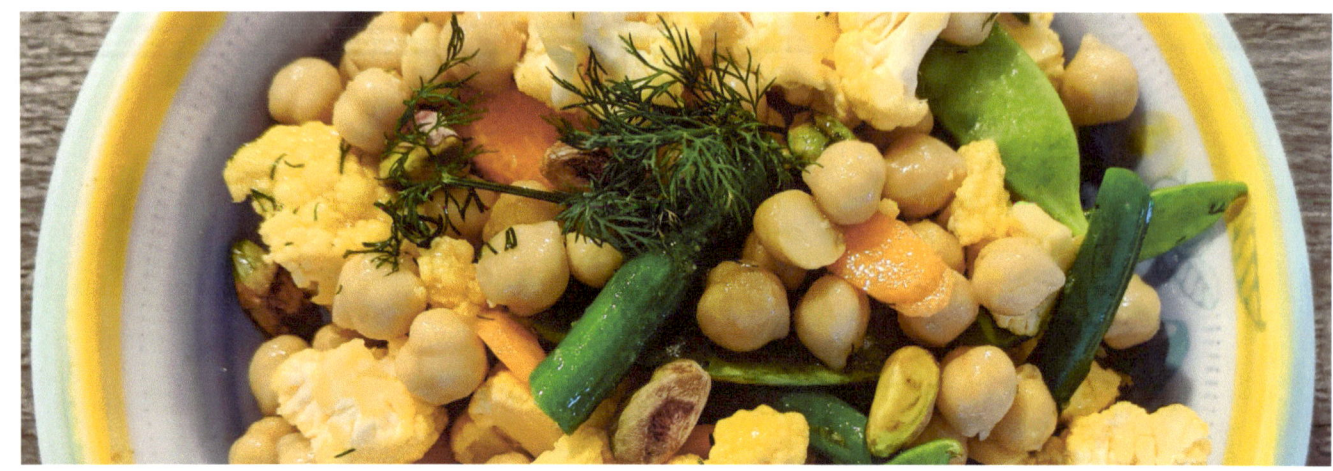

CAULIFLOWER CHICKPEA GREEN BEAN SALAD

Cauliflower come in four colors now – yellow, purple, green, and orange. The challenge for a spring dish is to prepare the cauliflower while preserving the magnificent color. Cauliflower florets capture surrounding ingredients inside their nooks and crannies, so the wrong ingredients could turn an orange cauliflower into a red or brown blob.

For a fresh veg salad, make it simple, and use bright colors. I went with orange and green colors, adding in a few chickpeas and a brushing of fresh dill dressing. What better herb announces late spring than dill?

Ingredients

For the Salad
- 2 cups orange cauliflower florets (about ½ inch pieces)
- 8-10 green beans; wrapped in wet paper towel, microwaved 90 seconds, rinsed, drained, halved
- 10 snow peas
- ½ cup canned garbanzo beans, rinsed and drained
- 1 small, narrow carrot; peeled, sliced thinly on the diagonal
- ¼ cup shelled pistachios

For the Dressing
- 1 tbsp olive oil
- 1 tbsp chopped fresh dill weed
- 1 tsp lemon juice
- ½ tsp grated lemon peel
- 1 tsp sugar
- Salt and pepper to taste

Instructions

Combine all the salad ingredients in a bowl. In a smaller bowl, mix all the dressing ingredients in a bowl. Toss the salad with the dressing.

Elevate This: This can be an elegant dish for an Easter or St. Patrick's Day meal. Serve the salad with a protein, or with other sides with your main dish. Keep the fresh herbs simple – just one or two. Try some mint and/or French tarragon. Be wary of adding other juicy or wetter vegetables that might color bleed, such as tomatoes, purple carrots, or beets. You want the colors in the dish to remain clean.

Serves 4 as a side dish or 2 as a main dish

FRONT RANGE NIÇOISE SALAD

The cookbook, Niçoise, is one of my favorite inspirational cookbooks. It is a beautiful cookbook and readers can easily feel transported to the sunny, Provence–Alpes–Côte-d'Azur region of France. Niçoise is the French word for "in the style of Nice." Traditionally these salads include black olives, tomatoes, beans, green vegetables, anchovies, and a lot of garlic. I'm sure we can accommodate that.

Niçoise salads are decomposed, meaning they are not tossed in dregs of dressing. Less is more. I chose to give the potatoes, lentils, and farro a bit of an herb and garlic flavor, and to allow that mixture to permeate the rest of the ingredients. Let's pull together our own version of a Niçoise salad with the goodness of Northern Colorado. French Tarragon grows beautifully, so let's be sure to add that to the vinaigrette.

Ingredients

For the Dressing
- 1 tsp minced shallot
- ½ tsp Dijon mustard
- ½ tsp chopped fresh tarragon (a little goes a long way)
- 1 tbsp white or champagne vinegar
- 2 tbsp olive oil
- Salt and pepper to taste

For the Salad
- ½ cup cooked French lentils
- ½ cup cooked farro
- ¼-½ tsp of Provence style or French herb mix (ie. thyme, basil, rosemary, tarragon, savory, marjoram, oregano, bay leaf)
- 1 garlic clove, minced
- Drizzle of extra virgin olive oil
- 4 baby potatoes, steamed (I used purple for more color)
- 2 cups fresh red or green lettuce (anything but Iceberg)
- 4-6 grape tomatoes, quartered
- 6-8 green beans; wrapped in wet paper towel, microwaved 2 min., rinsed, drained, dried
- 6-8 sugar snap peas; microwaved 90 sec. in bowl of water, rinsed, drained, cut on diagonal
- Anchovy fillets (optional)
- 1 egg (optional), boiled or soft-boiled
- Niçoise or any beautifully brined olive (I am hooked on Healthy Harvest black olives)

Instructions

Mix the first four dressing ingredients in a small bowl. Slowly whisk in the olive oil until emulsified. Mix the lentils, farro, herb mixture, garlic, and a drizzle of olive oil in a bowl. Salt and pepper to taste.

Mix half of the dressing ingredients with the potatoes. Artfully arrange the lettuce greens on a plate.

Place the lentil mixture, potatoes, tomatoes, green beans, sugar peas, and anchovies (if using) in separate sections over the lettuce.

Slice the hard-boiled or soft-boiled egg. Add to center. Drizzle remaining vinaigrette over the salad.

Elevate This: Experiment with different colored and textured lettuces. A grating of carrot will add color. Crispy Capers found in the *Elevations* section (p. 168) will add some salt, brine, and crunch.

Serves 2 as a salad dish

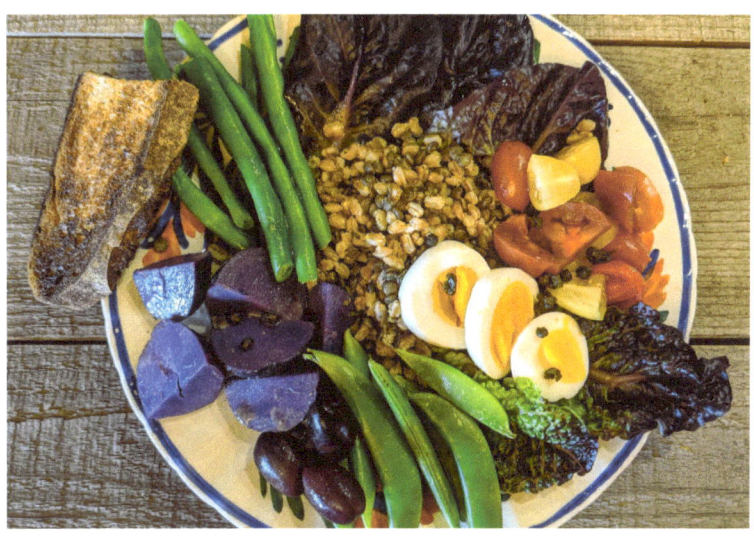

The Elusive Morel and More

My husband and I have always eaten mushrooms – usually as a small side, a mushroom sauce over a chicken breast, or in Beef Bourguignon. Mushrooms were rarely the main event, as we, like many, were mentally trained to look for the meat first, then everything else. For many years, the only types of mushroom you could find in the store were white button, cremini, portabella, and on occasion, shiitake.

When we moved to Colorado I met my friend, Camilla, who introduced me to not only beekeeping, but also foraging. We went foraging together in the Rocky Mountains and I was instantly hooked. I felt very European with my straw basket, gloves, cute hat, and a knife. I was determined to find the Colorado version of a European porcini. We found a few oddities, but nothing edible. From that point on, a basic, store-bought white mushroom never looked the same.

Another friend, Candy, accompanies me on an annual hunt for the elusive morel. Our first year foraging together, we found one sad morel, but we were thrilled beyond measure. We've been skunked since, but we keep the faith! Last season we moseyed into someone with a bag of golden morels they had found right along the Poudre River cottonwood bosques, less than three miles from my house.

During our third year of foraging, my friends and I day-tripped along the Poudre River and found an amazing assortment of mushrooms, including boletes. We could not have been happier. It was terribly exciting and on top of that we had a great friend day in the mountains.

For those interested, the Colorado Mycological Society has a very active page on Facebook. The better foraging appears to be in Southwest Colorado, as celebrated by the annual Shroomfest in Telluride. The group page is fun to follow. It's hard to not get excited about and a bit envious of some of the shroom loot posted by fellow Colorado foragers. There is a lot to study about mushrooms, so take your resource guide, and only eat what you 100% know is edible.

Throughout the year, I have my own shroomfest here with the wonderful local growers including Hazel Dell Farms, Hope Farms, and Willow Creek Farms. There is some cross-over, but each farm has a special niche for its customers. My favorites are King Trumpets from Hazel Dell, blue oysters from Willow Creek, and morels from Hope Farms.

I hope you enjoy these recipes—which add texture and umami to your dish—as you discover the most fabulous fungi in nature.

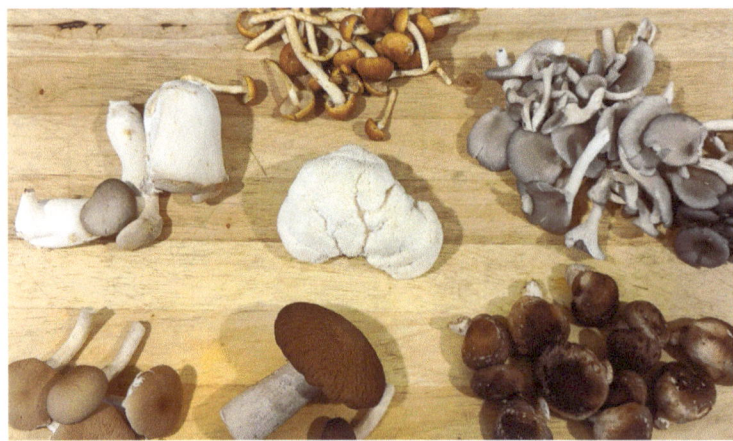
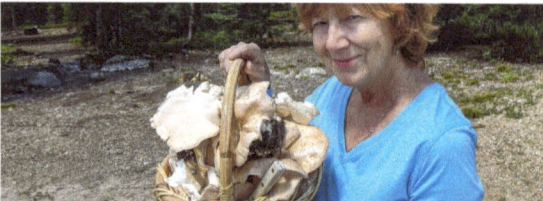
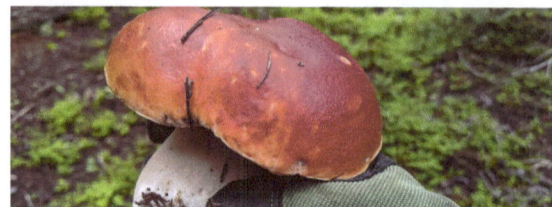

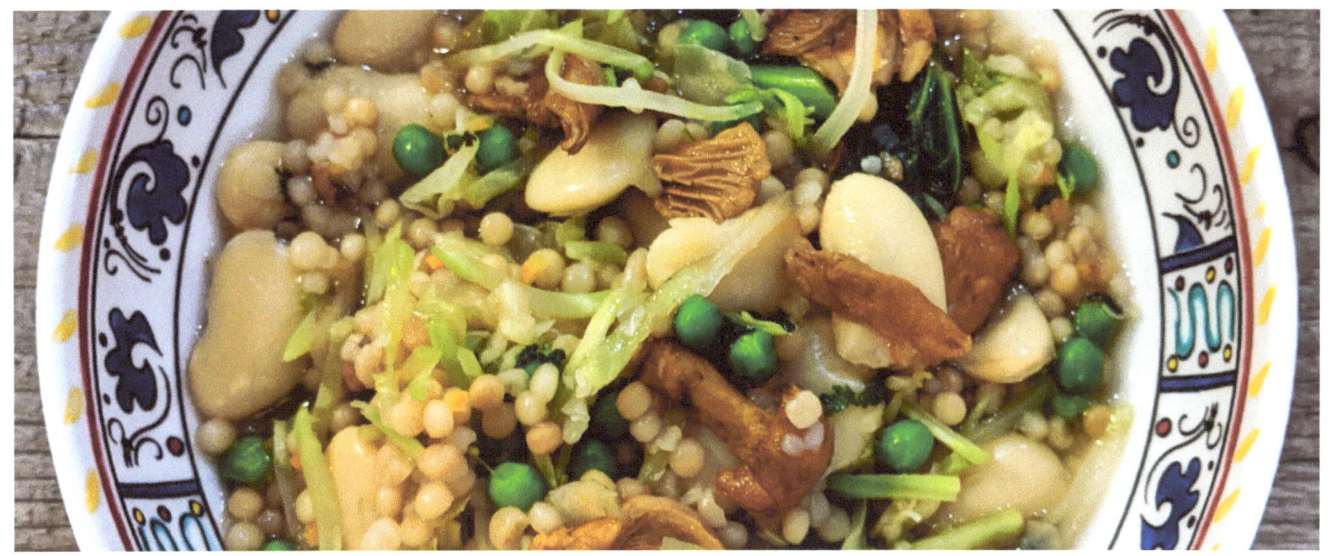

ISRAELI COUSCOUS MUSHROOM BEAN SOUP

This dish came together as I was trying to use up things I had in the pantry. It is also a big nod to Colorado mushroom foraging and the local retail mushroom farmers.

Every year during Lent, my husband Mike and I have a Lenten challenge. We attempt—and many times succeed—to use up what is in our fridge, freezer, and pantry. The rule: don't buy anything except perishables, and send cost savings to a favorite charity. One thing to know is that beans and mushrooms are a great marriage.

Ingredients
- 2 cups vegetable broth or chicken broth
- 1 tsp mushroom powder
- A couple cubes homemade frozen mushroom broth (p. 28) (about ½ cup)
- ½ cup Israeli couscous
- 1 can large butter beans
- Some frozen peas
- 1 cup sautéed mushrooms (mine were pre-sautéed and frozen)
- 1 cup mix veg from bag of sweet kale mix
- Dash of Maggi
- Dash of Marmite
- 1 tsp asafetida

Instructions
Make 2 cups of vegetable or chicken broth. Place in a saucepan and add 1 tsp mushroom powder for umami, and the mushroom broth if you have it. There is no magic here – use what you have.

Add Israeli couscous, cook for 5 minutes until al dente. Rinse and drain the butter beans. Add the beans, mushrooms, and greens (kale works great).

Add a dash of Maggi and Marmite, and 1 tsp of asafetida. Cook on low heat for 10 minutes.

Add the peas and cook for 3-4 minutes. You want them to be warm while staying a beautiful spring green. Divide into serving bowls.

Elevate This: Use chanterelles, shiitakes, or cinnamon cap mushrooms. Garnish the dish with grated carrot and/or any of the nutritional yeast mixes found in the *Elevations* section (p. 168). This is a mild soup. A little spice goes a long way.

Serves 2 as a soup dish

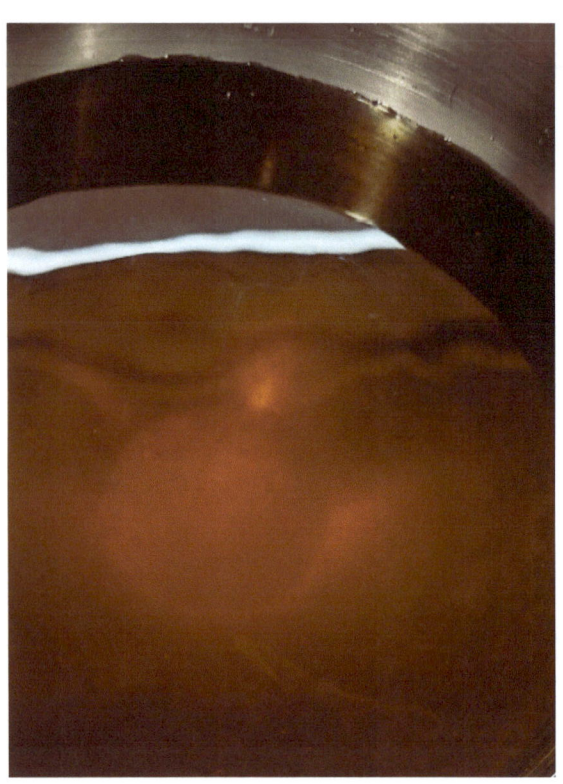
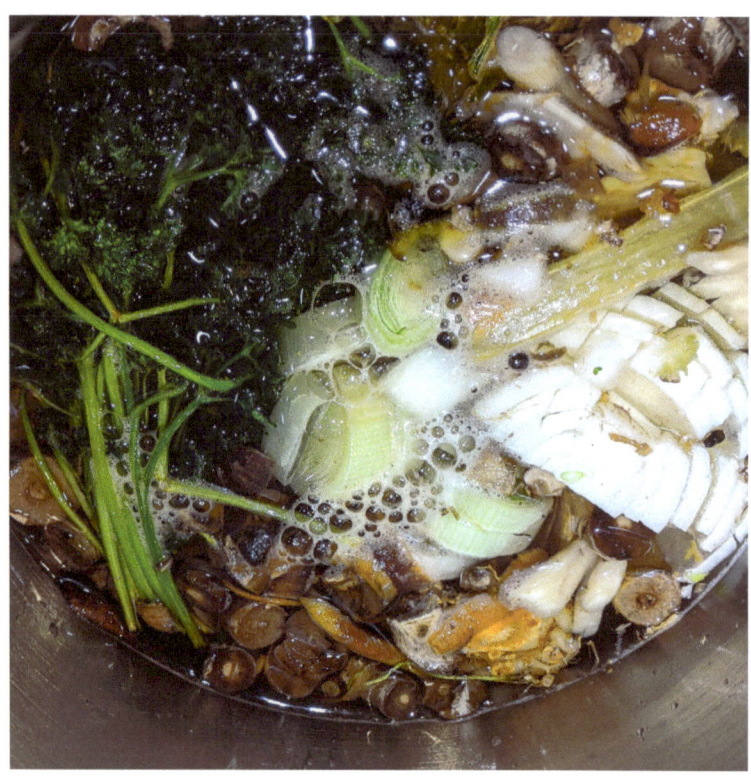

MUSHROOM STEM VEGETABLE BROTH

I love the art of vegetables simmering slowly to develop flavor, and learning how the flavors intensify, blend, complement, or sometimes literally, go to pot. There is such a thing as too much celery. Though my dad did say that you can never have too much parsley.

Mushrooms are a superb way to bring umami to a dish. Usually we simply cut, slice, sauté, or roast. Grocery stores now regularly carry button, baby bella, portabella, cremini and shitake, along with a smattering of smaller packages of cinnamon cap, Lion's mane, or other specialty mushrooms when available. Foraging is a marvelous way to experience even more mushroom varieties – just be careful, knowledgeable, and only eat those that you are 100% sure of their species.

As with every mushroom you are prepping, you may ask yourself, "What do I do with those stems?" I sometimes dry them in a dehydrator and use a coffee or spice grinder to grind them to a fine pulp. The powder adds a touch of umami to any dish.

Years ago, I started saving every scrap of vegetable in the freezer that was a fit for a soup base. Basic vegetables might include carrot scraps, carrot tops, onions, leeks, garlic, parsley, cilantro, and celery. Leeks are huge in size, and many times I have leftovers from a bunch, so I just clean, slice, and package to freeze. After all, any weepiness caused by freezing a leek doesn't matter when it is in a purée. Waste not, want not! Add mushroom stems and pieces to the freezer – don't bother to wrap them, just toss them in a plastic bag.

Helpful Tips

The following tips apply to any broth. Do not fast boil to get things done more quickly. A low simmer allows the vegetables to slowly release flavor without melting down into particulate matter. You will have a clearer broth in the final result.

Another thing to consider is to do what you can to avoid a tan or gray colored sauce. Creating a dish is like painting. You want to start with pure colors, like gold or brown. Build color into your dish by adding additional color varieties.

Aim to achieve a balance of sweet, savory, bitter, and salty, with some umami. A bit of tartness can brighten a broth. Carrots are sweet. Celery is sometimes bitter. Parsley is slightly bitter, but herby. Onions are savory, but can also be sweet, depending on the variety. Some people add fresh tomato at the beginning, or a bit of tomato paste at the end. A little goes a long way.

For this mushroom broth, our umami comes from the mushrooms, thus I do not add any tomatoes to the cooking process. There is a theory that when you combine two or three umami ingredients, the flavors are complementary rather than additive – so mushrooms, a splash of Maggi, and some miso in the soup will come together beautifully in a final dish.

Now, let's make the Mushroom Stem Vegetable Broth!

Ingredients
- 8 ounces mushroom stems and pieces (about 2 cups)
- 2-3 celery stalks
- 1 cup carrot peelings
- ½ onion, quartered
- ¼ cup sliced leeks (optional)
- 2 garlic cloves
- 1 handful frozen parsley or cilantro
- 1 tsp salt
- 3-4 peppercorns

Instructions
Place all ingredients in a stock pot and cover with water. Place over medium heat.
Bring to a slight boil, then immediately turn the heat down to low and simmer for 1 hour. Do not allow the vegetables to roll and touch each other – the slower the simmer, the better.
Allow broth to cool.
Strain through a sieve.
Strain again through a coffee filter.
Place back in saucepan and bring to a low simmer.
Reduce broth by ⅓ to concentrate flavors.
Cool and move to your storage.
Use the mushroom broth as a liquid with which to cook grains, or use it in a plant-based sauce or soup.

Note: You can try this recipe in an Instant Pot, but keep in mind that the recommended temperature and water movement should not be full simmer, nor should it be a slow-cook – it is somewhere in between.

Makes 2-3 cups

Age of Asparagus

I owe a debt of gratitude to Matt Martindale of Martindale Family Farms, and their FarmFresh CSA brand. In early May of 2020, Matt posted on Facebook Marketplace that his fresh asparagus was available, and *voilà* – I became a loyal customer of his, long into winter. I asked myself years ago if I would benefit from buying a CSA, as there would be produce in the batch that I would surely not use. Like eggplant and acorn squash – uh oh!

Martindale Family Farms has been farming in Gilcrest, about nine miles south of Greeley, Colorado for over 35 years. In 1976, the Martindales were hand-selected and invited to be one of five original farmers working directly with the Colorado Department of Agriculture, in an effort to pioneer a new concept for Colorado's very first farmers market. Keeping the tradition alive, Matt helps his parents with farming, marketing and the distribution of their produce through farmers markets and direct CSA pickups.

Participating in a local CSA got me down, green, and dirty (and healthier) with what the weekly or bi-weekly CSA boxes have to offer. One of my greatest culinary thrills was receiving the fresh asparagus. I had never eaten "field run" asparagus (I did not even know the term, "field run"). Along with the asparagus was a batch of sugar snap peas – another fantastic local find. Fresh, non-pre-bagged sugar pea pods provide a vegetable sweetness that is beyond measure.

I usually prepare asparagus by boiling, roasting, grilling, or broiling it. It's important to know what it should taste like with these different techniques. They shouldn't all taste the same. The crunchy caramelization makes a beautiful presentation, and a touch of lemon counterbalances any bitterness. Take note that overcooked asparagus will gain a bitter and sour taste that is hard to correct.

Let's experience the fresh, green, sweetness of asparagus. Enjoy the variety of upcoming preparations and recipes!

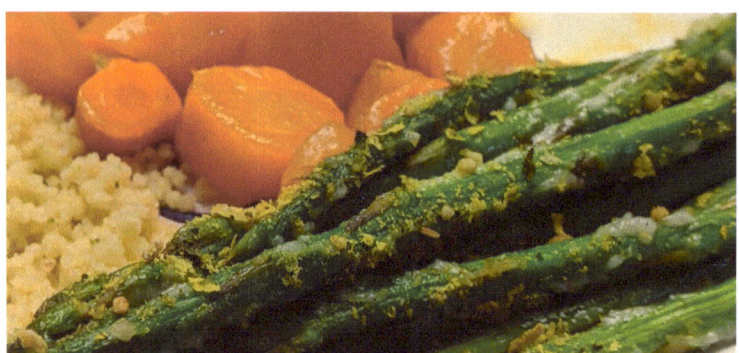
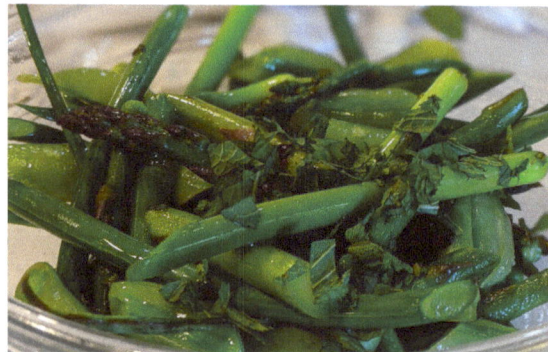
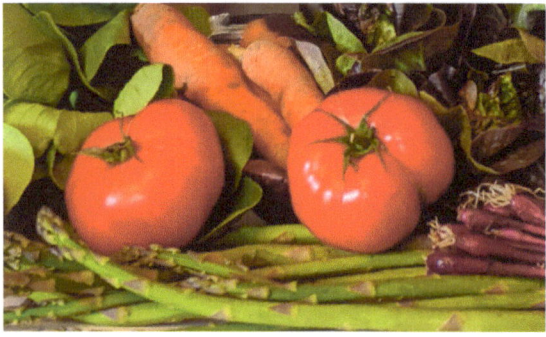
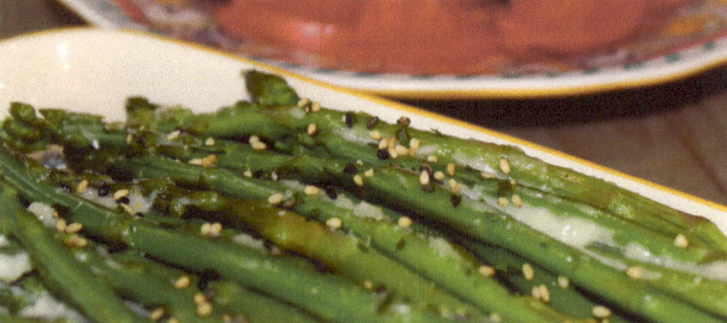

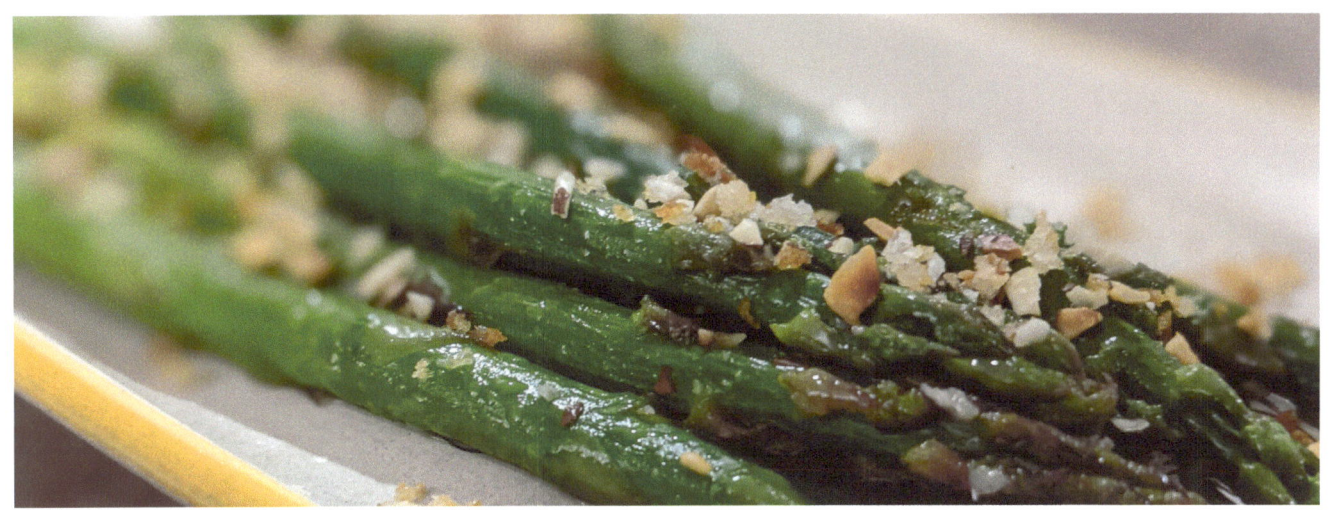

SKILLET ASPARAGUS WITH PANKO ALMOND CRUMBS

Don't get me wrong – I love grilled or roasted asparagus, but I don't always want to fire up the grill or wait for the oven to preheat. When I am short on time, my quickest technique is to parcook the veg by wrapping some spears in wet paper towels and microwaving them for 30 to 60 seconds, just until bright green (not done). Then rinse, drain, cool, and use promptly or keep in the fridge. Parcooking is also a good way to keep your asparagus (and broccoli) fresh for a couple additional days. The beauty of this dish is that the asparagus cooks without caramelizing on the stove top in about 6 minutes.

Ingredients

For the Asparagus
- ½ lb asparagus (8-10 spears), 1 inch cut off the bottom
- 2 tsp butter (dairy or non-dairy)
- 1 tbsp water
- 1 garlic clove, mashed with ½ tsp oil and ¼ tsp sea salt

For the Panko Almond Crumbs
- ½ cup panko bread crumbs
- 4 cups sliced almonds
- 1 tsp olive oil
- Salt and pepper
- Spice or herb mixture of choice

Instructions

For the Panko Almond Crumbs
In a small skillet, heat the oil over medium low heat. Add the rest of the ingredients and stir until bread crumbs and almonds are golden. Pour into a dish to cool.

For the Asparagus
Over medium heat, melt the butter in a skillet large enough to accommodate the asparagus.
Add water, garlic and salt. Stir well.
Add the asparagus. Cover and let steam for 2 minutes. Uncover and cook another 2-3 minutes, until skillet is almost dry and you can pierce the asparagus with a paring knife with some resistance.
Transfer to a serving dish and garnish with the Panko Almond Crumbs from above.

Elevate This: Sprinkle 1 tbsp nutritional yeast into the bread crumbs for umami and a cheesy taste.
Add local honey or Toum (p. 130) for a flavor burst.

Serves 2 as a side dish

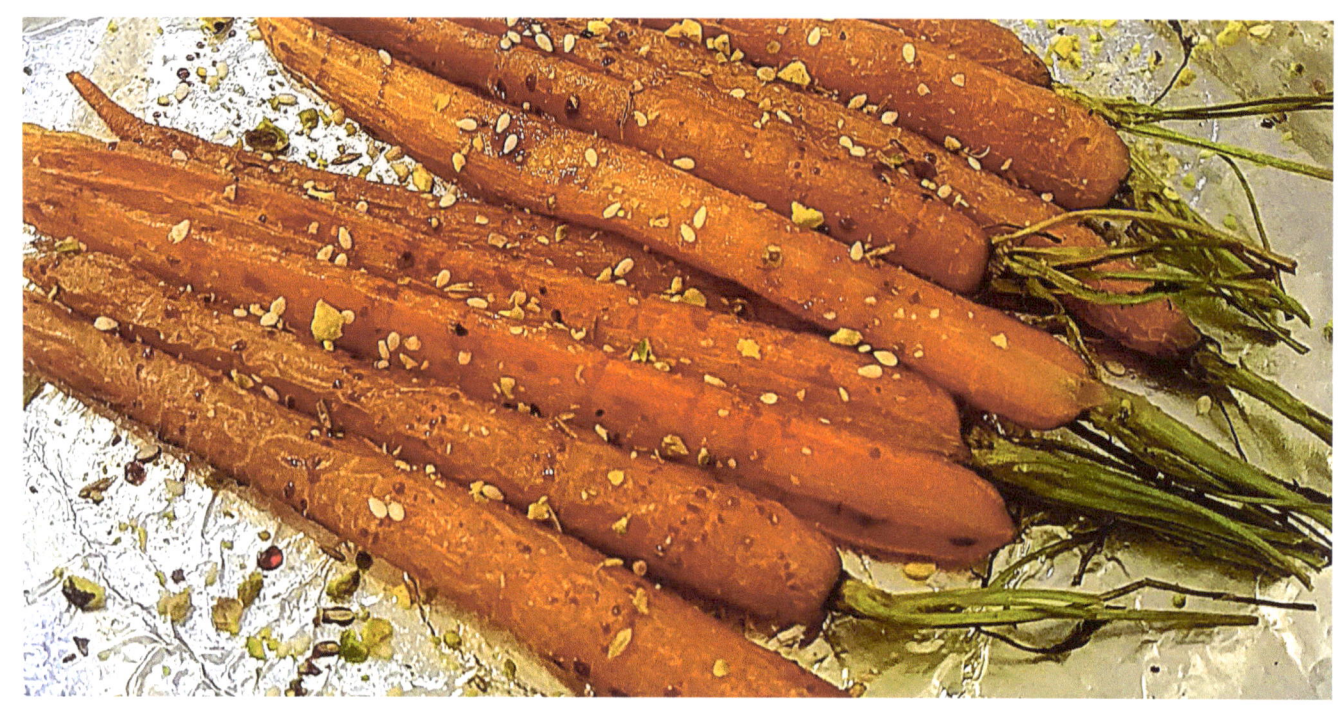

ROASTED CARROTS WITH FURIKAKE

This is a great technique that I have seen in multiple cookbooks including America's Test Kitchen *and Marcella Hazan's* Essentials of Classic Italian Cooking. *Keep this technique within your veg prep and cooking skills pack. You are basically steaming the veg in the oven in a covered vessel (aluminum foil pan or cast-iron skillet), then uncovering for the last 5-10 minutes to roast. How easy is that? This technique works for other vegetables – you will just need to adjust the initial steaming time.*

Ingredients
- 6-8 carrots; whole or sliced lengthwise (depending on the size)
- ½ cup water
- 1 tbsp oil
- Furikake sprinkles (quick mix instructions found in the *Elevations* section, p. 168)
- Toasted sesame oil

Instructions
Preheat the oven to 400°F.
Place the carrots on a sheet pan or cast iron skillet. Add the water and oil. Cover with aluminum foil.
Bake for 10-15 minutes or until carrots are almost fork tender. A little resistance is okay.
Remove the foil and roast for 5-10 minutes or so, until the water is evaporated and the carrots caramelize. Remove from the oven and place in a serving dish. Sprinkle with furikake and a small drizzle of sesame oil.

Elevate This: Use any of the cuisine mixtures in the *Elevations* section (p. 168). Think toasted pistachios and dukkah. Go Mediterranean or French. Add a drizzle of local honey, thyme lavender butter, or Toum (p. 130).

Serves 2 as a side dish

PERFECT GREEN BEANS

Green beans can be challenging to cook. Either they are undercooked and squeak against your teeth when you eat them, or they are floppy when overdone. The key to perfection is using a paring knife to test your green beans to see if they are cooked. When pierced, you should be able to insert a paring knife easily into the bean, pick the bean up, and it should slide off the knife easily. If there is resistance, it is not done.

Beans are fairly perishable in my opinion, so if I am not going to use the green beans in a few days, I do the microwave parcook trick – I trim the beans, wrap them in a wet paper towel, and microwave them for two minutes. They will not be fully cooked, but they will be a brighter green and resistant to perishing. Rinse, drain, dry, and store in the fridge. This will buy you time.

You now have a fool-proof recipe to cook market fresh beans that you might find at a vendor such as Miller Farms. So now, when you go to stuff your Miller Farms bag full of veg for $10 at their farmers market booth, you may add in some additional green beans!

Ingredients
- ½ lb fresh green beans, stems removed
- 1 tsp oil, or butter (dairy or non-dairy)
- ¼ tsp salt
- ½ cup water

Instructions
Place the green beans in a skillet large enough so they all fit nicely in the bottom of the skillet.

Add the oil or butter, salt, and water. Bring the pan to a boil, then reduce the heat to medium low, cover, and let simmer for 5-10 minutes or until you can pierce the green beans with some resistance.

Remove the lid and continue to cook the beans until the water is evaporated and you can pierce the beans easily with a paring knife.

At this point, if you want to leave them in the pan and brown a bit, that is nice too. But now you should have brilliantly green, cooked green beans – ready to eat alone or with a topping.

Elevate This: Sprinkle with fresh herbs and a nutritional yeast blend recommended in the *Elevations* section (p. 168). Almonds are traditional, but pistachios will work too. Think different cuisines! Pair with the Quinoa Millet Pea Bowl (p. 23) or a soup recipe from this section.

Serves 2 as a side dish

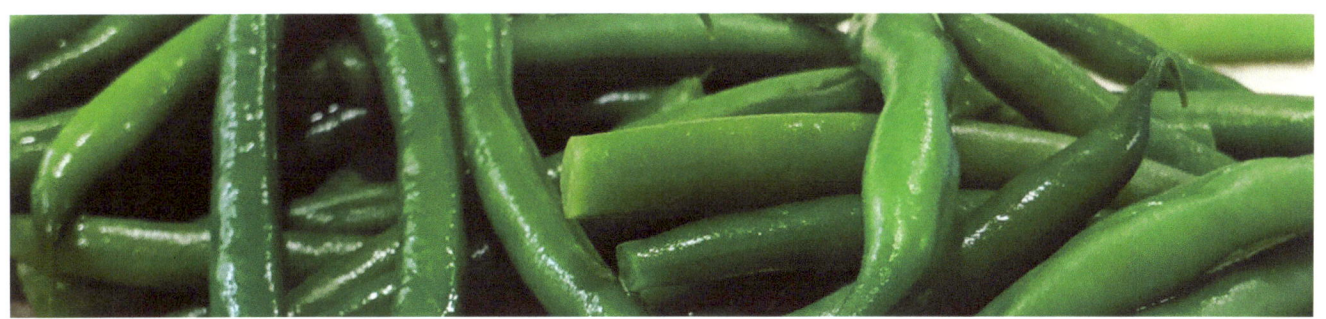

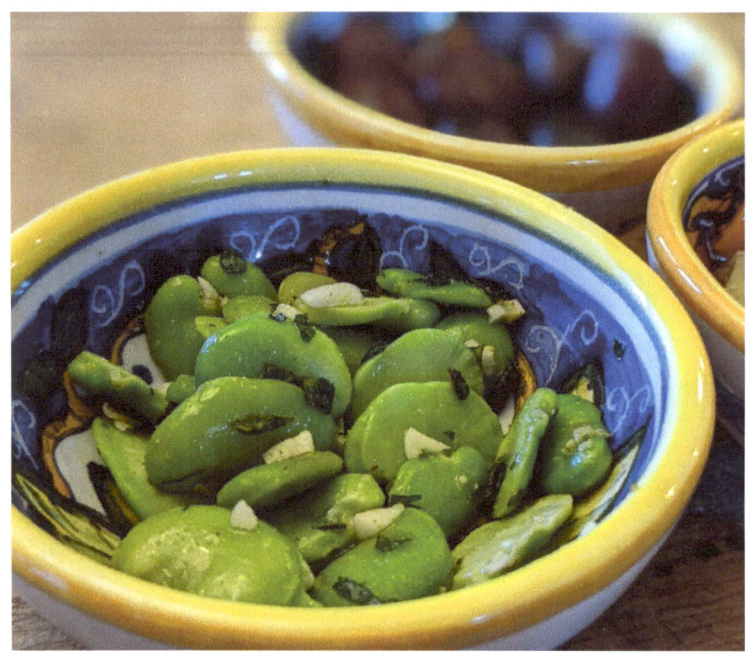
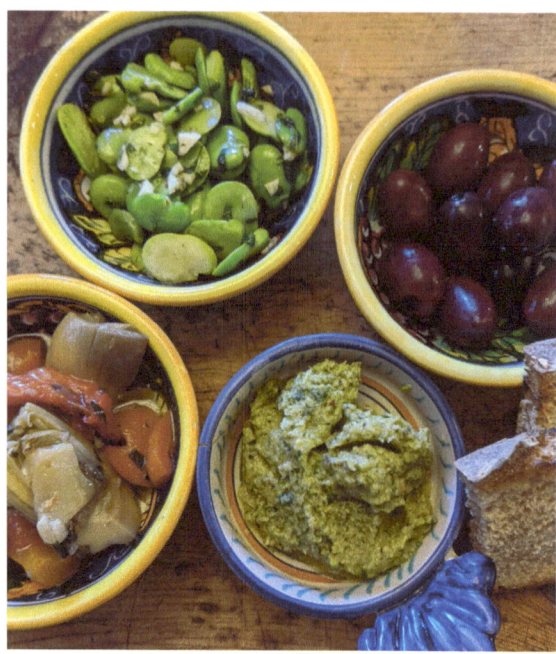

FRESH FAVA BEANS WITH GARLIC, MINT, AND CUMIN

Fava beans cross multiple cultures. They are a tasty bean that has two layers of shell – a thick outer layer and a thin inner layer that need to be removed before you can enjoy the soft lusciousness of the bean.

In warmer regions, fava beans are in season in May. But here in Northern Colorado, we are barely ready by then to get our plants in the ground, so we seek alternative sources for specific products. Thankfully, we have a great little local Mediterranean market, Olive Tree Market, that carries fresh fava beans. I no longer order them online as frozen, and then double-peel the little rascals (however therapeutic it feels to get close to nature with that process). The beans arrive at the store double-peeled and ready to enjoy. Yeah!

The owner of Olive Tree Market wanted me to try these double-peeled beans with cumin and mint, and I added the garlic. Easy, yum. Fava beans are also great stirred into risotto, or mashed into a dip or hummus. If you don't have access to fava beans, soybeans are a good substitute.

Ingredients
- ½ tsp cumin
- 1 tsp of chopped fresh mint
- 1 garlic clove, minced
- 1 tsp oil
- 1 cup fresh fava beans (or frozen, double-peeled fava beans, thawed in microwave for 2 min. Do not overcook the beans so your dish will stay bright green.)

Instructions
Mix the first four ingredients in a bowl. Add the beans and marinate at room temperature for about 20 minutes. Salt and pepper to taste.

Elevate This: Stir into cooked risotto or orzo at the last minute for a more substantial dish. Create a local antipasto tray with Giardiniera (p. 63), Healthy Harvest olives, and Shak Shouka's dips or sauces.

Serves 2 as part of an antipasto tray

CINNAMON CAP MUSHROOM VEGETABLE MEDLEY

This recipe came together after a fantastic trip to Hazel Dell Mushrooms after which I left with a collection of beautiful mushrooms. Curious as to what can be created with bits and pieces of fresh ingredients found in the fridge, this recipe came alive with both sweet and savory veg – and a bit of vermouth.

Serve this medley alone or over your favorite grain or pasta. A helpful hint I learned from Nigella Lawson: Vermouth is an easy substitute for dry white wine. It has the same characteristics as white wine, but doesn't go bad as quickly.

Ingredients
- ½ tbsp butter (dairy or non-dairy)
- ½ tbsp olive oil
- 1 shallot, minced
- 8 baby Dutch potatoes; steamed, cooled, quartered
- 1 cup cinnamon cap mushrooms
- 2 tbsp vermouth
- 1 cup sugar peas
- 1 cup green beans; trimmed, microwaved for 90 seconds, flash-cooled
- 1 carrot; cut into batons, microwaved for 2 minutes, flash-cooled
- 1 cup vegetable broth, preferably a vegetable glace for added glossiness
- Pea shoots
- Salt and pepper to taste

Instructions
Heat oil and butter in a skillet over medium high heat.
Add the shallots and saute until golden.
Add the potatoes and cook 2 minutes.
Add the mushrooms and cook 2 minutes.
Push the vegetables to the side. Add the vermouth to deglaze the pan.
When liquid is reduced by half, add the sugar peas, green beans, and carrots. Cook for 2-3 minutes.
Add the vegetable broth and reduce pan sauce to half, or until you can run a spoon across the bottom of the pan and leave a streak in the pan.
Salt and pepper to taste.
Serve and garnish with pea shoots.

Elevate This: Sprinkle with dried herb mixture, bread crumbs or a drizzle of balsamic vinegar.

Serves 2 as a main dish

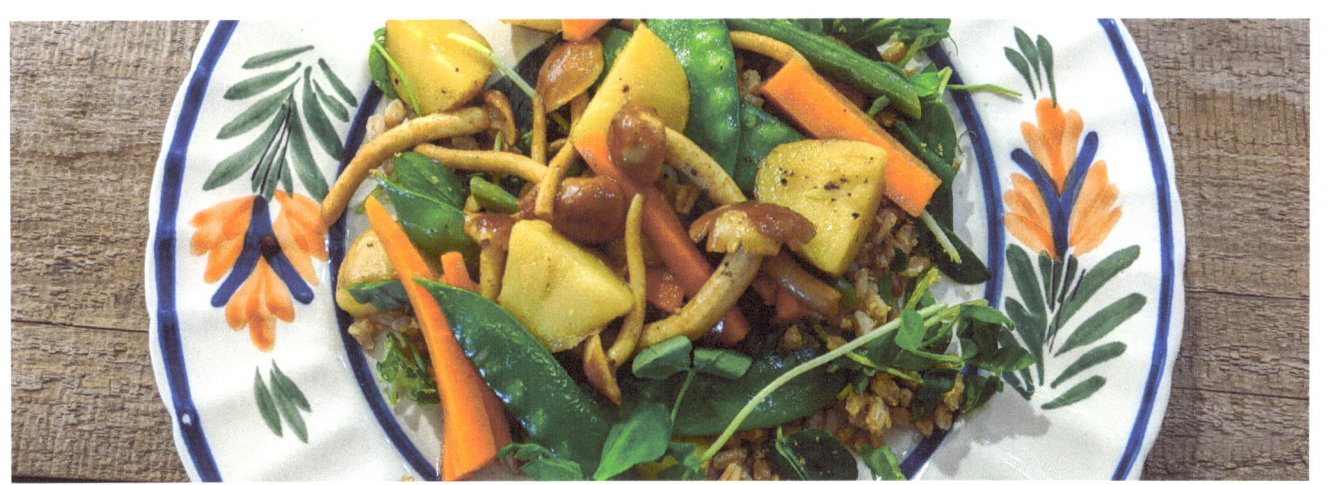

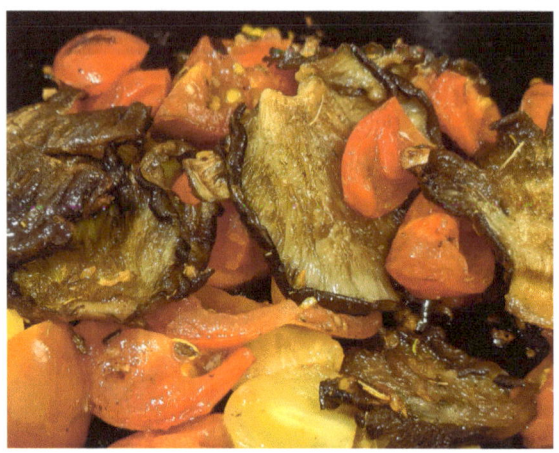
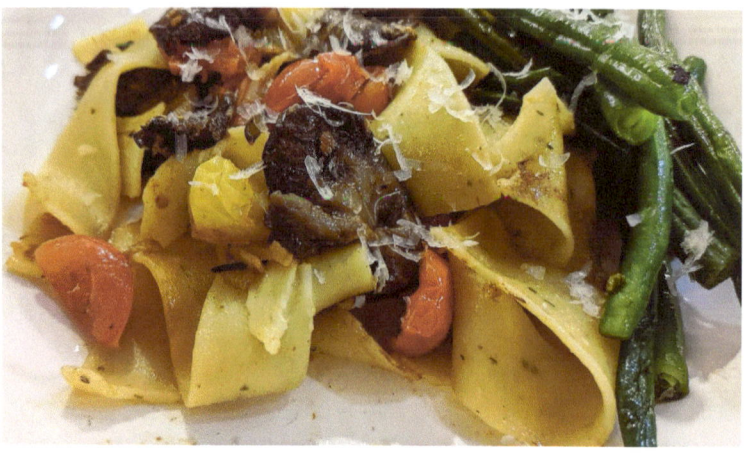

ITALIAN GRILLED OYSTER MUSHROOMS WITH GARLIC CHIVE PAPPARDELLE PASTA

This dish was prepared on the stovetop with a cast-iron grill pan. The grill pan helps elevate the oysters so they stay drained while caramelizing. I recommend trying this on a well-seasoned outdoor grill with large oyster mushrooms.

Ingredients
- 1 tbsp avocado oil
- 1 tsp chile flakes
- 1 tsp whole fennel seeds
- 1 garlic clove, smashed
- Salt and pepper
- 8-10 large oyster mushrooms, stems removed
- 8-10 grape tomatoes, halved
- 8 ounces garlic chive pappardelle, or other wide pasta

For the Garnish
- Grated parmesan (dairy or non-dairy)

Instructions
In a large bowl, combine the first 5 ingredients and mix well. Add the oyster mushrooms, and turn to thoroughly coat the mushrooms with the oil mixture. Place the tomatoes in the oil mixture to pick up any remaining oil mixture ingredients.

Lay mushrooms on grill pan on medium high heat. Place a skillet on top of the mushrooms to flatten them. Grill mushrooms for 5 minutes until browned on one side. Turn and repeat the process. Push mushrooms aside. Place tomatoes to one side of the grill pan. Turn off heat and let tomatoes continue to cook.

Boil pasta as directed. Drain and save pasta water. Add the pasta, mushrooms, and tomatoes to a separate skillet on low heat. Add 2 tbsp pasta water. Cook for 5 minutes until the pasta water is absorbed. Garnish with parmesan (dairy or non-dairy) and serve.

Elevate This: Add some baby spinach leaves, toasted bread crumbs, a sprinkle of Italian seasoning, a drizzle of extra virgin olive oil, crispy sage leaves, or a few toasted pine nuts. Serve with Perfect Green Beans (p. 33).

Serves 2 as a main dish

CONICAL MORELS IN WHITE WINE CREAM SAUCE

May signals morel season in Colorado. Ah, the elusive morel which I have yet to find more than three of, but have eye-witnessed bags of morels from other foragers. Technique and luck, I guess. Fortunately, we have a local supplier of dried morels, Hope Mushrooms, that offers other dried as well as fresh mycological delights. Brandy or vermouth works nicely in this dish.

I made this dish plant-based, but feel free to substitute cream or half and half for the plant-based milk, cashew cream and nutritional yeast.

Ingredients
- 4 ounces (about 12) dried morels
- 2 tbsp butter (dairy or non-dairy)
- 2 garlic cloves, minced
- ½ small shallot, minced
- 1 tsp sea salt
- ½ tsp white pepper
- ½ cup dry white wine
- ½ cup non-dairy milk
- ¼ cup cashew cream
- ¼ cup nutritional yeast
- ½ lb cooked pasta of choice

For the Garnish
- Chopped parsley

Instructions
Place the morels in a bowl and cover with hot water. Soak morels for 30 minutes. Strain through a cheesecloth and reserve liquid. Rinse the morels well and cut lengthwise.

Heat the butter (dairy or non-dairy) over medium heat in a small skillet. Add shallots, garlic, and salt, and sauté until golden soft. Add the morels. Sauté 2 minutes. Add the wine to deglaze the pan. When the sauce thickens, add the milk, cashew cream and nutritional yeast. Lower heat and cook for 5 minutes or until sauce thickens further.

Add pasta to pan. Stir until pasta is coated with sauce. Place in bowls and garnish with chopped parsley.

Elevate This: Experiment with a very gentle drizzle of truffle oil or truffle salt, or fresh cracked smoked black pepper. Add some red pepper flakes, freshly chopped thyme, or garlic herb parmesan crumbs. A side of asparagus always complements morels.

Serves 2 as a main dish

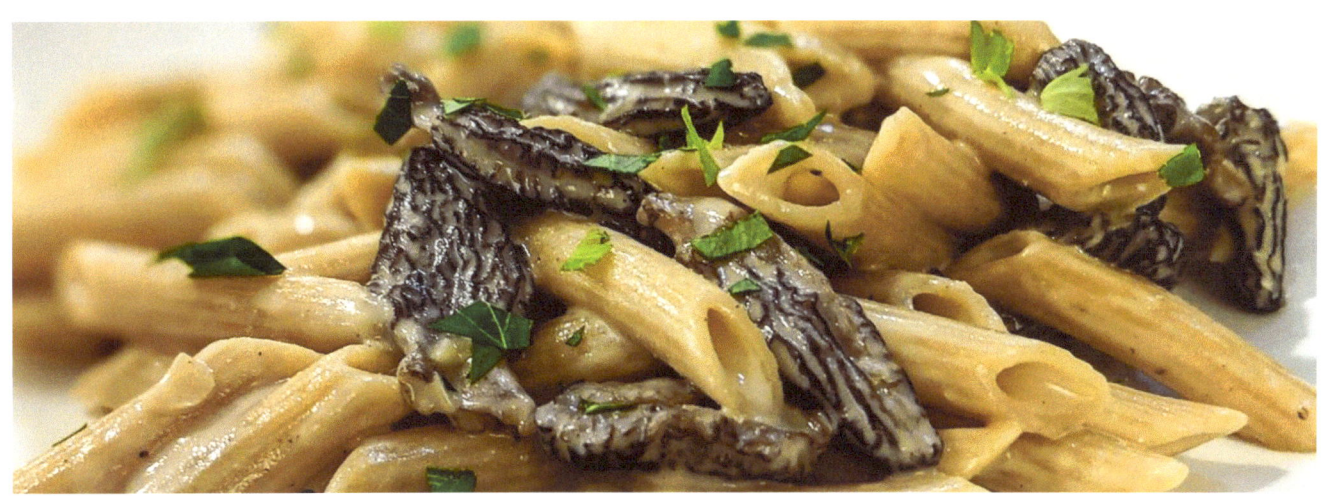

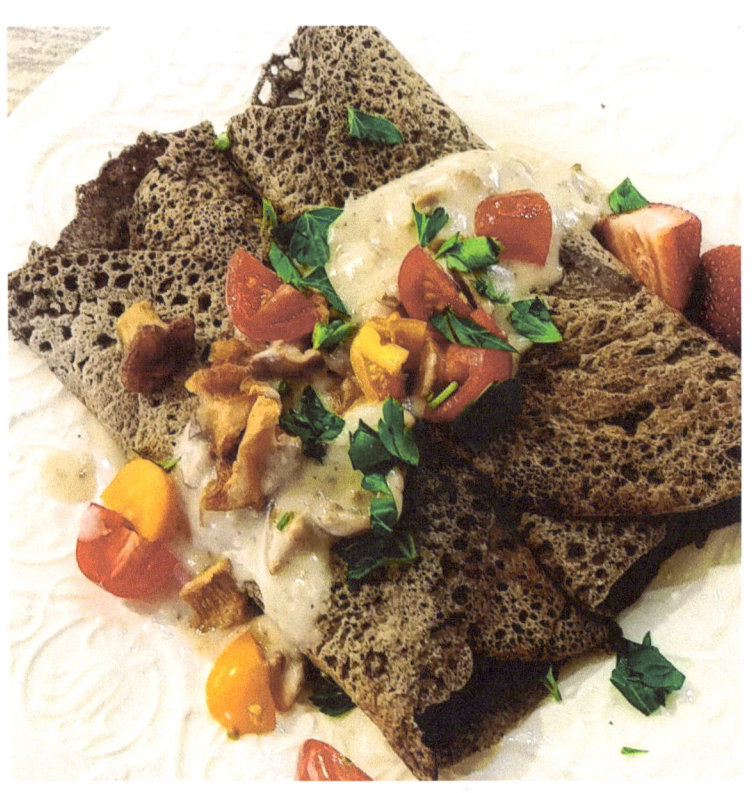 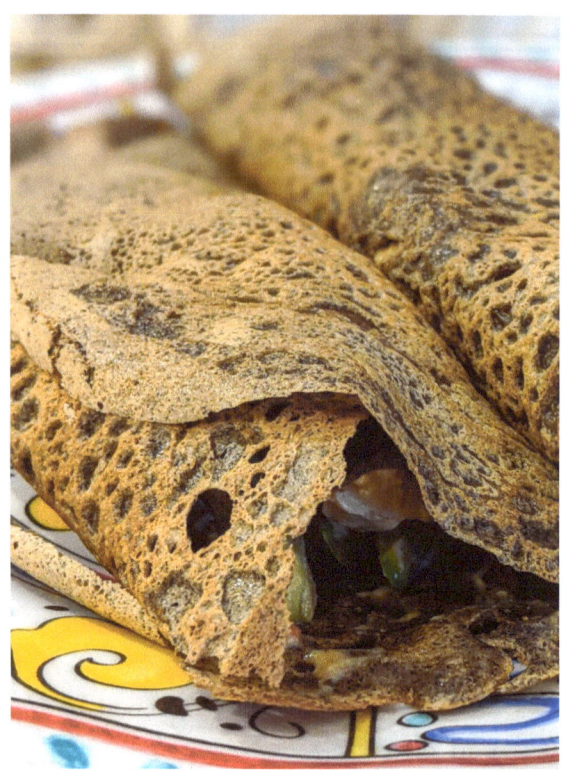

BUCKWHEAT CRÊPES WITH MUSHROOM ASPARAGUS CREAM SAUCE

There is a flatbread or wrap for every cuisine – be it pancakes or Indian dosas. We humans seem to enjoy wrapping our fillings in some kind of batter that may have a flour, sourdough, or chickpea base. In this case, it's buckwheat – a pseudocereal or seed that is consumed as a cereal grain, but doesn't grow on grasses like wheat, oats, or barley. Wraps are a great way to use up a few vegetables that can be pulled together for a beautiful main dish.

We have a lovely French café in Fort Collins called La Creperie. When I want a French staycation, this is my "go to" place to enjoy regional food treats from Brittany, and take home some macarons and crusty French bread. La Creperie buckwheat crêpes are folded in a traditional four-corner method. My skillet is smaller, so I fold in the more Americanized way – in thirds. It is worth purchasing an inexpensive crêpe spreader, but you can also use the dosa technique, as described in the recipe instructions. This is a lovely dish for a Spring holiday event.

Ingredients

For the Crêpes
- 1 cup buckwheat flour
- ½ cup egg substitute (ie. JUST Egg), or 2 eggs
- 1 cup water
- ½ tsp salt
- Oil or butter for skillet

For the Filling
- 2 tsp oil
- ½ shallot, minced
- 4 ounces cremini mushrooms, sliced
- 8-10 grape tomatoes, halved
- 2 tbsp vermouth
- ½ cup non-dairy milk or half and half
- 4 asparagus spears; ends cut off, wrapped in wet paper towels, microwaved for 30 seconds, cut into thirds
- 1 cup baby spinach
- ¼ cup sliced chicken breast or similar meat substitute (optional)

Instructions

For the Crêpes
Blend all of the crêpe ingredients in a blender until well incorporated. Refrigerate for at least an hour.
Heat a 12-inch skillet or crêpe pan over medium heat and coat the pan with ¼ tsp oil or butter (dairy or non-dairy). I use a silicone brush to spread it around. (Alternatively, you can save your dairy or non-dairy butter stick papers, and use those to coat skillets when needed.)
Test your skillet with a drop of water. You do not want the pan too hot – you want a gentle sizzle.
Pour ¼ cup crêpe batter into the pan while gently tilting or swirling the pan. Using the crêpe spreader, gently place the spreader on the batter and twirl it to thinly spread the batter in the pan. Or, using the dosa technique – starting at the center, use the bottom of a soup ladle to move the batter around the pan to as thin a layer as possible. Small holes will appear just as with regular pancakes, and you can dab a bit of batter into any gaping holes.
Allow the crêpe to completely brown on one side. The edges will crisp up and you will be able to tuck your pancake flipper underneath the crêpe.
Flip the crêpe and cook the other side.
Repeat the process with the remaining batter.

For the Filling
In a skillet, heat 2 tsp oil over medium heat.
Add the shallots and sauté until very soft.
Add the mushrooms and sauté until soft.
Add the tomatoes and cook for 1 minute.
Add the vermouth to deglaze the pan. Scrape off the bottom of the pan. Cook until vermouth is evaporated.
Lower the heat and slowly add the milk product.
Stir the mushroom mixture periodically until it thickens.
Add the asparagus and spinach (and cooked meat or meat substitute, if desired).
Continue to cook on medium low until mixture is thick enough to mound a bit (not runny).
Place ¼ of the mixture into the middle of one crêpe, then fold the outside edges in.
Top the crêpes with some of the filling, and serve.

Elevate This: Add a few green peas. Sprinkle roasted pine nuts, a bit of Microgreen Pesto or Microgreen Pistou (p. 129), or serve with the Earth Day Three Pea Salad (p. 19). Substitute oyster, shiitake, or chanterelle mushrooms for a softer approach to the funghi.

Makes 4 crêpes. Serves 2 as a main dish

BRUSSELS SPROUT ASPARAGUS SUGAR PEA STIR FRY

This recipe combines all the green and beauty of Spring in one dish. It also highlights the super quick method to prep asparagus for an easy meal. Don't faint at using coconut oil – it is a small amount, and is the secret ingredient in this dish.

Ingredients
- 10 stalks fresh asparagus, bases trimmed
- 5-6 Brussels sprouts, thinly sliced
- 10-12 sugar snap peas, cut in half on the diagonal
- 2 garlic cloves, minced
- 1 tsp coconut oil
- 1 tsp white sesame seeds
- 1 tsp black sesame seeds
- 1 tsp Nigella seeds
- ½ tsp crushed red pepper
- sliced almonds, toasted

Instructions
Wrap the asparagus in a wet paper towel and microwave on high for 90 seconds. Run cool water over the asparagus, drain, and let dry. Cut in half on the diagonal – this can be done ahead of time.
Heat the coconut oil in a skillet over medium heat. Add the garlic, seeds, and red pepper, and cook for 20 seconds.
Add the Brussels sprouts and asparagus, and cook for 2-3 minutes.
Add the sugar peas and cook for 1 minute.
Sprinkle with toasted sliced almonds and serve.

Elevate This: Serve over brown rice, glass noodles or ramen. Sprinkle with furikake seasoning or just a bit of smoked soy sauce for added flavor.

Serves 2 as a main dish

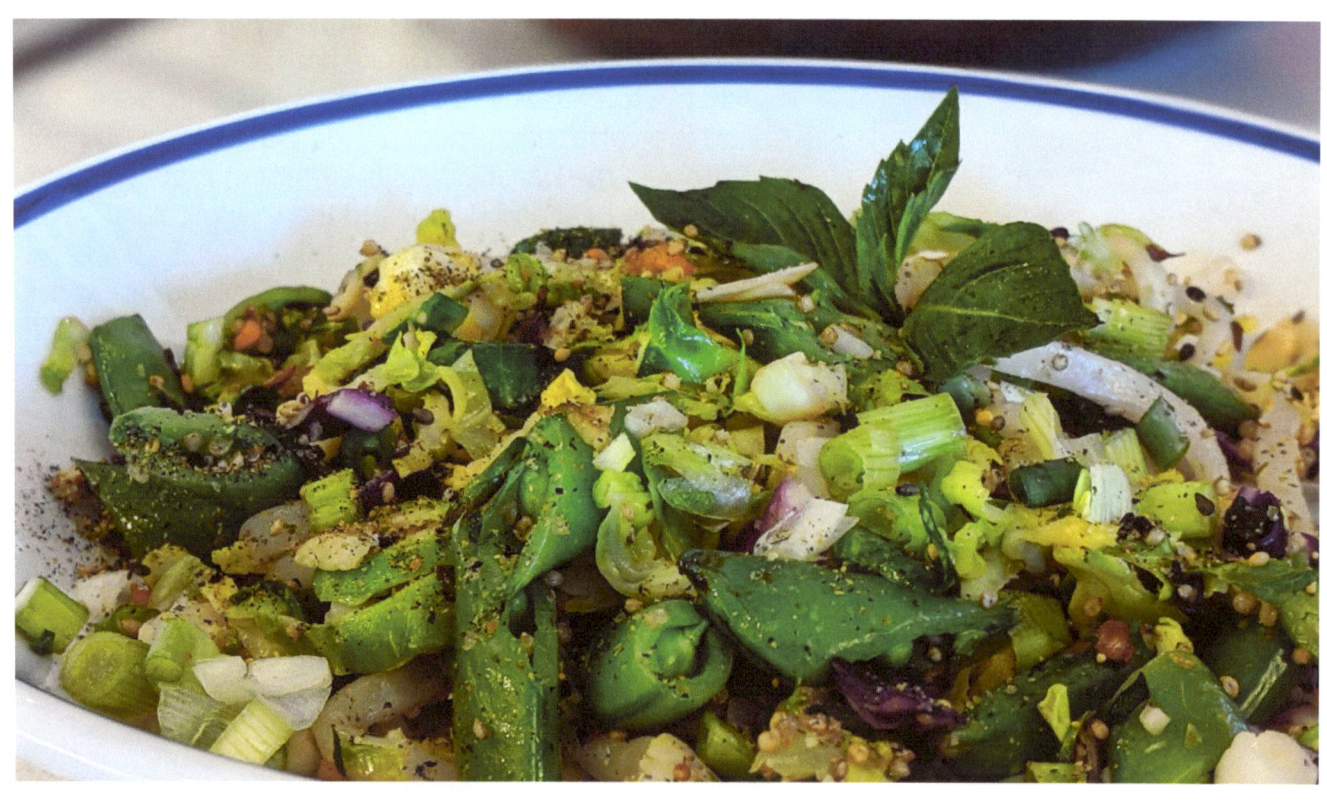

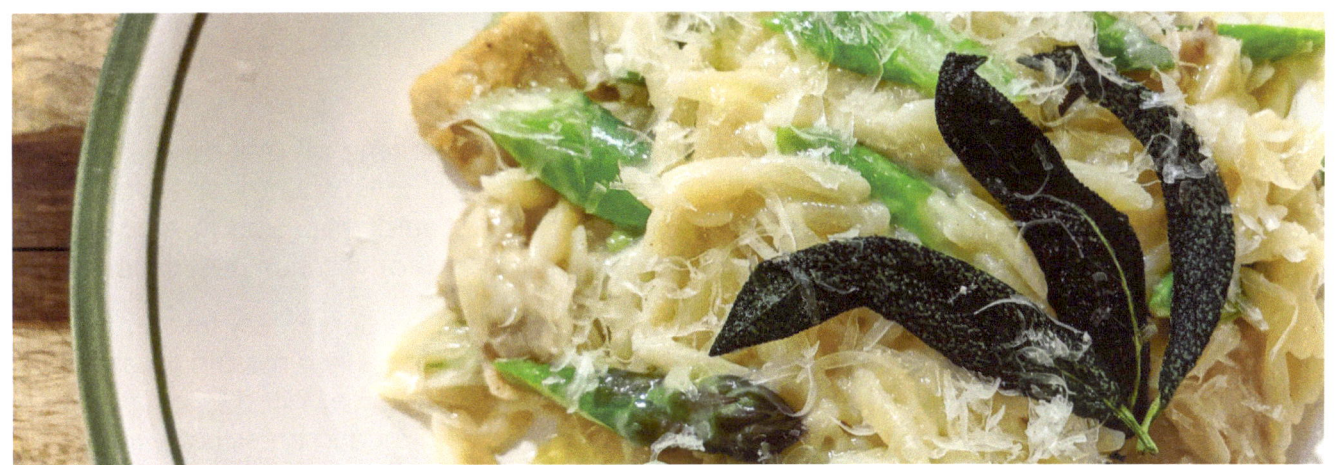

CREAMY SAGE ORZO WITH ASPARAGUS AND PEAS

I learned to make creamy orzo from Rachel Ray. Part of the creaminess comes from the orzo absorbing all the pasta water. It pairs well with sage, which grows wonderfully here in Northern Colorado. I have multiple bushes, and I enjoy using it in dishes, or just walking by and rubbing my hands against it to capture its scent. Sage is known to ease negative moods and fatigue by cerebrally, emotionally, and spiritually stimulating and clarifying the mind, while exhibiting a balancing, uplifting, soothing, and strengthening sense of being. One can only hope!

Ingredients
- 1 tsp oil
- 1 tbsp minced shallots
- 1 tsp minced garlic
- 1 cup orzo
- ¼ cup dry Vermouth
- 1 ¾ cup vegetable broth or chicken broth
- 8 sage leaves, divided
- ¼ cup parmesan (dairy or non-dairy)
- 6 asparagus spears; microwaved in wet paper towel for 2 minutes, rinsed, drained, cut on diagonal into 2-inch pieces
- 8-10 sugar peas; microwaved for 90 seconds, rinsed, drained, cut in half on diagonal
- Pinch of salt

For the Garnish
- Crispy sage leaves

Instructions
In a large sauce pan, heat the oil over medium heat.
Add the shallots and sauté until golden.
Add the garlic and sauté 30 seconds.
Add the orzo and sauté for 2 minutes.
Add the vermouth and allow sauce to reduce down.
Add the vegetable broth and 4 sage leaves. Cover and allow orzo to absorb the liquid – about 15 minutes. Stir occasionally. The mixture should look like a thick soup. Uncover. Add the dairy or non-dairy parmesan. Cook on low until mixture reduces and resembles risotto.
Stir in the asparagus and peas.
Place the remaining 4 sage leaves and oil in a small bowl. Coat the sage with the oil and add a pinch of salt. Microwave at 1-minute intervals until sage is crispy. Plate the orzo in bowls. Garnish with the crispy sage.

Elevate This: Play with herbs –you may enjoy mint and thyme. Add a small white bean or your preferred protein. Mushrooms are always a match. English peas or diced carrots will add color and sweetness.

Serves 2 as a main dish

Picnic on the Poudre

For a long time, we have enjoyed staycations as part of our regular time-off scheduling. It has been educational and entertaining to use these special "trips" to study a country or region, its history, wine or beer, and of course the food. On the patio, or at the river's edge, a good imagination can turn a simple picnic into a breezy visit to a hoped-for vacation destination spot.

Picnics do not need to be comprised of a hotdog, sandwich, hamburger or easy takeout food. It is entirely possible to grab leftovers in the fridge and—in this case—a little mashing makes a picnic an extra special event. As I write this, I am reminded of when we visited Denmark for our family heritage tour, there were Smørrebrød (open face butter and bread) offerings everywhere, alongside herring and other specialties. We longed terribly for a hamburger! Fast forward to 2021, and a beautifully staged Smørrebrød might now be our preference!

Bread helps give foundation to leftovers. The Italians might use crostini. We used my husband Mike's sourdough. You may choose a toast of some nature. Toasting is the operative word, although the Danish do not toast their brown bread, and they—gasp—use a fork and a knife. It works for them.

While scouring the fridge and pantry for ingredients, we discovered the following leftovers and spice mixes from The Spice and Tea Exchange®:

Ingredients
- 4 steamed purple potatoes
- ½ cup of mashed yellow lentils and garbanzos
- Healthy Harvest olives
- Carrots
- Sugar snap peas
- 8 grape tomatoes
- 5 Yukon Gold baby potatoes
- Blueberries
- Blackberries
- Microgreens
- 1 handful spinach
- Crispy Capers (p. 168)
- Pickles
- 1 bottle French Ginger Lemonade

This picnic became Provence-style with a nod to Tuscany. Mashing was the easy prep option. Purple potatoes mashed with garlic and a touch of olive oil and salt. Lentils and garbanzos were mashed with Garden Mirepoix Sea Salt Mix. Grape tomatoes were blended with olive oil and Tuscany Spice Blend. Yukon Golds were mashed with Black Truffle Salt and a bit of vegan butter. We packed it all up in a basket with some pretty towels and utensils, and set off to a picnic on the Poudre. In case you were wondering – no beer or wine on county park property.

As stated in the *How To Use This Cookbook* section, a spice shop is your best friend to up the ante of adding veggies to your lifestyle. Use the spices and herbs you have, or visit your local spice shop for cuisine-related spice blends.

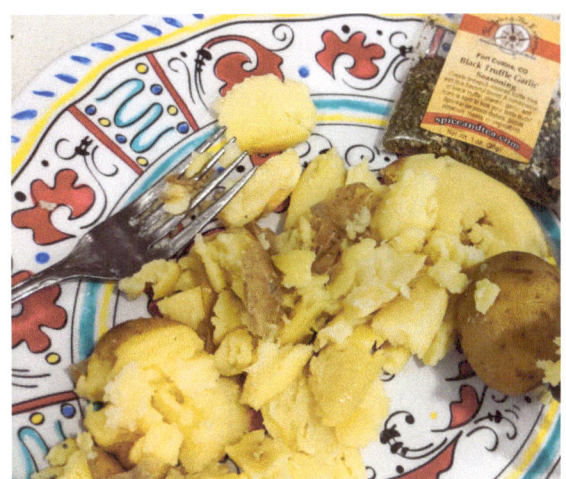
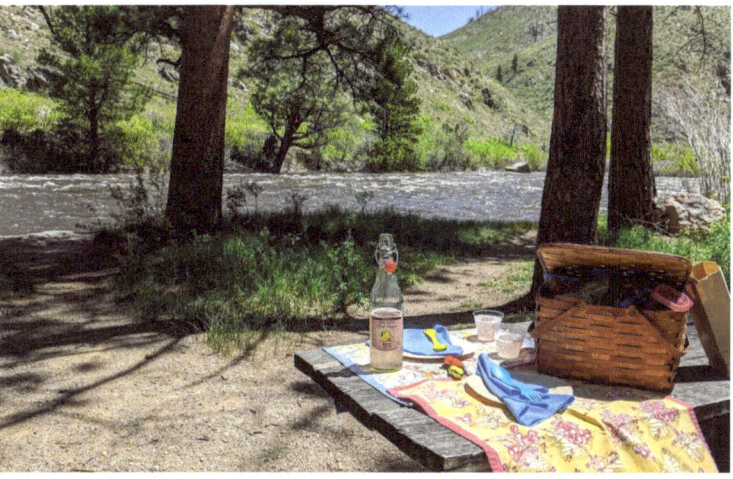
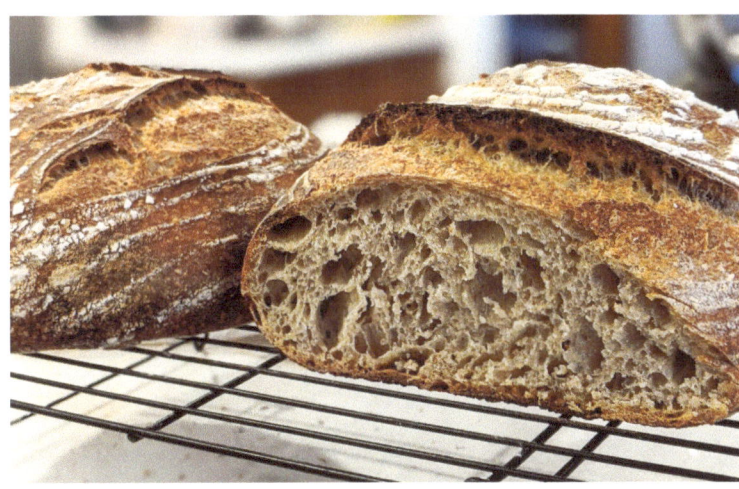
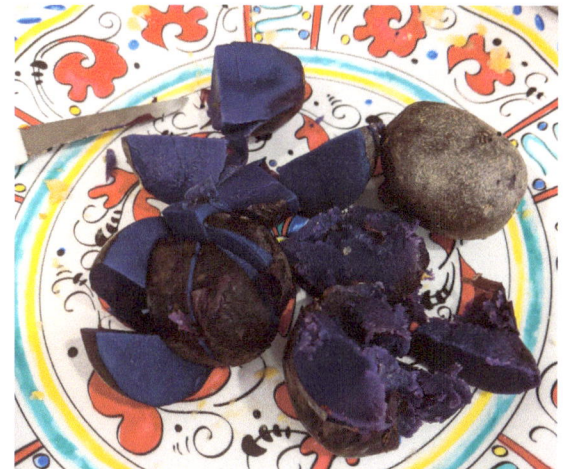

43

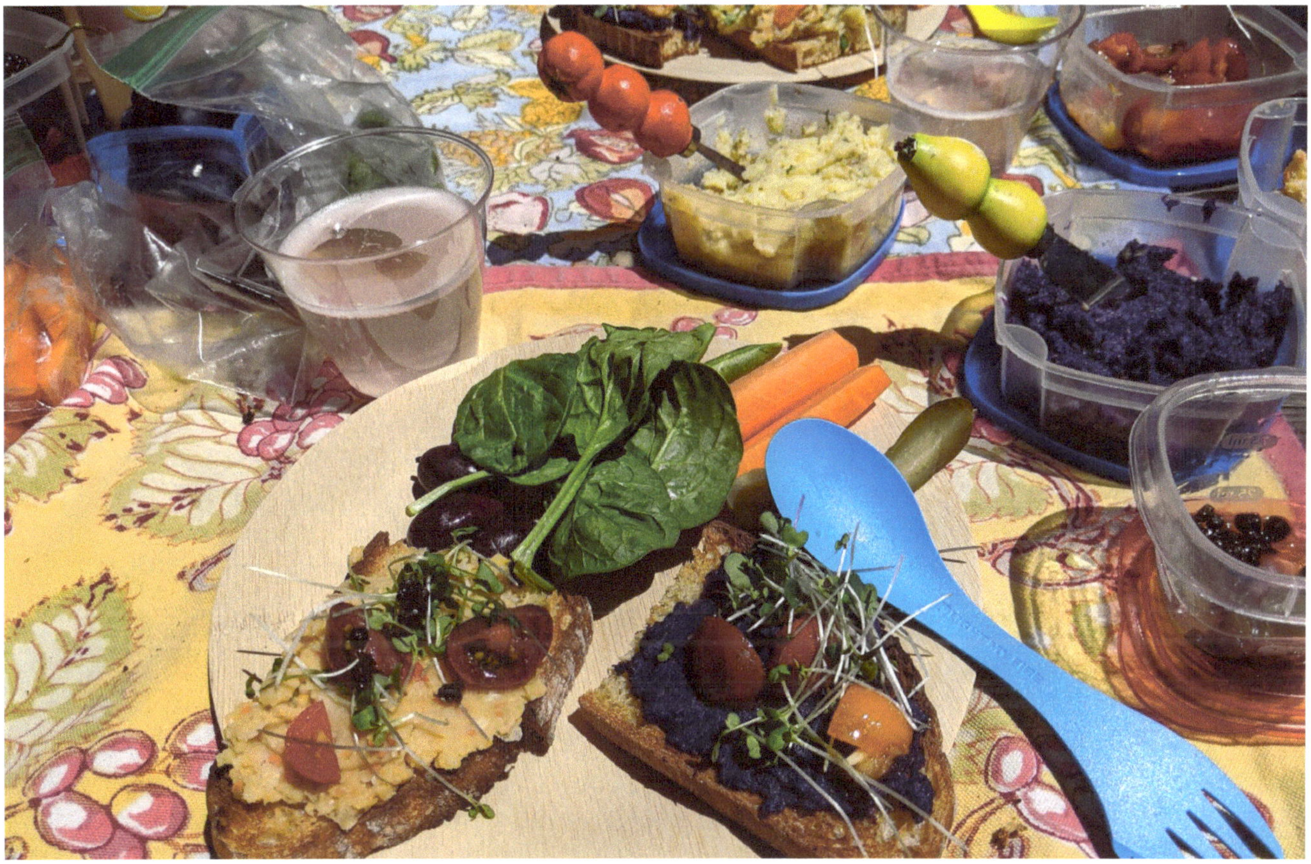

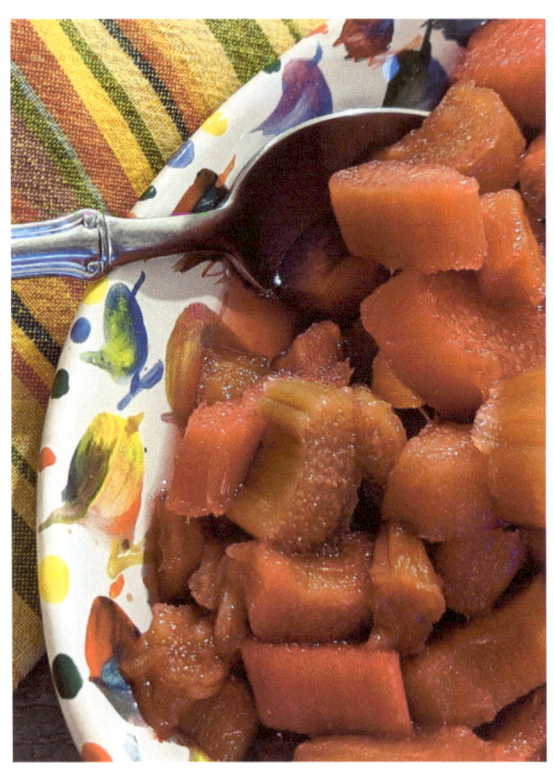 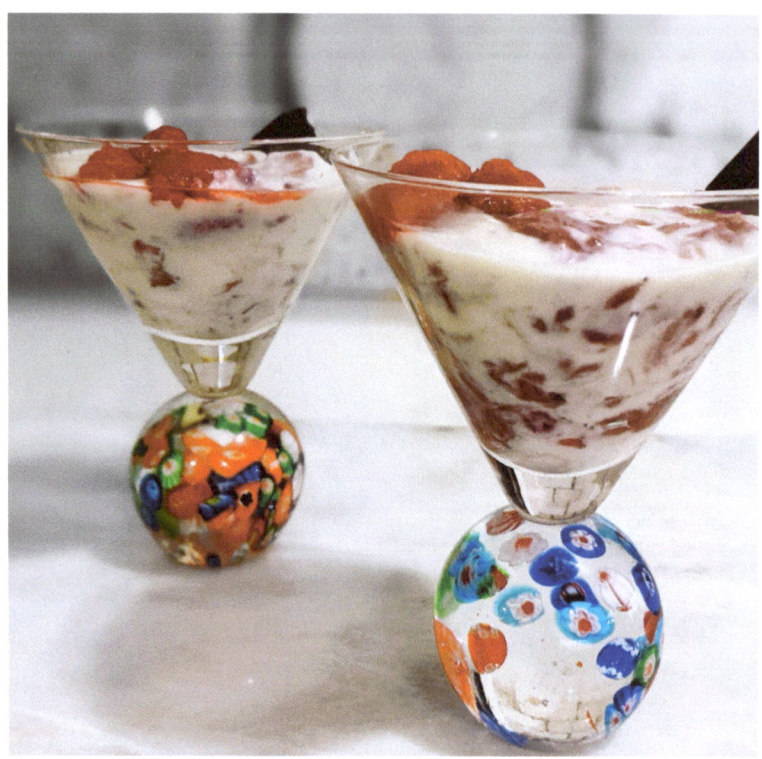

RHUBARB TWO WAYS

Who doesn't love that first little green curl of rhubarb leaf as it emerges from the soil in early spring? It is a sign of hope! Rhubarb is tart. It can be eaten raw, dipped in a sweetener, or as many of us do, made into a baked dessert dish. Crumble, pie, and tart recipes are readily available. An interesting find is a Romanian soup with tomato and rhubarb – perhaps I'll share the recipe in my next cookbook.

Rhubarb is such a lovely, brilliant color, but it turns a bit gray when cooked too long. Some cooks add red food coloring—gasp!—while others add another red berry. It's always nice to have a backup plan for a cooking error. Here are two ways to cook rhubarb – a savory side dish and a dessert, depending on how long you cook the rhubarb.

SPICED RHUBARB

Ingredients
- 1 ½ cups of 1-inch pieces of chopped rhubarb stems – the redder, the better
- 3 green cardamom pods
- ½ tsp ground cardamom
- 2 tbsp thinly sliced crystallized ginger
- 1 tsp dried orange peel, or ½ tsp freshly grated orange rind
- ½ cup sugar, or more to taste
- 1 tbsp water

Instructions
Place all the ingredients in a saucepan and cook on medium heat until the rhubarb is fork tender – a little resistance is okay. We want the rhubarb to stay red and hold its shape.
Scoop out the rhubarb chunks and reserve in a bowl. Bring the remaining sauce to a boil, then lower the heat and reduce sauce down to a syrup.
Remove the cardamom pods.
Gently stir the syrup over the rhubarb chunks.
Serve as a side or dessert bite.

Serves 2 as a side dish or dessert

RHUBARB FOOL

Use the ingredients for the Spiced Rhubarb, but cook the rhubarb to a softer stage. If you can mash with a fork, it's perfect. Swirl in ¼ cup fresh raspberries or strawberries. Let cool.

For the plant-based cooks – make a stabilizer by melting 1 teaspoon of plain gelatin or agar-agar powder with 2 teaspoons hot water. Let the stabilizer cool a bit to thicken. Whip together 1 cup of silken tofu, ½ cup powdered sugar and the stabilizer. Chill the tofu mixture for 1 hour, then swirl in the rhubarb mixture.

If you prefer to use dairy products, use whipping cream whipped with a bit of sugar to stabilize, a frozen whipped dairy product, Greek yogurt, or a home crafted simple custard.

Garnish either option with more berries.

Elevate This: Think crunch and think complementary. Add a small piece of dark chocolate, a sprinkle of salted caramel sugar, or a mini ginger cookie bite.

Serves 2 as a dessert

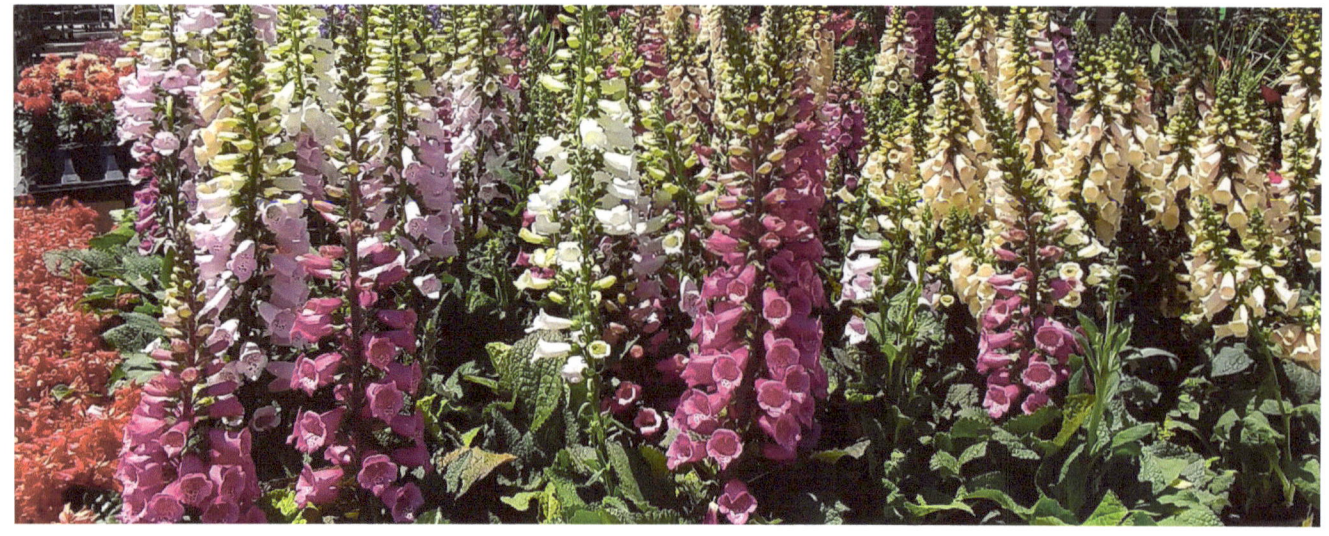
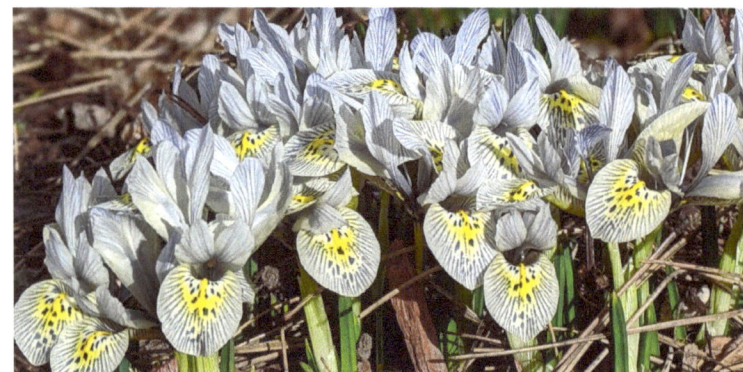
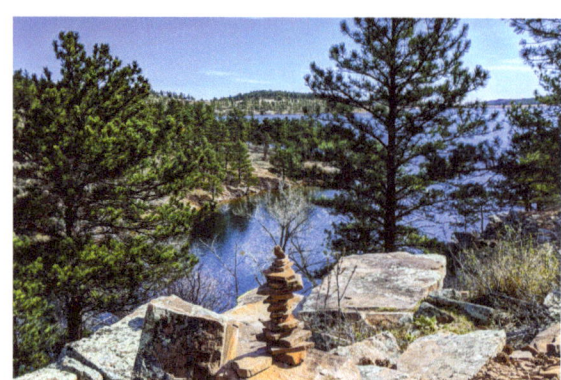
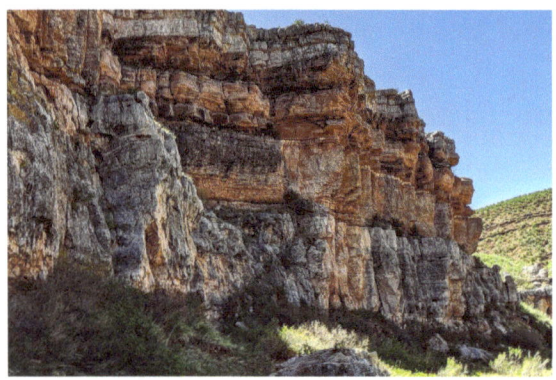
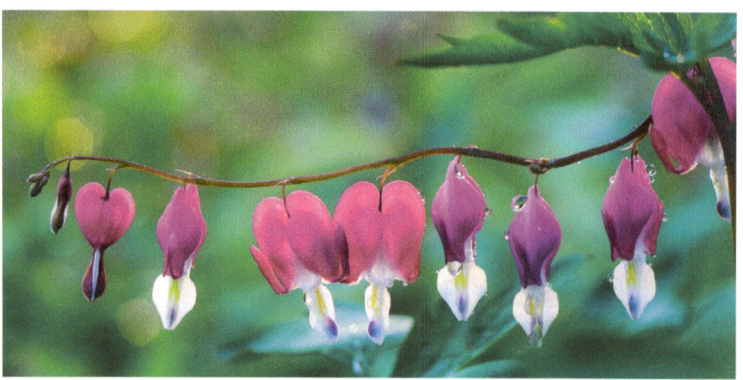
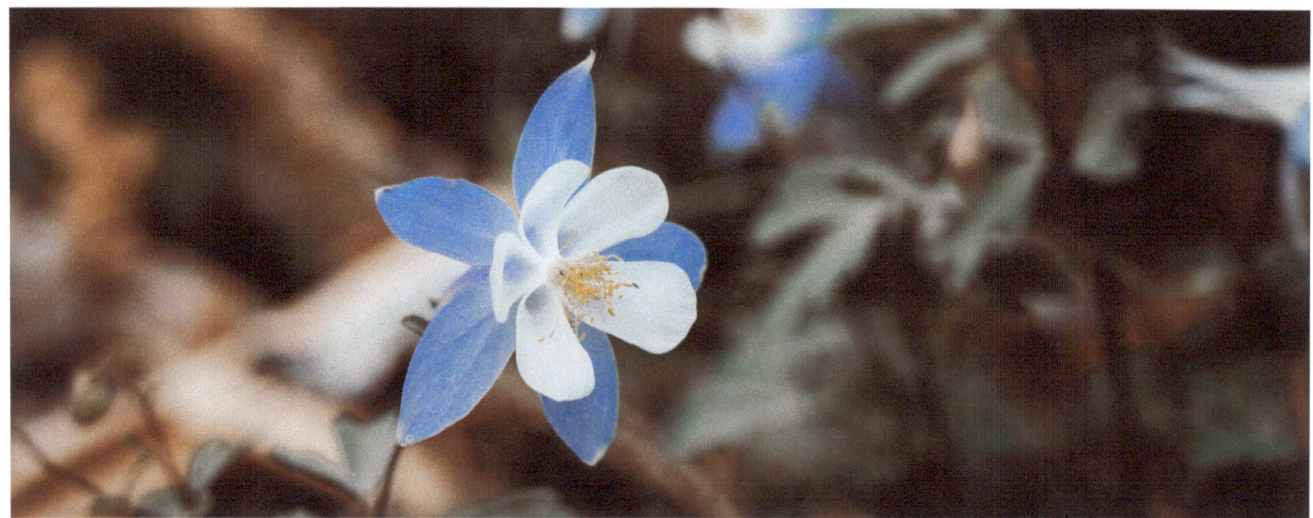

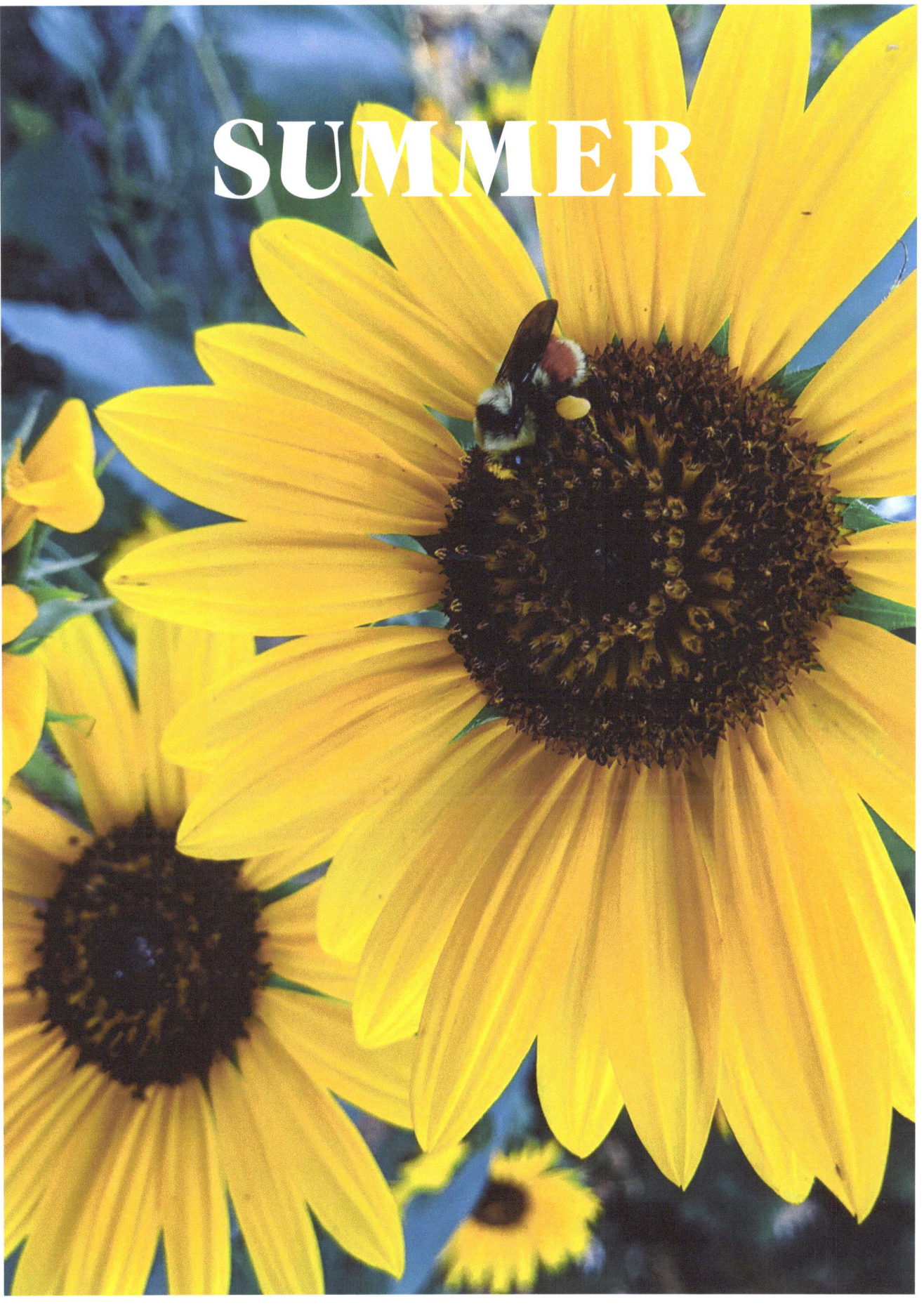

SUMMER

Nature's abundance is truly upon Northern Colorado in July, August and part of September. The planting that began in May is beginning to bear fruits (and veg!), and we are reaping the rewards of the summer harvests.

Warmer weather vegetables arrive at the farmers market and in the community and personal gardens. Beans, root crops, tomatoes, peppers, corn, squash, herbs – anything that loves a long summer day and a cool night to flourish, arrives at our table. The entire region is alive with produce and goods. Fort Collins, Longmont, Boulder, Loveland and more – every town, and sometimes each of the counties, has at least one weekly market, if not two, in the summer. Customers can walk past, pause, almost gasp in amazement at the beautiful offerings, chat with growers, and buy anything from herbs, flowers, vegetables, and fruits, to specially roasted and ground coffees, hand crafted pastries, eggs, dairy, and other meat products.

Later in the summer, the Rocky Ford melons, Palisade peaches, sweet and sour cherry varieties, and Olathe corn are transported to our area from other parts of Colorado. The selection seems endless for several weeks more. But we know it will be gone at first frost, so we are busy freezing, canning, and of course eating, the goodness of Colorado.

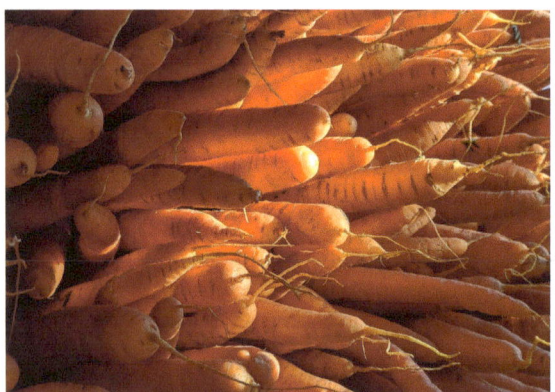
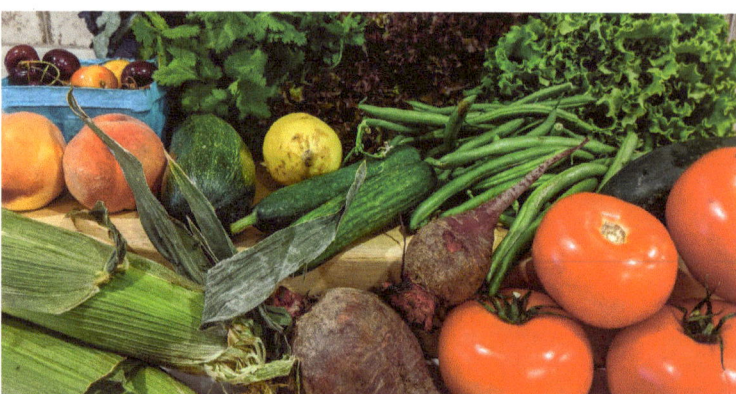
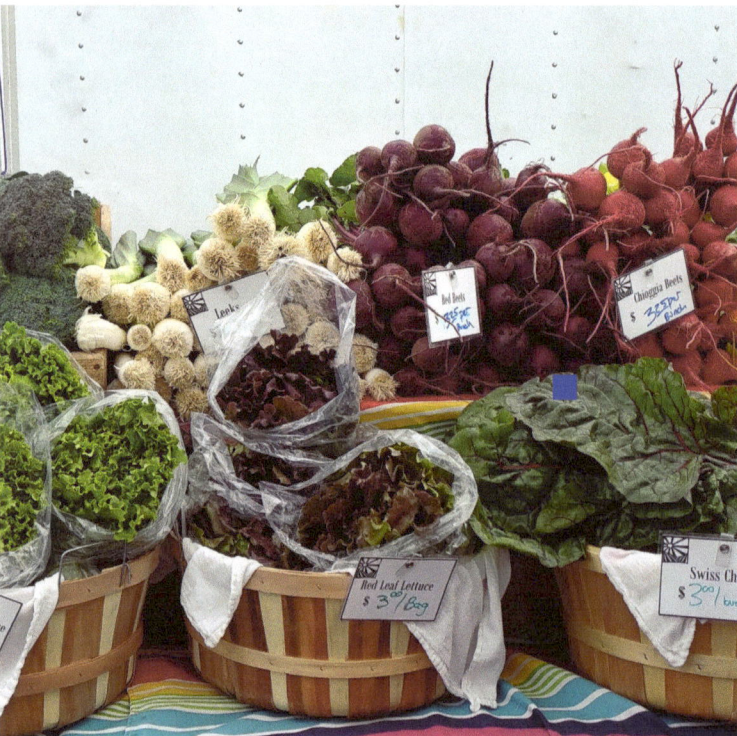
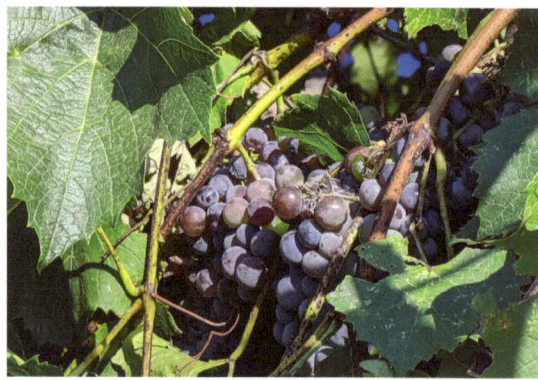
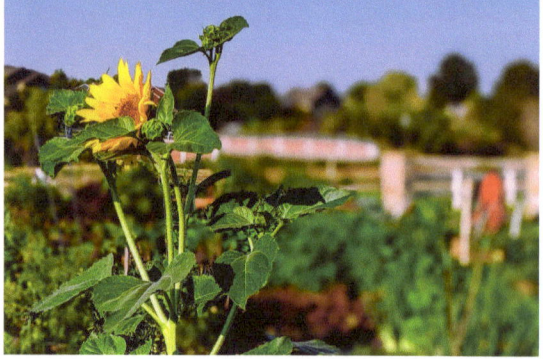

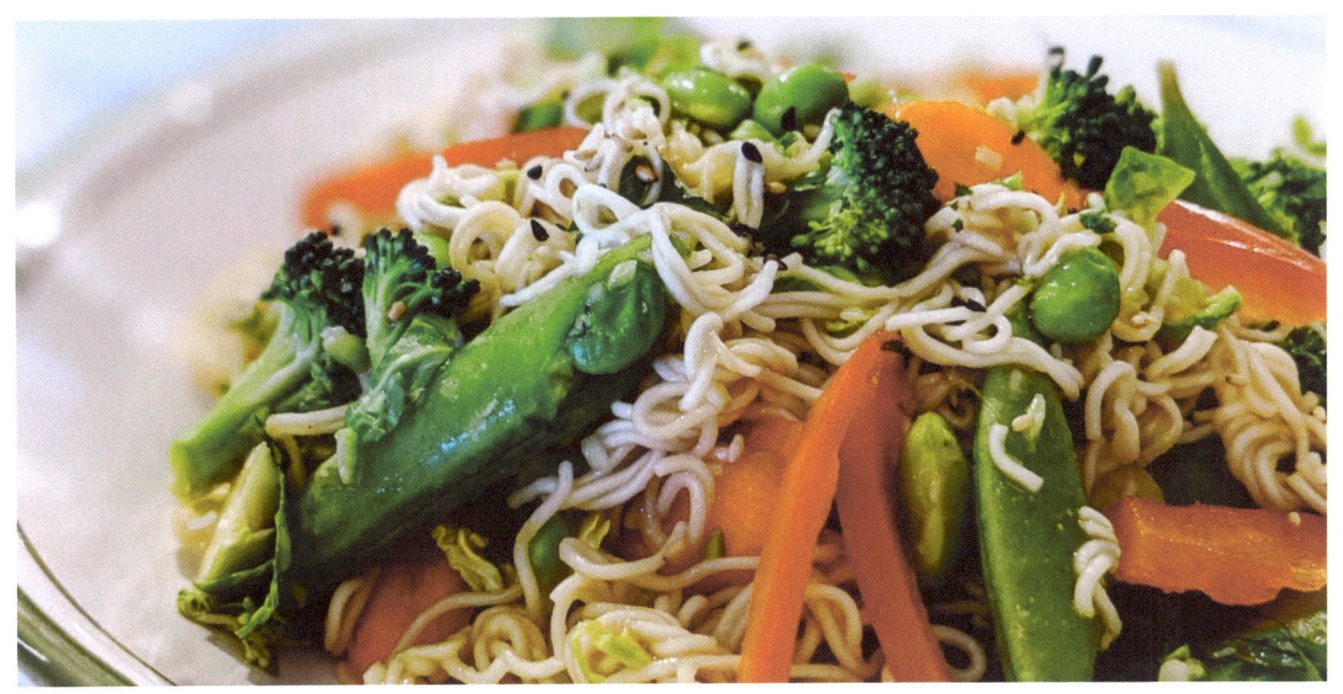

RAMEN NOODLE REVIVAL

Ramen is not passé! You can now find millet ramen, brown rice ramen, even beautiful black, forbidden grain ramen. There are even ramen food trucks now. This dish celebrates the cusp of spring and summer with a bit of fresh, whatever you have on hand, from the CSA or market. In this case, it was peas, carrots, broccoli, Brussels sprouts, green onions and more. This is a fresh and light summer salad, so have some fun elevating this basic dish into something you will enjoy again and again.

Ingredients
- Millet or mixed grain ramen noodles (or ramen of choice)
- 2 tsp peanut or canola oil
- 2 tsp mirin, rice vinegar, or soy sauce (or a little of each!)
- 1 cup of broccoli florets, microwaved 90 seconds in water
- Broccoli stems from the florets, grated into small pieces
- 6 Brussels sprouts, thinly sliced
- 1 carrot, sliced on the diagonal
- 6-8 sugar peas, sliced on the diagonal
- 2 tbsp chopped green onions

For the Garnish: Chopped cilantro, toasted sesame seeds, slivers of red bell pepper, drizzle of sesame oil

Instructions
Place noodles in a bowl and cover with hot water. Set aside for 5 minutes. Drain noodles while reserving ¼ cup noodle water in a separate bowl.
Add ramen noodle spice mixture (if you have it) to the water and stir. Add oil and mirin, vinegar, or soy sauce. Mix well and add the liquid back to the noodles.
In a large bowl, combine all the vegetables, add the noodles, and toss well. Add the garnishes and serve.

Note: If your ramen does not come with a spice mixture, combine ½ cup vegetable broth, 1 tsp soy sauce, 1 tsp red miso paste, and 2 tsp cornstarch in a bowl. Microwave until mixture thickens.

Elevate This: Try Yakisoba or Pulmuone noodles from the market or switch noodles for vegetarian potstickers. Add ½ cup frozen edamame (microwaved 90 seconds in water) for protein. Add almonds for crunch.

Serves 2 as a main dish

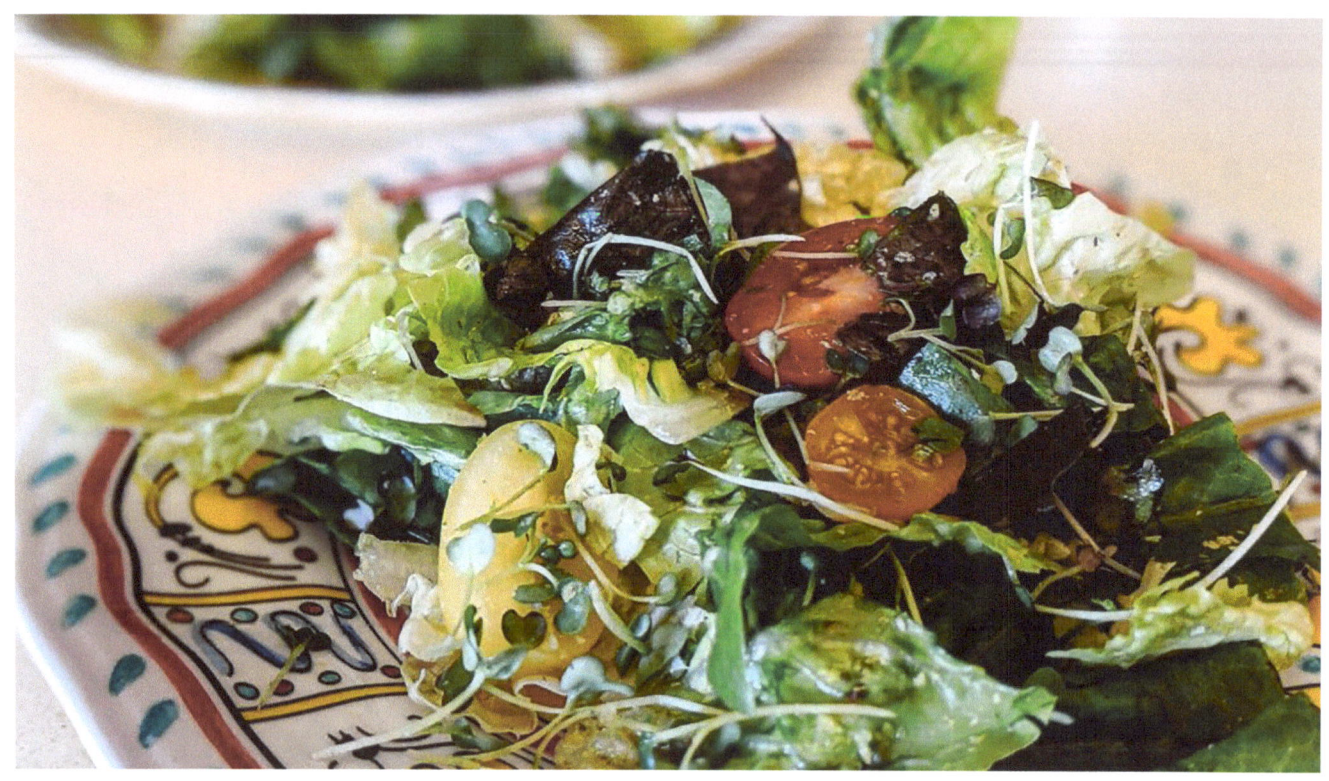

SIMPLE SALAD WITH GRATED GARLIC DRESSING

Bags of baby greens seem to be the norm these days in the grocery stores. Of course, they are easy and pre-washed. No prep required. They are perfect for a busy lifestyle. Yet, beyond the Simpson Red and Romaine, there are a myriad of head lettuces to explore within our plant-based lifestyles.

Local growers in Northern Colorado are raising fantastic varietals such as Four Seasons (sounds so much better in French! - Merveille de Quatre Saisons), Austrian Speckled Trout, and Italian Passion Brune. If you can't find them, maybe plant a few seeds in a pot during your own lettuce growing season!

This is our go-to dish and my husband has learned to make it. I enjoy mixing the salad with clean hands. It is a very tactile experience of connecting with the food goodness. There is only one tablespoon of oil in the salad, so use your best extra virgin olive oil.

Note: *The grater can be found online or at specialty cooking stores.*

Ingredients

For the Salad
- 1 head of tender green or red lettuce – such as Butter, Red Oak, or Merveille de Quatre Saisons
- ½ cup of spicy microgreens
- 10 grape tomatoes, halved

For the Dressing
- 1 garlic clove, peeled
- 1 tbsp extra virgin olive oil
- 1 tbsp nutritional yeast
- Sea salt and pepper to taste

Instructions

Wash, spin, and tear the lettuce into a bowl.
Add the spicy microgreens and tomatoes.
Grate the garlic clove on a garlic grater.
Add the olive oil into the grater bowl, mix in with a soft spatula, and let stand for 5 minutes to infuse the flavor.
Pour the infused oil (garlic bits and all) over the lettuce.
Sprinkle the nutritional yeast and mix with your hands.
Salt and pepper to taste.
Plate and serve.

Elevate This: Less is more. Add pine nuts, a small bit of feta (dairy or non-dairy) or a few sunflower seeds to make this dish worthy of company.

Serves 3-4 as a salad dish

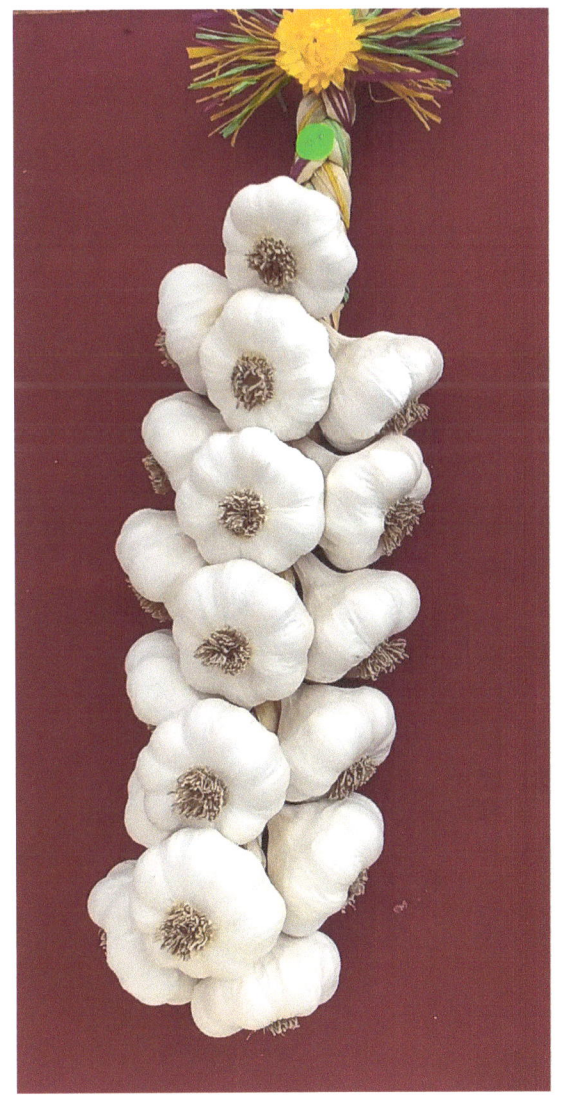
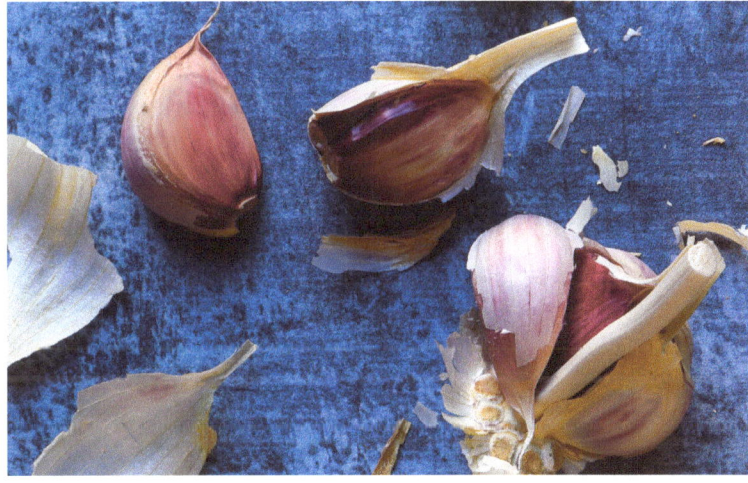
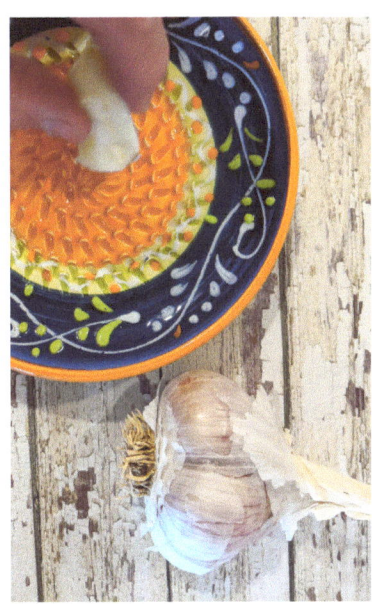
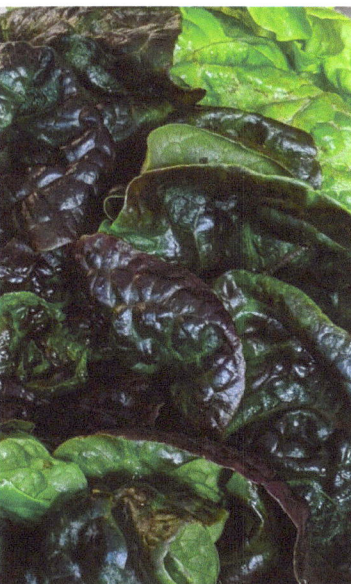

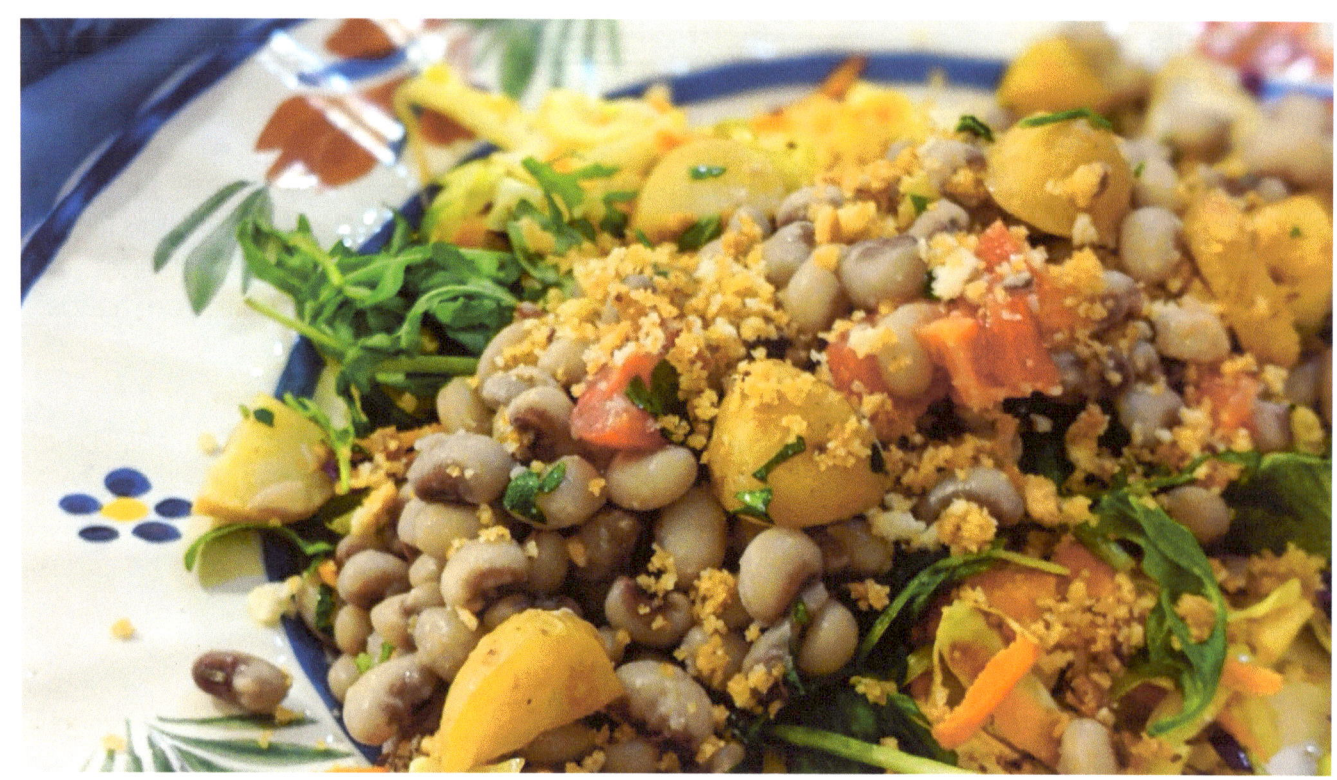

BLACK-EYED PEA SALAD WITH CABBAGE

An unusual find in Northern Colorado is locally grown black-eyed peas. On the Vine at Richmond Farms had their first pea harvest in 2019, and much to my dismay, I was too late to get some fresh peas. It will definitely be on my future radar.

Having grown up in the South, I did my fair share of shelling peas. They were not my favorite pea to cook and eat, as the broth turned an ugly gray color. But after reading Dan Buettner's Blue Zone® longevity research, in which the Ikarians eat an exceptional amount of this pea in their diet, I was inspired to rethink this Southern specialty. This dish is a great way to use up straggling leftover veg. Enjoy this Greek version of the black-eyed pea. If you can find the conehead cabbage, that's a bonus.

Ingredients

For the Peas
- 2 cups cooked or 1 can black-eyed peas, rinsed and drained
- 1 steamed Yukon potato, cubed
- 1 garlic clove, grated into 1 tbsp olive oil
- 1 tsp Greek seasoning
- 8 grape tomatoes, halved lengthwise
- Salt and pepper to taste

For the Cabbage
- 2 cups sliced conehead or Napa cabbage
- 2 garlic cloves, minced
- 1 tbsp oil
- 1 tsp celery seed
- ½ tsp caraway seed
- 1 tsp white pepper
- Salt and pepper to taste

For the Garnish
- Toasted breadcrumbs
- Chopped parsley

Instructions

Combine all the pea ingredients in a bowl, and let sit for 15 minutes to meld.
Salt and pepper to taste.
Heat the oil in a skillet over medium heat. Add the cabbage and garlic and sauté for 2-3 minutes, just until it begins to wilt.
Push the cabbage aside, and place the celery, caraway seeds and white pepper in the middle of the skillet. Warm the seeds then push the cabbage back to the center and cook on low for another 3-5 minutes.
Place the cabbage mixture into bowls and top with the peas.
Salt and pepper to taste.
Garnish with breadcrumbs and chopped parsley.

Elevate This: Add a spicy green such as fresh arugula or sunflower shoots and a touch of grated carrot for more color.

Serves 2 as a main dish

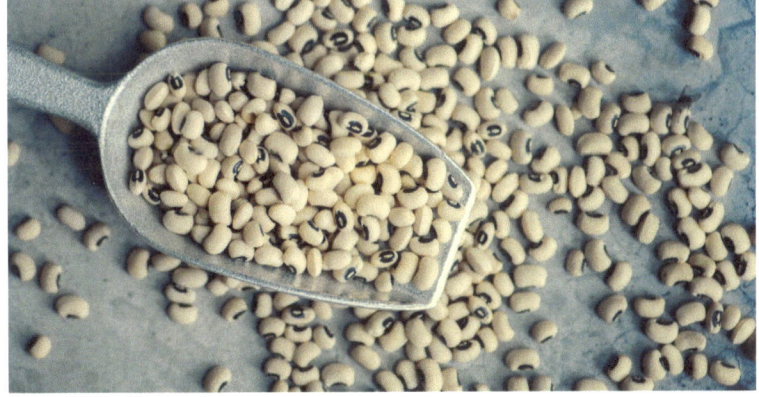
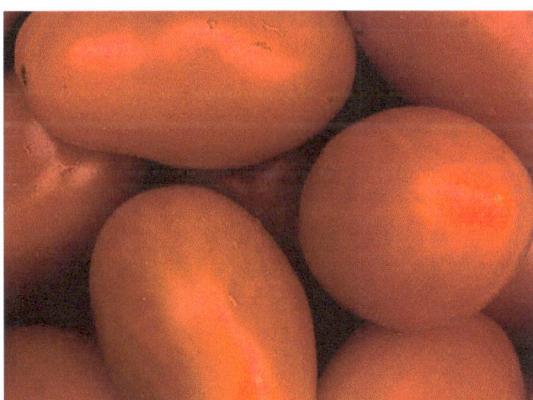
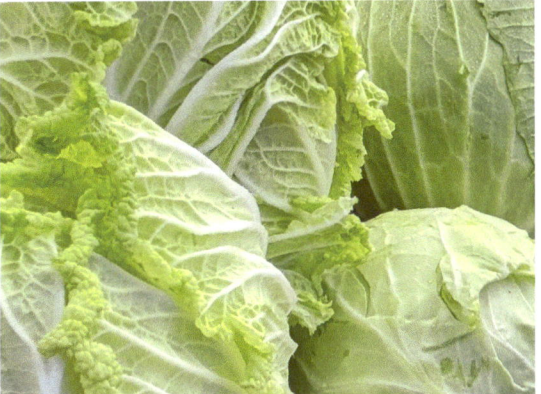
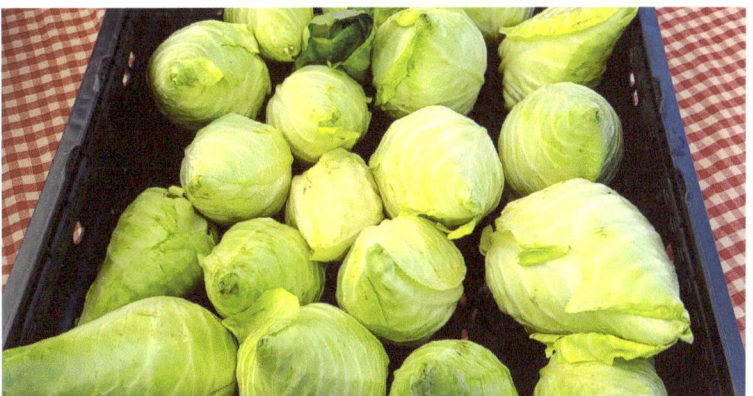

Strawberries 101

I love strawberries, but not the gigantic, red, white and green berries we usually get in grocery stores that sometimes don't look quite normal. You know the ones I am talking about – when you slice the berry, you almost need a bread knife. Strawberries that are so big that you can put only two or three in your palm. Those berries we think are so wonderful dipped in dark chocolate, but when you bite into them, there is a gaping canyon – what is up with that?

I prefer small to medium sized, beautiful, glossy, all-over ruby fruits sprinkled with little brown seeds, with no hint of white, off white, cream, sand, or alabaster near their crowns, or green variations near their stems. The ones that come, say, 15-20 to a pint. Berry size is a source of contention for me. In the 1960s and 70s, you could buy pints of small, sweet strawberries. The only way to buy strawberries now is in quart containers, because—you guessed it—the strawberries at the grocery store are modified to be huge. And they are tasteless.

The short strawberry season here in Northern Colorado starts in mid-June and lasts about three weeks. Then, depending on the berry variety, the plant will host a second short season again in August. There are multiple pick-your-own strawberry farms in the area, including On the Vine at Richmond Farms and Garden Sweet Farms. One can spend a joyful hour picking the most luscious, delightful, red, juicy strawberries ever!

Once you have eaten a locally grown strawberry, you really will want to rely on the strawberry zen you'll experience directly from the farm – but, in a pinch, it is possible to find good strawberries at your local grocery store. With that said, I elected not to include a cooked strawberry recipe in this collection. Fresh sliced strawberries accompany anything from lettuce greens to ice cream. Macerate the berries in some sugar for an hour to tease out the juices. Or, just eat the strawberry whole. Experiencing a little playful mindfulness while savoring the fruit will enhance the eating experience.

So, how do you keep your berries lovely for several days so you can enjoy a daily pleasure moment of real, juicy strawberries? I did some research. Keep the moisture out. Remove the mold spores. Store flat if possible. Reusable fruit and vegetable bags, such as Green Bags, work great. Some experts propose a vinegar wash, but I did not find the vinegar taste satisfying.
If you have time, try this tip:

1) Prepare a solution of 1 tbsp lemon juice (out of a bottle) and 1 cup cold water.
2) Place strawberries in a colander. Sprinkle the lemon juice over the berries to coat. Drain.
3) Allow to air dry and place back in the fridge in a flat storage container if possible.

Of course, there is the distinct possibility you will eat your strawberries very quickly, and storage will not be an issue.

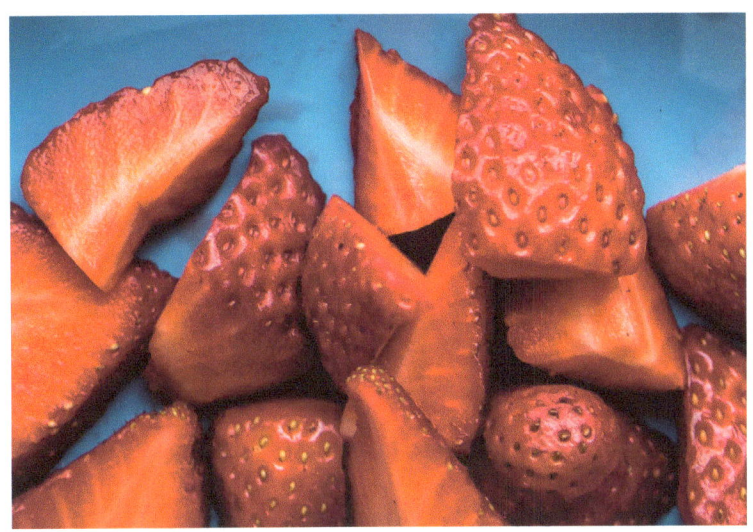
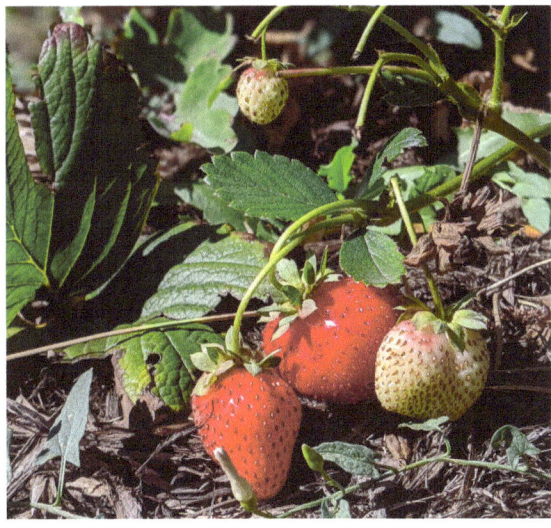
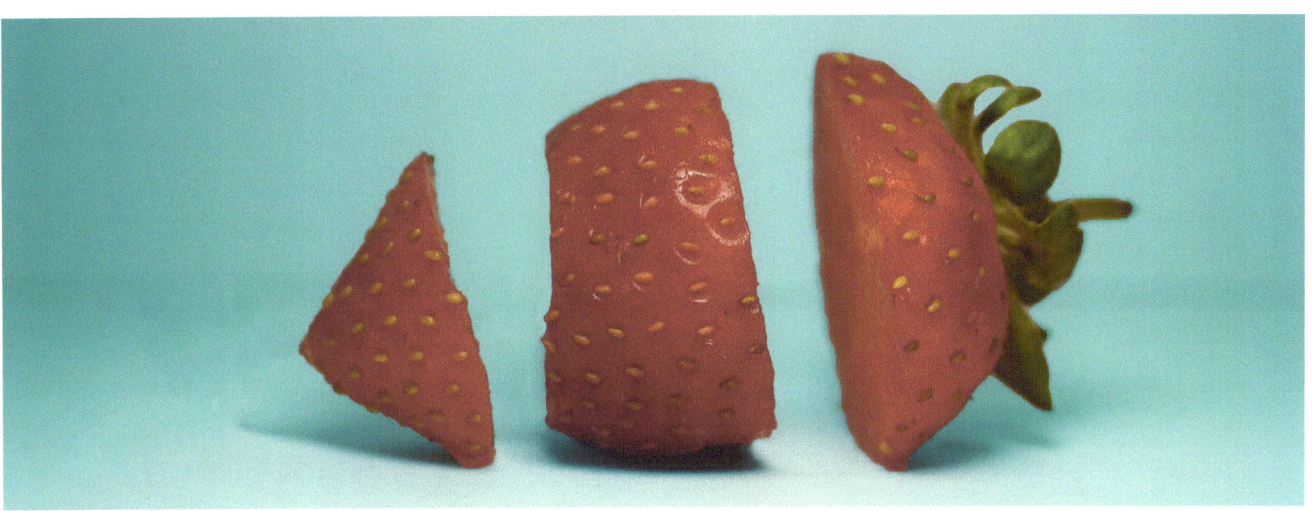
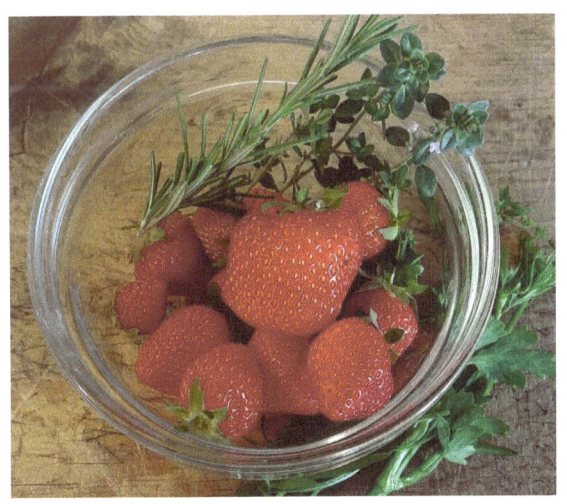
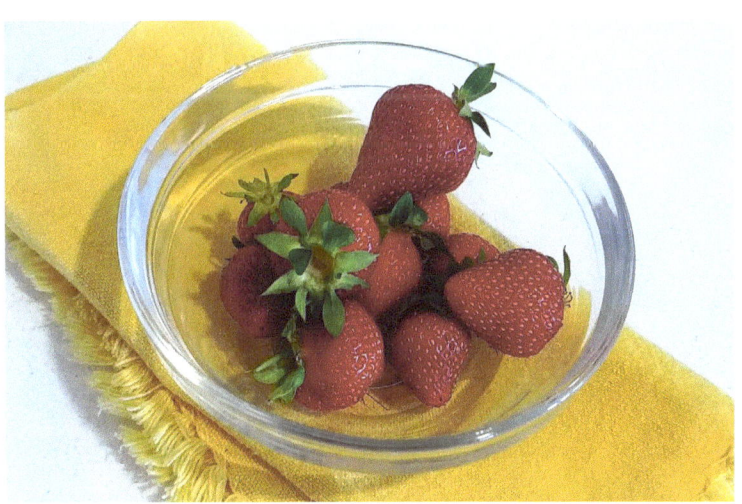

HEIRLOOM TOMATO SALAD

We eat with our eyes. I believe the more we see what freshness looks like, the more we train our inner selves to appreciate and want to eat plants.

Sometimes easy is best. A salad doesn't always have to be hand-pulled chopped lettuce, mixed greens, and tossed with a heavy dressing. Consider allowing the whole veg or a slice of a veg to take center stage.

This luscious heirloom tomato lays gracefully on a few leaves of beautiful dark green French lettuce. A sprinkling of microgreens, strips of fresh basil, a drizzle of good olive oil, and you have a lovely al fresco summer salad.

Ingredients
- 1 heirloom tomato
- A few large leaves of beautifully green lettuce
- Microgreens of choice
- Fresh basil
- Extra virgin olive oil
- Sea salt and pepper to taste

Instructions
For each serving, artfully assemble a few large lettuce leaves on a beautiful plate in a style you prefer.
Slice the tomato and layer a few slices on the lettuce.
Sprinkle on the microgreens, and drizzle with olive oil.
A sprig of basil is a final touch.
Salt and pepper to taste.

Elevate This: A few pine nuts or good quality olives on the side will give a bit of umami.

Serves 1 – multiply the recipe for as many salads as you'd like to create.

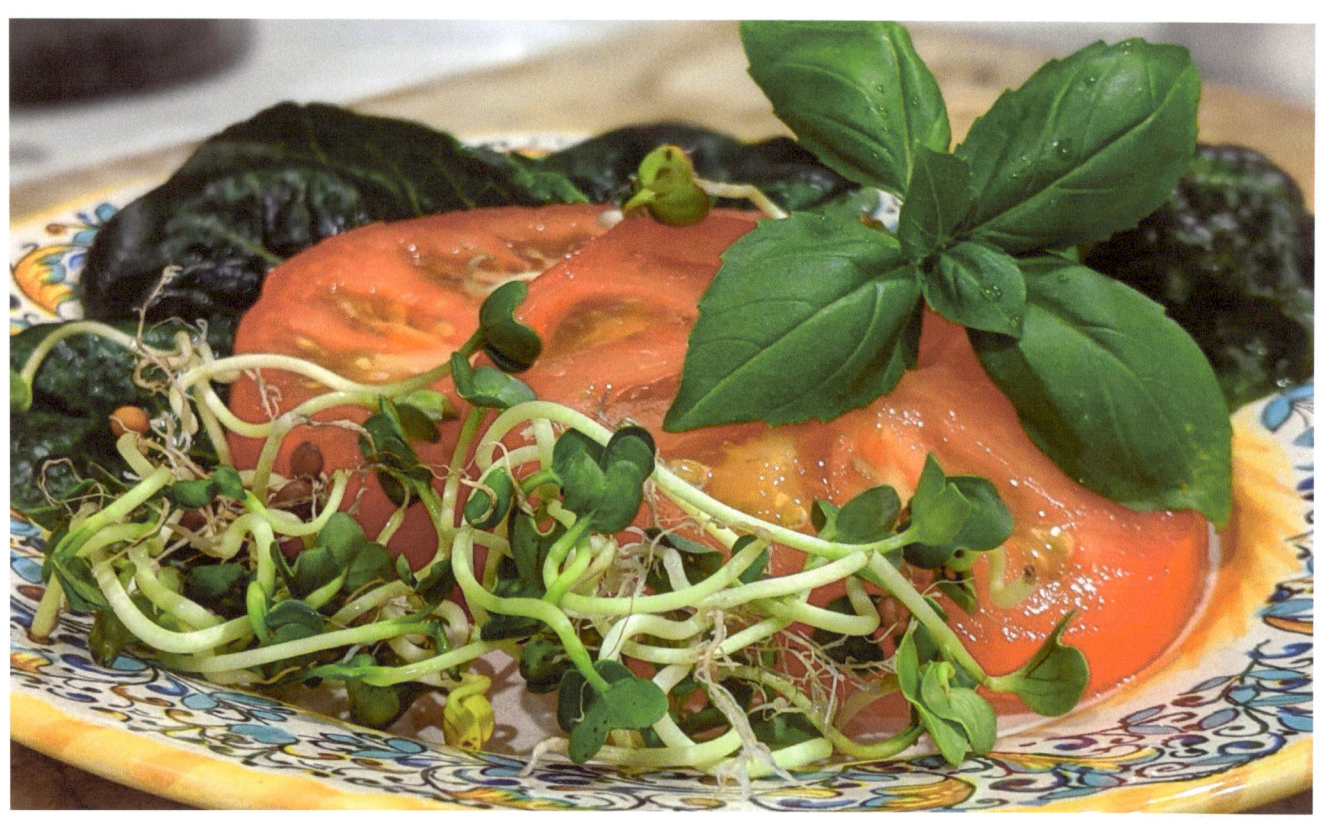

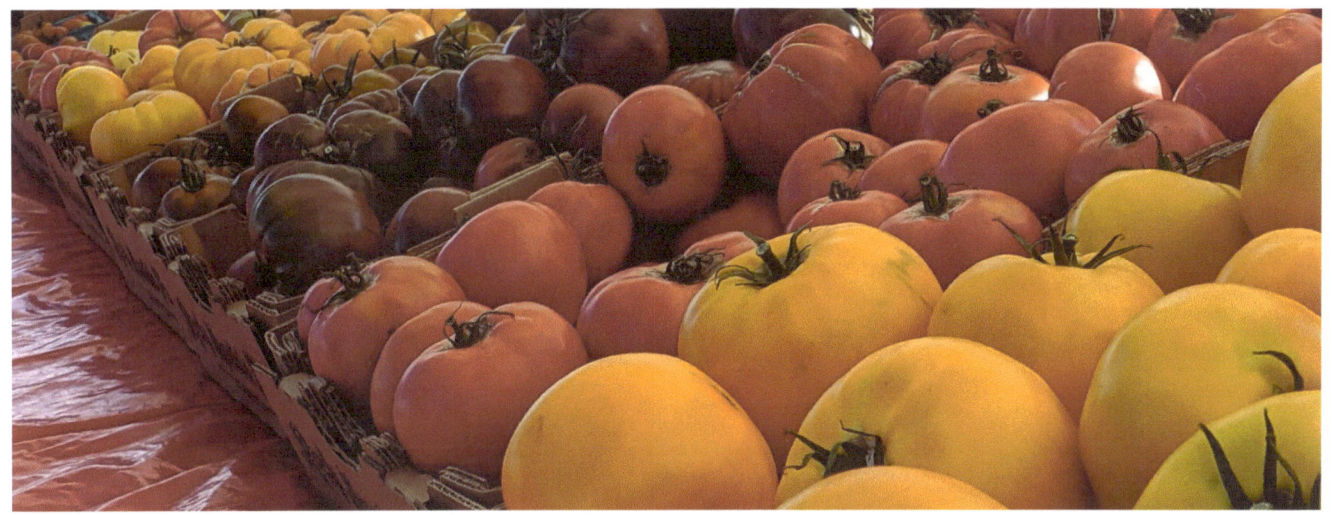
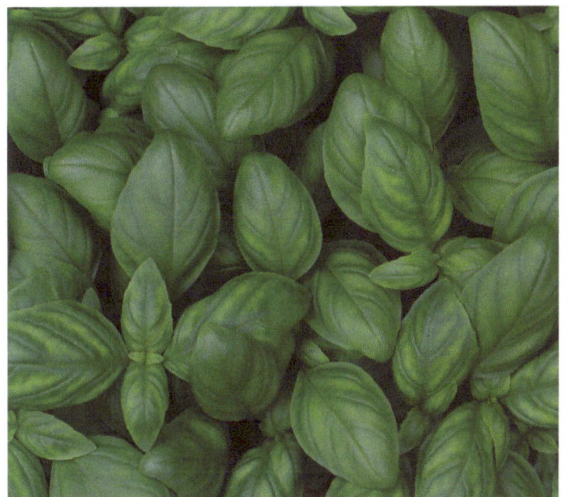
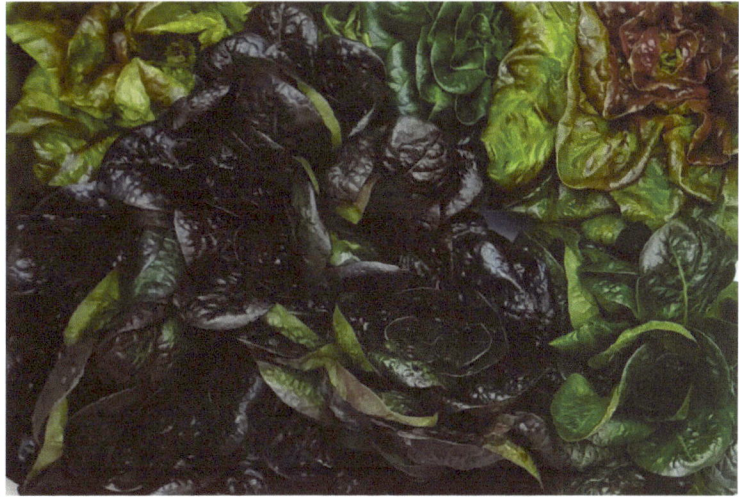

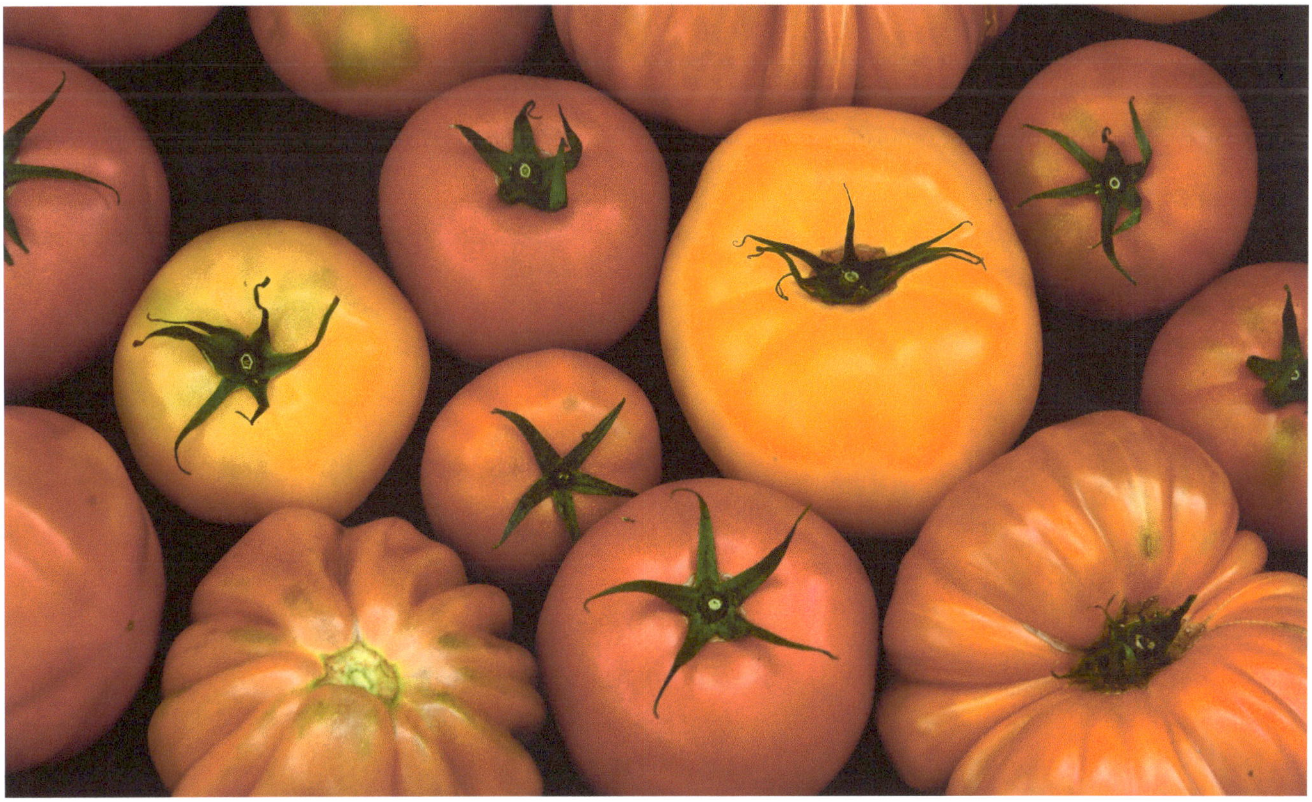

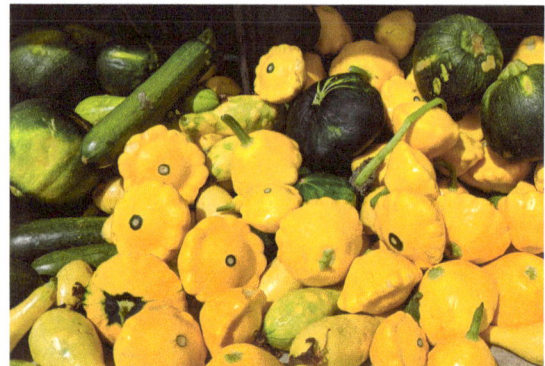
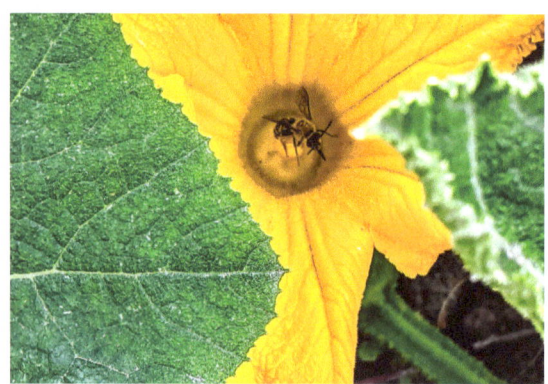
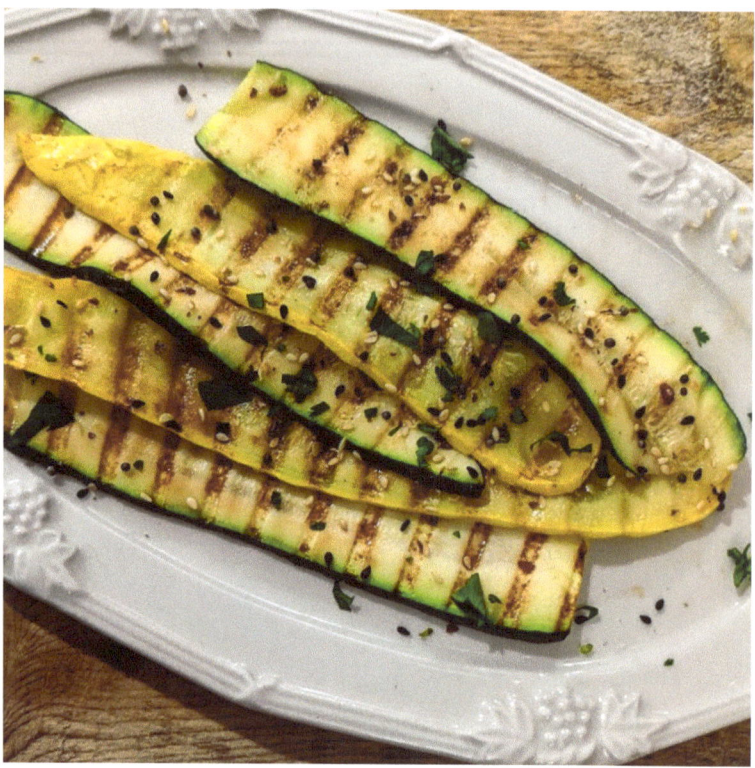

GRILLED SQUASH WITH MISO AND SESAME GLAZE

This is a beautiful way to add a Japanese boost to what could be a rather boring vegetable. Really fresh squash can weep moisture when cut, creating a soggy dish, so take the time to remove the moisture from the squash.

Ingredients
For the Glaze
- 1 tbsp water
- 2 tbsp white miso
- 1 tbsp rice vinegar
- 1 tbsp sugar
- 1 tsp soy sauce (smoked soy sauce preferred)

For the Squash
- 1 lb zucchini or yellow (crookneck) squash, sliced ¼ inch thick lengthwise
- 1 tsp salt
- 1 tsp white sesame seeds
- 1 tsp black sesame seeds
- 1 tsp black mustard seeds

Instructions
Salt the squash. Place the squash slices between 2 paper towels. Allow towels to absorb extra liquid for 15-20 minutes.

Heat the grill. Mix all the glaze ingredients in a bowl. Combine all the seeds in a skillet and gently toast the seeds until aromatic. Remove the pan and cool.

With a pastry brush, spread glaze on both sides of the squash. Reserve 1 tbsp glaze for finishing the dish. Grill the squash until fork tender, but not too soft. Move the squash to a serving plate. Paint the slices lightly with the remaining glaze, sprinkle with the seed mixture, and serve.

Elevate This: Squeeze a bit of lime or grate some lime zest over the squash. Some crushed Sichuan pepper would add a bit of zing and color.

Serves 2 as a side dish

CHUPE DE ELOTE Y PAPAS

(Peruvian Corn and Potato Chowder) *This recipe combines the best of fresh summer corn, the cobanero pepper offered through farmers market vendor Green Belly Foods, and the Peruvian beans found at the Pope Farm booth. One of my favorite spices is paprika. Be sure to use smoked for this recipe, but keep sweet, smoked, hot smoked, and bittersweet in your pantry!*

Ingredients
- 1 tbsp oil, or butter (dairy or non-dairy)
- ½ cup diced onion
- 3 garlic cloves, minced
- 1 dried Guatemalan cobanero chile pepper, crushed (½ dried chipotle pod can substitute)
- 1 tsp smoked paprika
- ½ cup aquafaba or water
- ½ cup vegetable broth
- 1 large potato, steamed, peeled and cubed
- 1 ear of corn, shucked and cut into ¾-inch pieces
- ½ cup milk or cashew almond milk
- Salt and pepper to taste

For the Garnish
- Cilantro, sweet paprika, and grape tomato leaves

Instructions
Heat the oil or butter (dairy or non-dairy) in a medium stock pot.
Add the onions and sauté until soft and golden.
Add the garlic, chile and paprika. Sauté until fragrant, about 30 seconds.
Add the aquafaba or water, and the broth, potato and corn. Cook until corn is tender and broth thickens.
Turn down the heat to low and add the milk (dairy or non-dairy). Cook until mixture thickens.
Salt and pepper to taste.
Place in serving bowls and garnish with cilantro, sweet paprika and grape tomato halves.

Elevate This: Sprinkle a mixture of nutritional yeast, cumin, salt, pepper, garlic on top. Serve over a grain of your choice. Farro or barley will both work great, as well as brown rice. Try a dash of Green Belly's Guatemalan Hot Sauce for a flavor boost.

Serves 2 as a soup dish

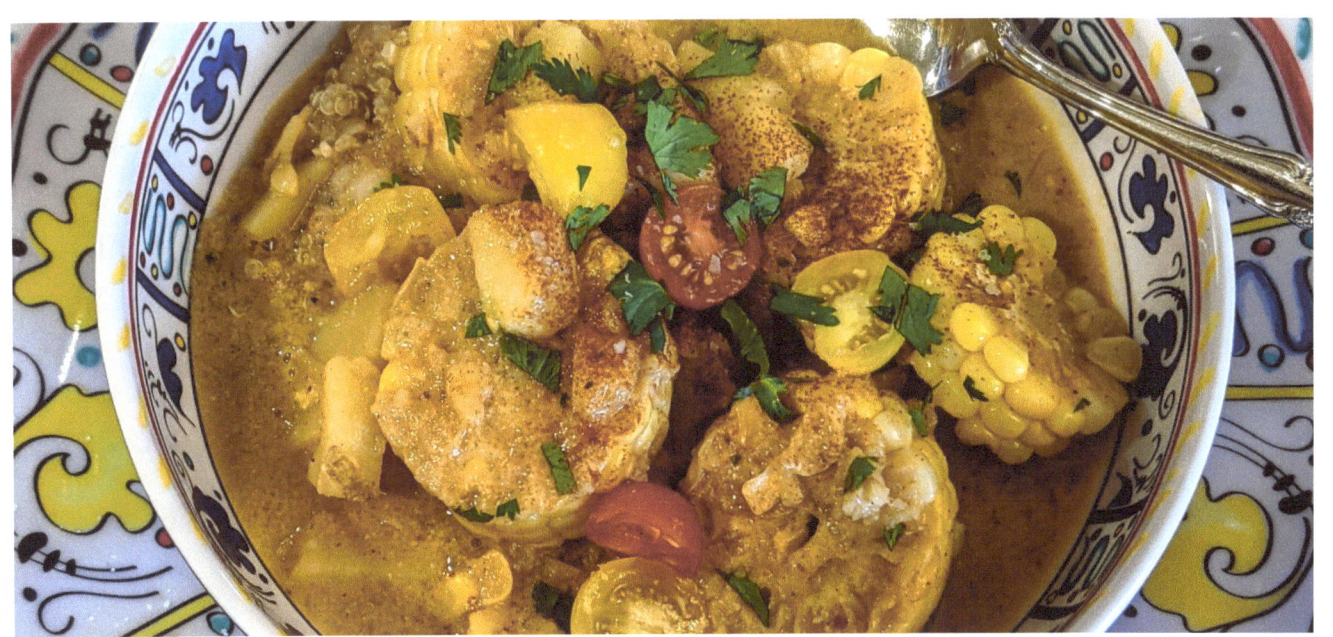

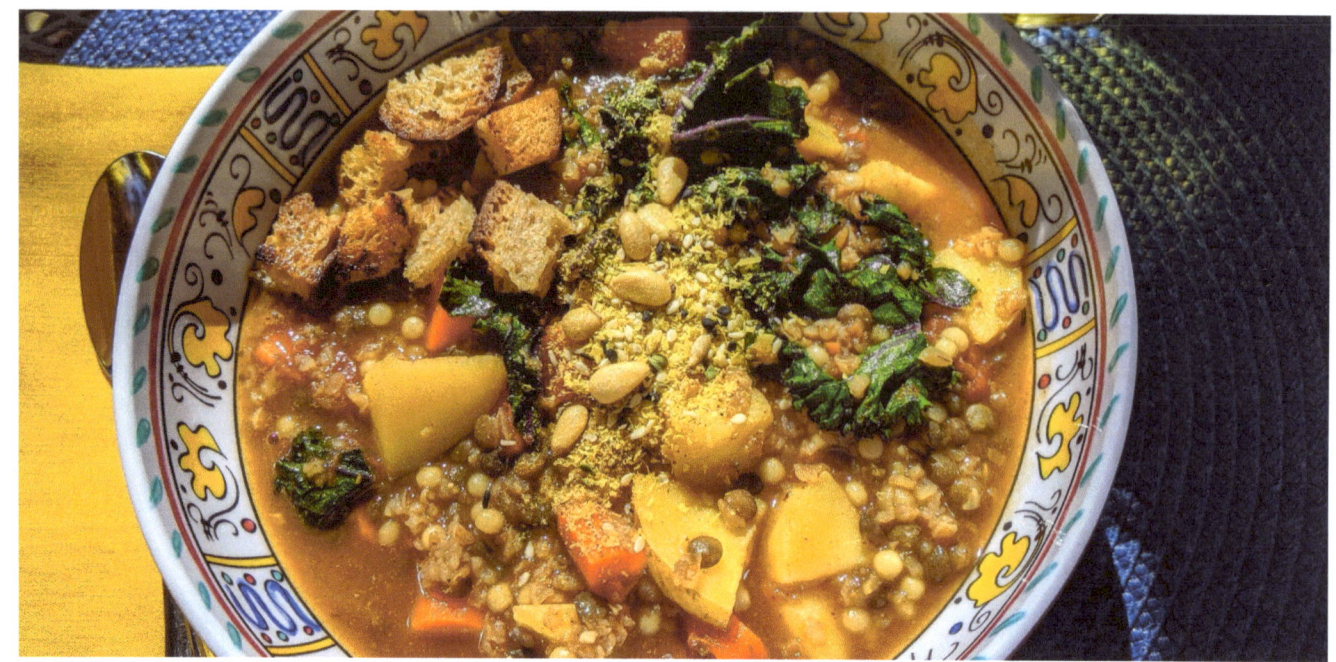

SARDINIAN SAFFRON FREGOLA WITH POTATOES AND PEAS

This recipe was another course I served as part of the The Spice and Tea Exchange® Fort Collins tasting. Fregola is a toasted, round, bead-sized pasta from Sardinia. It is similar to couscous, but it is toasted for added flavor. The toasting also helps hold its shape within your dish. If you cannot find fregola or sarda, Israeli couscous makes a reasonable substitution.

There may seem to be a lot of ingredients, but pulling it together is quite easy! As you can see from several dishes made with saffron in this cookbook, it is the magic in a dish. After you make this dish, you will want to add saffron to other dishes for that little je ne sais quoi – that indescribable thing that truly elevates your dish!

Ingredients

- 5 small baby red potatoes, cleaned and cubed (or 2 large red potatoes, cleaned and cubed)
- 1 tbsp oil
- 1 tbsp chopped shallots
- 2 garlic cloves, chopped or smashed
- 1 cup vegetable broth
- 1 cup hot water infused with ½ tsp or 8-10 saffron threads (this is the magic of this dish)
- 1 tsp of your favorite Tuscan Spice mix seasoning (or ½ tsp each of thyme, oregano, rosemary and parsley to taste)
- ½ tsp dried chile flakes
- 1 cup fregola or sarda
- 1 cup frozen peas
- 1 tsp lemon juice

For the Garnish
- 2 tbsp chopped parsley (or your choice of chopped herbs)
- Bread crumbs

Instructions

To speed things up, place the potatoes in a microwave safe bowl. Add enough water to cover the potatoes and microwave on high for 2 minutes until a knife slightly pierces the potatoes. Drain and reserve the water.

Heat the oil over medium heat in a large sauce pan with a lid.

Add the shallots and sauté for 2 minutes until soft.

Add the garlic and sauté for 30 seconds, until fragrant, not burned.

Add the vegetable broth, saffron water, Tuscan spice mix, and dried chile flakes. Bring to a slight simmer.

Add the potatoes, cover the pot and finish cooking the potatoes until a paring knife pierces the potato, about 5 minutes.

Add the fregola and cover the pot. Cook the fregola until it is tender. About 10 minutes.

Add an amount of reserved potato water for your desired consistency. The broth should become slightly cloudy and the mixture should thicken.

Add the peas and cook for 5 minutes. Cook and stir occasionally until the fregola is tender and the liquid is almost evaporated.

Add the lemon juice and stir.

Serve in a bowl and garnish with parsley, or your choice of chopped herbs, and bread crumbs.

Elevate This: Add a bit of kale, garnish with croutons and pine nuts, or substitute lentils for green peas for additional protein (as pictured).

Serves 2 as a side dish

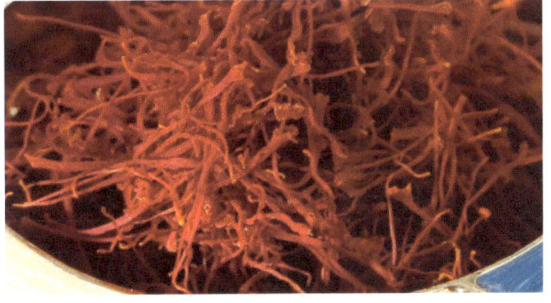
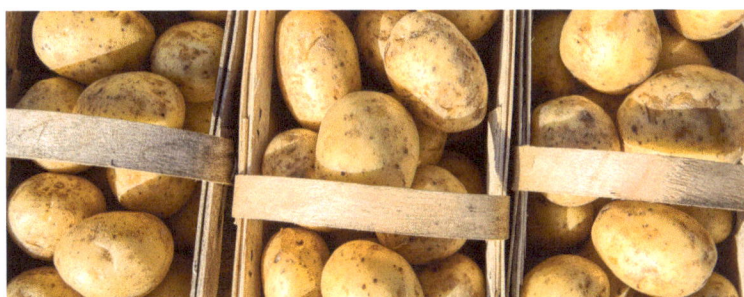
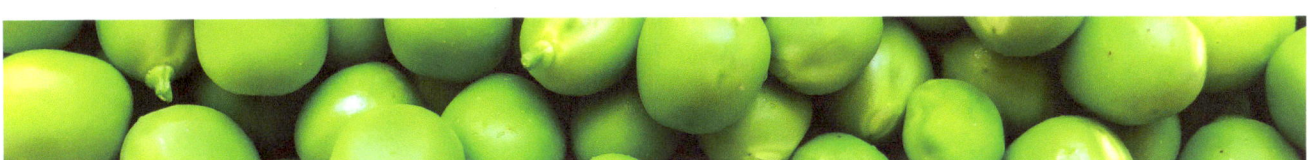

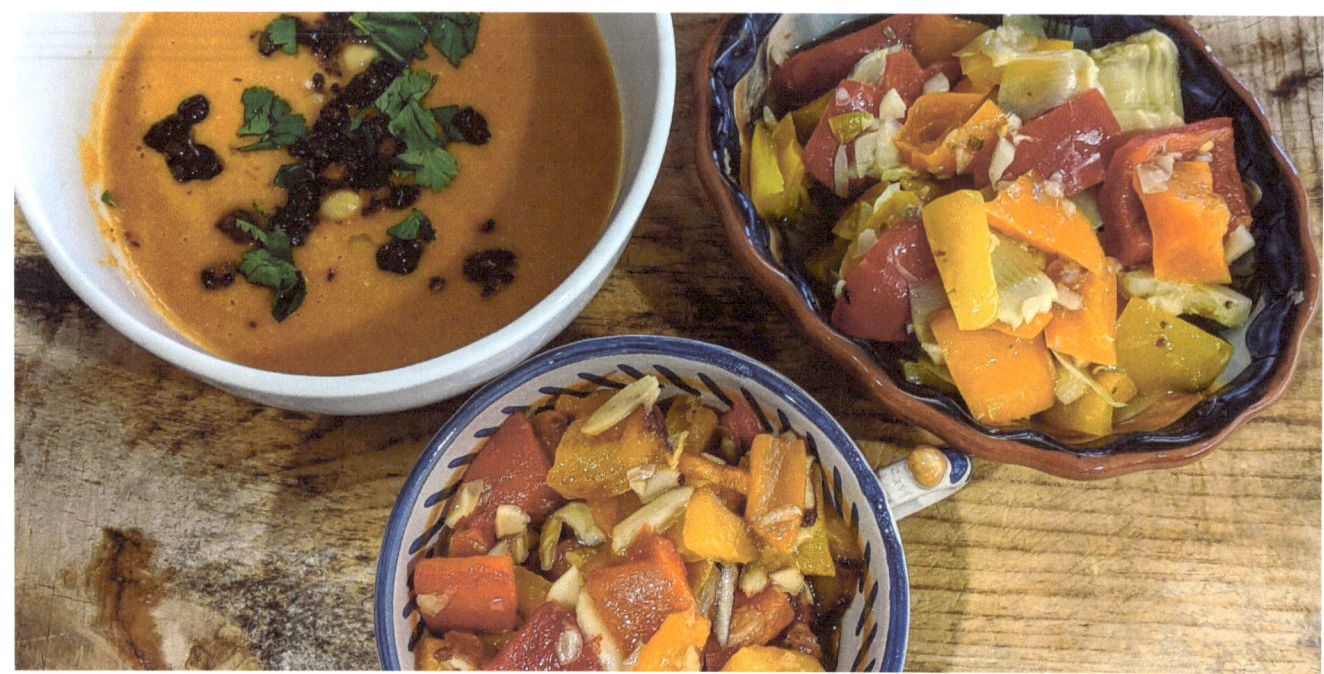

TRI-COLOR PEPPERS THREE WAYS

In the summer, Pope Farms in Greeley brings colored peppers to market along with an assortment of Italian and New Mexico varieties.

Roasting is a great way to create a base for other dishes. Just cut the peppers in half, take out the seeds, lay them flat on an aluminum foil sheet and roast at 400°F until the skins wrinkle a bit and char. Using tongs, place the hot peppers in a plastic bag until cool, then remove the skins. Or you can always just buy a jar, but fresh is always better.

Here are three quick recipes for those lovely peppers – roasted and fresh.

ETHIOPIAN ROASTED RED PEPPER & CHICKPEA SOUP

Ingredients
- 1 red pepper, roasted
- 1 can chickpeas; rinsed, reserve liquid
- 1 cup vegetable broth
- 1 tsp berbere powder (more if you like spicy)

For the Garnish
- Chopped cilantro
- Smoked mushrooms or bacon bits
- Crispy Capers
(see *Elevations* section, p. 168)

Instructions
Blend the pepper, chickpeas, and broth in a blender or in a saucepan with an immersion blender. Add the berbere seasoning. Heat until warm. Add reserved bean liquid to adjust to desired consistency.
Serve over a grain such as farro, barley, or brown rice. Garnish with chopped cilantro, smoked mushrooms (or bacon bits), and Crispy Capers.

Elevate This: A topping blend of nutritional yeast, toasted pine nuts, and dukkha or za'atar will add interest. Pomegranate seeds are really nice on this dish as well.

Serves 2 as a soup dish

ROASTED PEPPERS WITH SHERRY, HONEY & ALMONDS

Ingredients
- 1 tbsp dry Spanish sherry
- 1 tbsp local honey
- 3 tbsp olive oil
- 1-2 roasted, colored peppers, chopped into 1-inch pieces
- 2 garlic cloves, minced
- ½ cup sliced almonds, toasted
- Salt and pepper to taste

For the Garnish
- Chopped parsley

Instructions
Combine the first three ingredients in a bowl and whisk well. In a serving bowl, combine the sherry sauce and the remaining ingredients.
Marinate for 30 minutes.
Salt and pepper to taste.
Garnish with chopped parsley and serve.
This is a lovely Spanish dish to add to an antipasto tray.

Serves 4 as an antipasto dish

GIARDINIERA

Ingredients
- 1 each red, yellow, and orange fresh pepper; cored, seeds removed, and cut into 1-inch chunks
- 5 garlic cloves, minced
- 1 tbsp Kosher salt
- 5-6 jarred pepperoncini peppers, sliced
- 1 tbsp chopped fresh oregano
- 1 can artichoke hearts, drained, quartered
- 1 tsp chile flakes
- ½ cup good olive oil
- 3 tbsp brine from jar of pepperoncinis

Instructions
Place the fresh peppers, garlic and salt in a plastic container and fill with hot water. Allow the water to cool, then cover and place in the refrigerator overnight.
Drain the water and reserve the peppers and garlic.
Rinse for a few minutes to remove some salt.
Place the soaked peppers and garlic into a bowl.
Add the pepperoncini, oregano, chile flakes, and artichoke hearts to the bowl.
In a separate small bowl, whisk the olive oil and pepperoncini brine until thick. Pour the oil and brine mixture on top of the bowl of vegetables and stir.
Allow to marinate for a few days before using.
Serve as a part of an antipasto ensemble, an element on an arranged salad, or as a condiment with pizza (my personal favorite).

Makes 3 cups

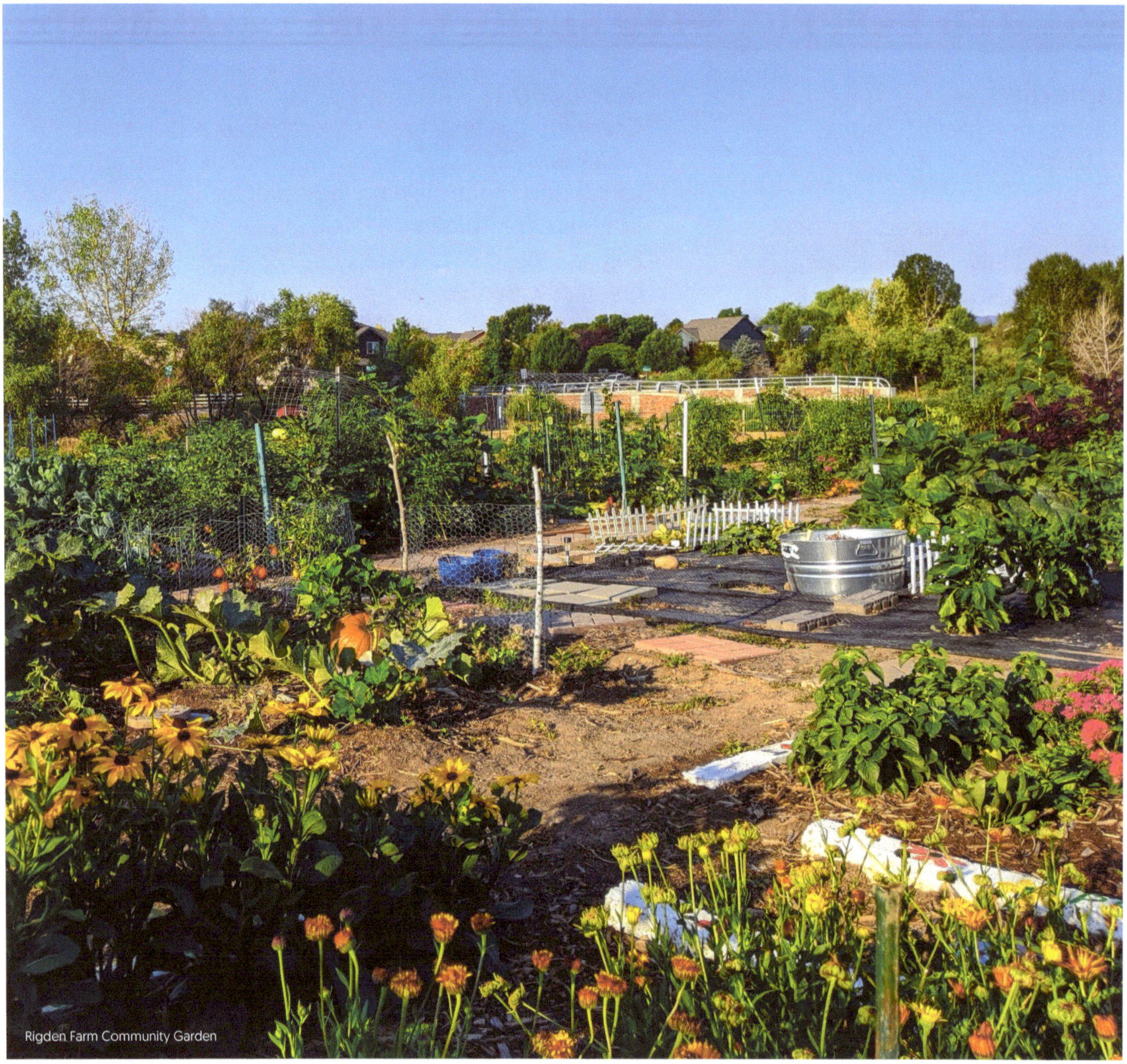

Rigden Farm Community Garden

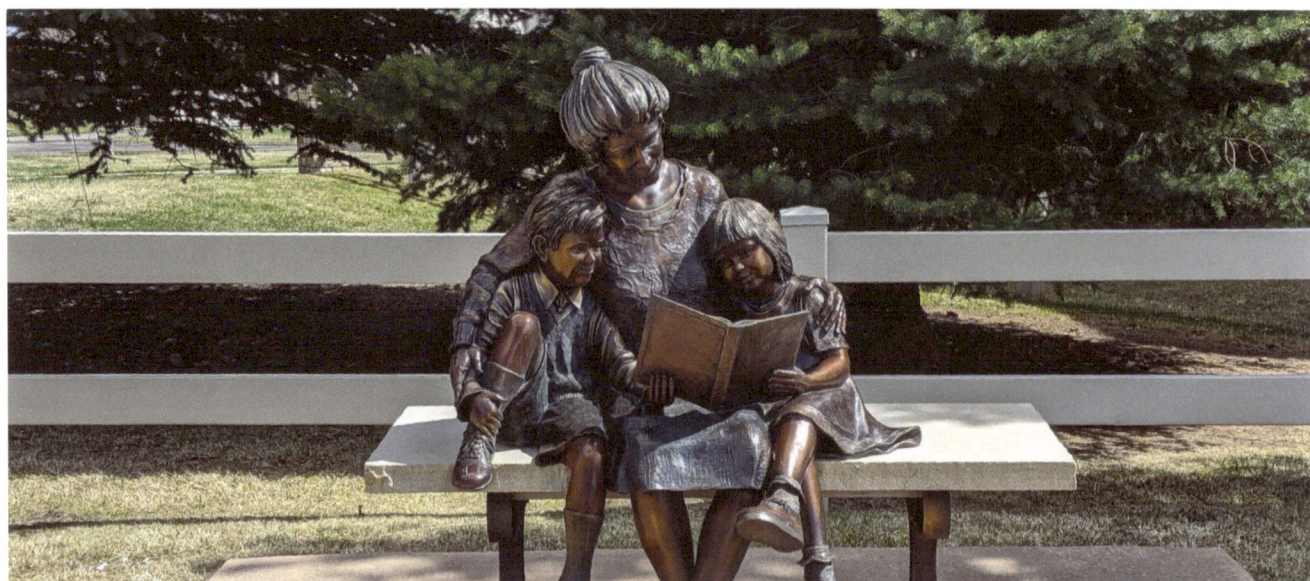

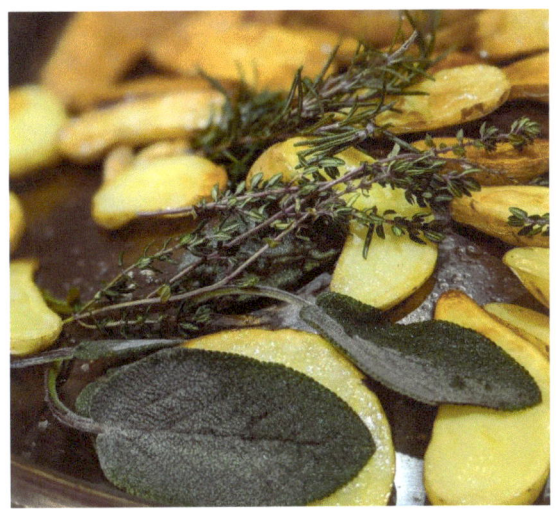
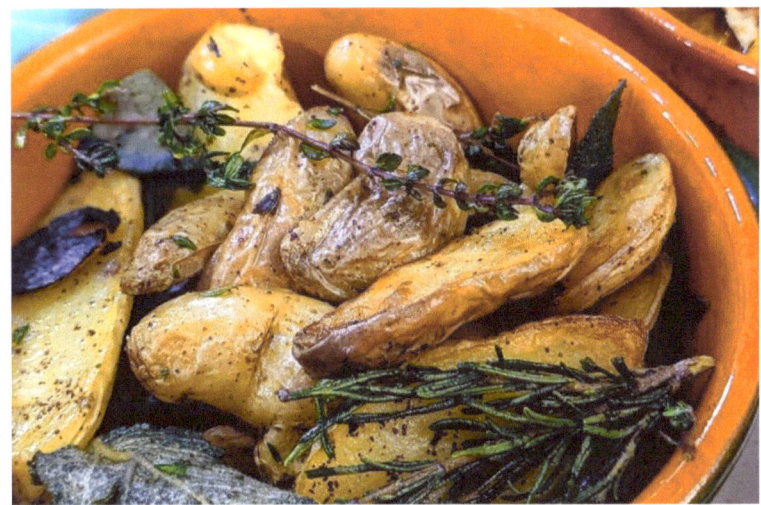
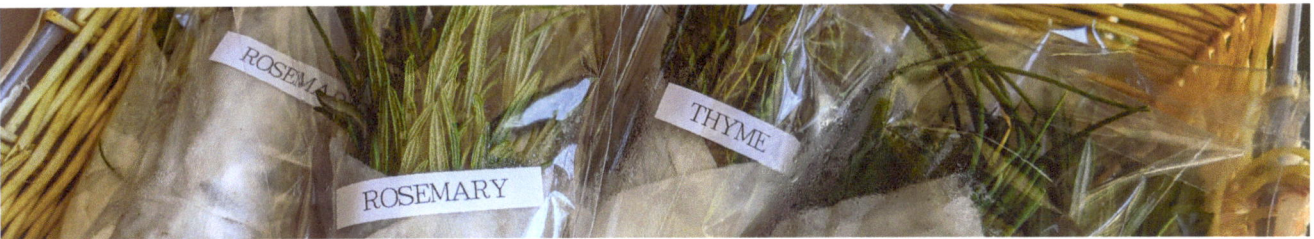

THREE HERBS AND SUMAC POTATOES

Sumac is an interesting spice. The name sumac comes from the Aramaic word "summaq" which means "dark red." The sumac berries are ground up into a beautiful dark burgundy powder about the size of very fine sea salt. The taste resembles lemon without the sourness. This dish is inspired by Yotam Ottolenghi, a favorite chef whom I follow for Middle Eastern cooking. I like crispy sage so I added it to this version. Cook the potatoes slowly so the garlic caramelizes gently.

Ingredients
- 1 lb fingerling potatoes, sliced lengthwise
- 2 tbsp oil
- 1 sprig of rosemary
- 1 sprig of thyme
- 6 sage leaves
- 5 garlic cloves, peeled and cut lengthwise
- 1 tsp sumac

For the Garnish
- Pan-fried sage

Instructions
Heat the oil in a large skillet over medium heat. Arrange the potatoes cut side down in the pan and sprinkle the garlic cloves in the oil. Pan fry 15 minutes or until the potatoes just begin to become golden. Flip the potatoes and add the herbs. Be sure the herbs are touching the oil in the bottom of the pan.
Cook 15 more minutes or until potatoes can be easily pierced with a fork.
Sprinkle with the sumac and toss.
Place in serving bowls and garnish with pan-fried sage.

Elevate This: The sumac is the main character of this dish. Consider something crunchy, like chopped toasted pistachios or almonds.

Serves 2 as a side dish

POTATOES WITH FENNEL AND ONION

Most of us think of licorice when we think of fennel. But when the bulb is gently sautéed, the familiar licorice taste dissipates, and a more gentle and kinder version of fennel emerges. This dish comes together quickly if you have a batch of baby Dutch potatoes steamed and ready to go for the week.

Ingredients
- 8 baby Dutch golden potatoes; steamed, cooled, and cut into ½-inch pieces
- 1 tbsp oil
- ½ fennel bulb, washed and thinly sliced
- ¼ medium yellow onion, thinly sliced (about ½ cup)
- Salt and pepper to taste

For the Garnish
- A few fennel fronds

Instructions
Heat the oil in a skillet over medium heat. Add the fennel and onion and allow to sauté until soft and golden. Do not burn.
Add the potatoes to warm them, and coat with the fennel and onion mixture.
You can add a touch of water to deglaze the pan.
Salt and pepper to taste.
Garnish with a few fennel fronds.

Elevate This: Consider including other root vegetables such as parsnips or kohlrabi. A sprinkle of finely minced, toasted almonds would add some crunch without overpowering the fennel.

Serves 2 as a side dish

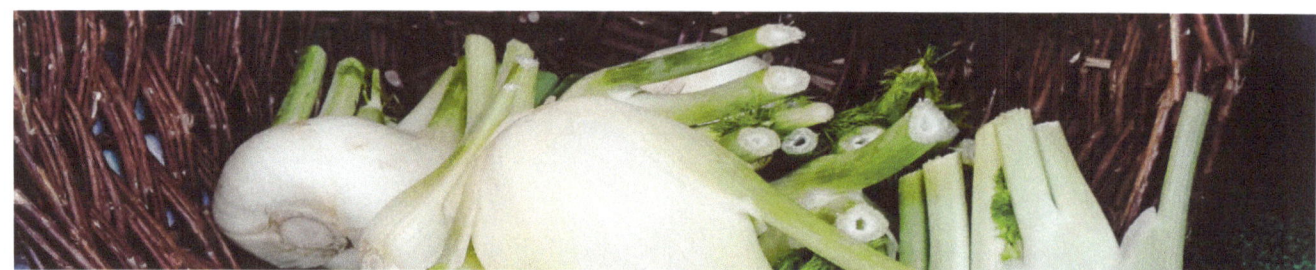
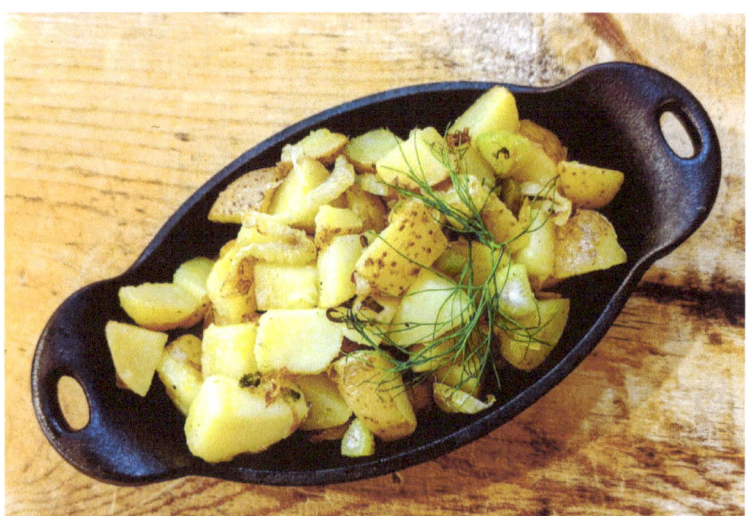
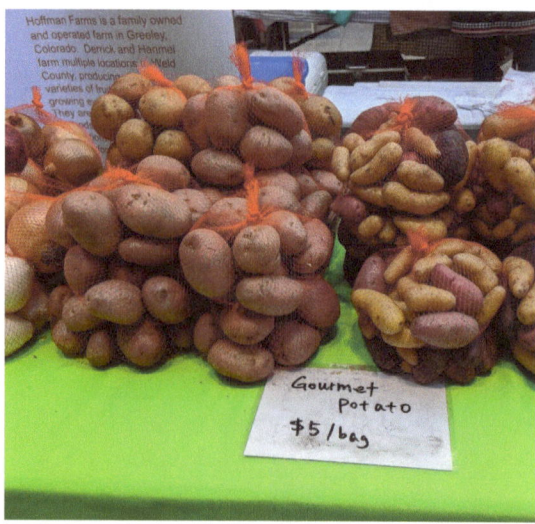

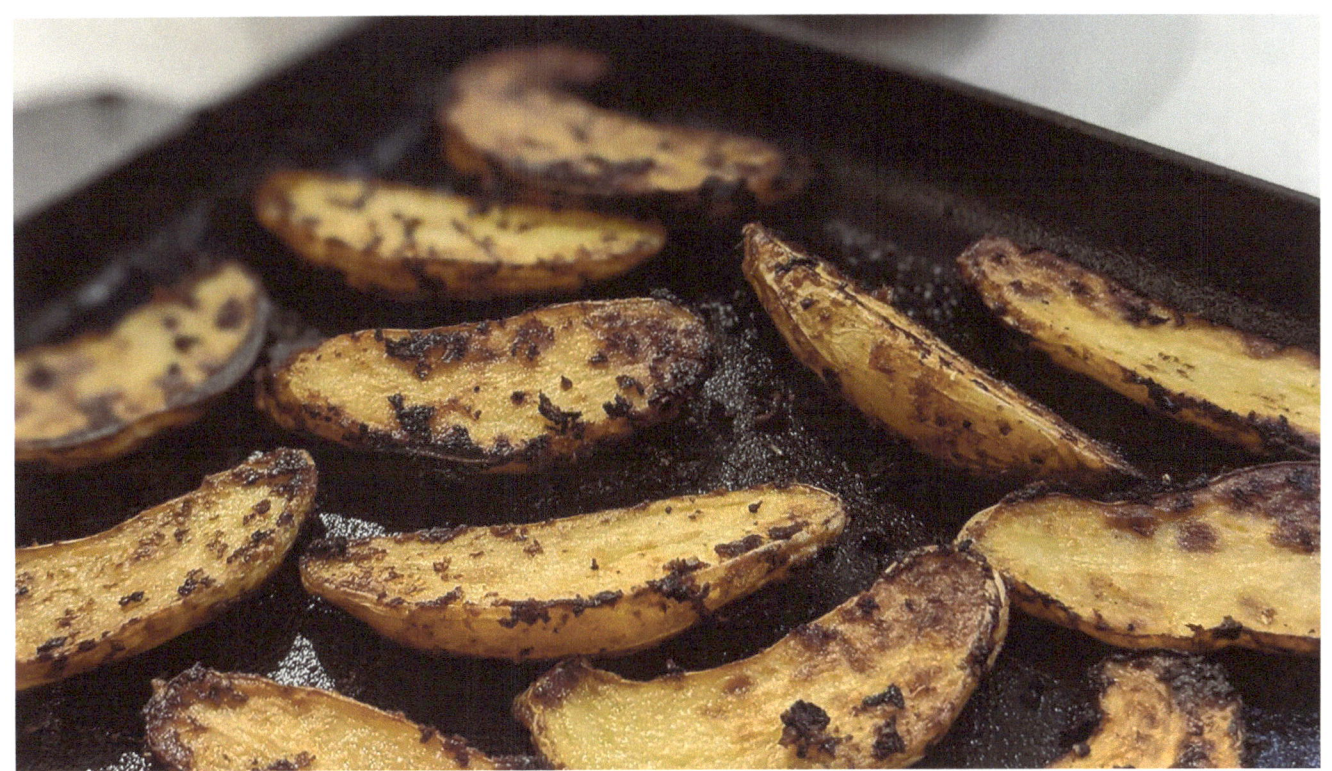

MISO PEPPER POTATOES

Miso is a fermented soybean paste that adds salty umami to Japanese dishes. In this case, it elevates the already wonderful and nutritious potato to a whole new level of yum. Red miso is generally saltier than light yellow and white miso, and has a more assertive, pungent flavor. The nice thing is, miso has a great shelf life and can be used to add oomph to any dish.

Your new ingredient to use is the Sichuan peppercorn, available at most spice shops. Its unique aroma and flavor is not hot or pungent like black, white, or chile peppers. Instead, it has a slight lemony overtone and creates a tingly numbness in the mouth that sets the stage for hot spices.

Ingredients
- 1 tbsp white miso
- 1 tbsp red miso
- 1 tbsp butter (dairy or non-dairy), melted
- 1 tsp crushed Sichuan pepper
- 1 lb fingerling potatoes

Instructions
Preheat the oven to 400°F.
Prepare a baking sheet with aluminum foil and non-stick spray.
Combine the first four ingredients in a bowl and mix well.
Add the potatoes and toss to coat.
Spread on the baking sheet and roast for 20-30 minutes until fork tender.

Elevate This: Sprinkle lightly with smoked soy sauce.

Serves 2 as a side dish

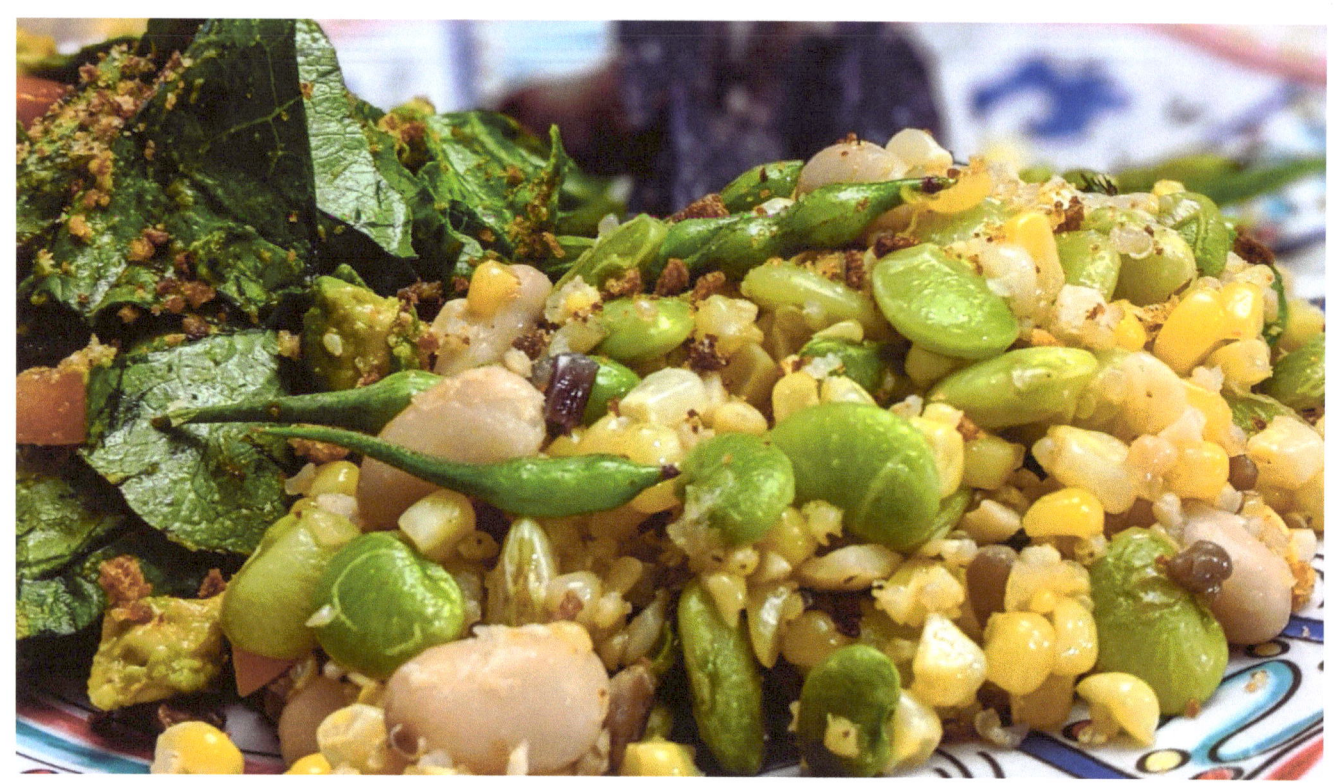

SUCCOTASH WITH A TWIST

As a nod to my Southern heritage, let's enjoy a succotash. This is a southern succotash I made with fresh Olathe corn, sugar peas, a bit of quinoa, millet, cannellini beans, and a special topping of radish seed pods I was gifted from a community gardener. What a treat!

Experiment and create your own. Think sweet, savory, and herby!

Helpful Tip: Batch cook different grains and save in the recently available reusable, stand-up freezer containers. Freeze in 1 cup portions and pull out just what you need – even if just ¼ cup of millet to add variety to a dish. Consider tubed lemongrass paste and ginger paste, found in the produce department. It keeps for a long time and is perfect when you want to add interest to a dish.

Ingredients
- 1 tbsp oil
- 1 small shallot, sliced thinly
- 1-inch tubed lemongrass paste
- 2 garlic cloves, minced
- 1 ear of corn, kernels cut from the cob
- 10-12 sugar peas; microwaved for 2 minutes, cooled and sliced on the diagonal
- ¼ cup cooked millet
- ¼ cup cooked quinoa
- ½ can cannellini beans, drained and rinsed
- Salt and pepper to taste

For the Garnish
- Radish seed pods, pea or Diakon radish shoots

Instructions
Heat the oil over medium heat.
Add the shallot and sauté until soft.
Add the lemongrass and garlic and cook 30 seconds until fragrant.
Add the corn and sauté until kernels become soft and a little caramelized (not too much – you don't want them burnt.)
Add the rest of the ingredients and cook 3-5 minutes until reheated. Sugar peas should stay crisp and bright green.
Remove from heat. Salt and pepper to taste.
Garnish with radish seed pods, pea or Daikon radish shoots – something with a little bite to it!

Elevate This: Add halved fresh grape tomatoes. Sprinkle with your favorite herb of choice.
Garnish with nutritional yeast blend, parmesan (dairy or non-dairy), or goat cheese (dairy or non-dairy).

Serves 2-3 as a side dish

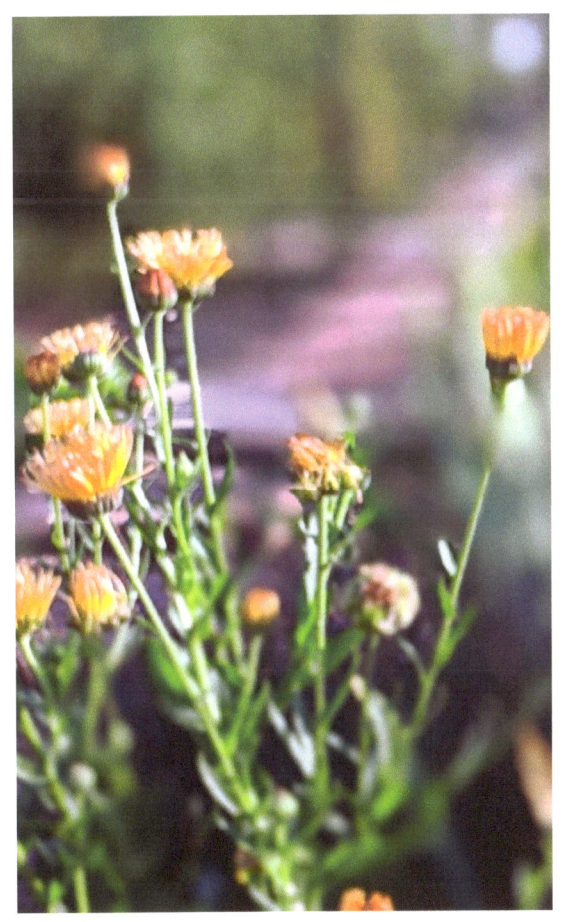
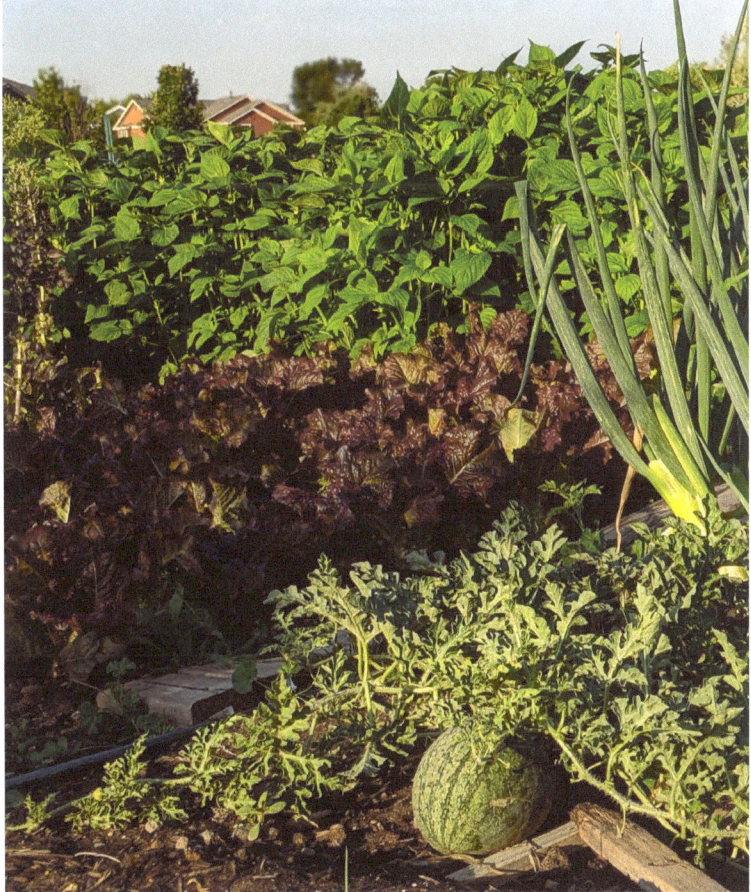

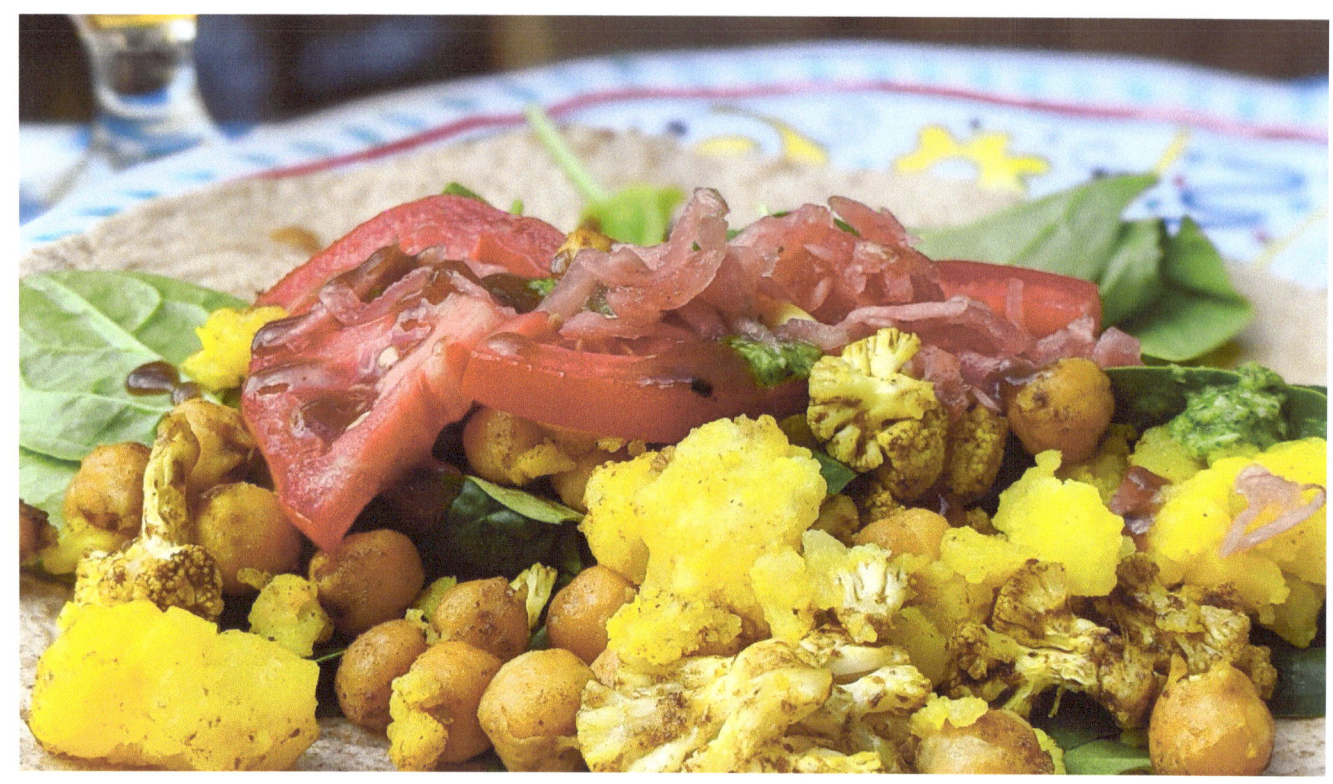

SMOKED CAULIFLOWER AND CHICKPEA SPINACH WRAP

In my wildest dreams, I never would have thought I would get a cauliflower almost every week in my CSA from July to September, so I had to start getting creative. The electric smoker was a lifesaver, as I could just put my test items in the smoker with mesquite chips and see what happened. Rarely did anything fail, including smoking tofu. And cauliflower.

If you don't have a smoker, you can just add one or two teaspoons of liquid smoke to your regular roasting routine, depending on your taste. The smoke elevates cauliflower to a whole new level. I personally prefer the smoker, as the cauliflower keeps its vivid color, but certainly roasting is a superb alternative.

Ingredients
- ½ head of cauliflower, cut into small florets
- 1 can chickpeas, drained
- 1 tbsp of your favorite Indian curry spice mix
- 1 tsp turmeric
- 1 tsp garam masala
- 1 tbsp oil
- 1-2 tsp of liquid smoke (if not using a smoker)
- 1 tsp salt
- 1 tsp black pepper

For the Wrap
- Tortillas or pita bread pockets (or the pumpkin flatbreads, p. 107)
- 1 beautiful, perfect summer tomato, cut in chunks or slices
- Baby leaf spinach
- Coconut Cilantro Chutney (see *Elevations* section, p. 168)
- Tamarind Sauce (see *Elevations* section, p. 168)

Instructions
Preheat smoker at 225°F, or preheat the oven at 375°F if roasting indoors.

Prepare sheet pan with foil and non-stick spray.

Mix all the ingredients in a bowl and spread onto your sheet pan.

Smoke for 60-90 minutes, or roast in the oven for 20 minutes.

Use the smoked cauliflower, chickpeas, and wrap ingredients to create your wrap. Drizzle the chutney and tamarind sauce to your preference.

Note: The chutney and tamarind sauces have long shelf lives in the refrigerator. I keep them in squeeze bottles in the fridge for quick access to enhance a dish.

Elevate This: Add a bit of hummus, Toum (p. 130), or fresh chopped cilantro. Some grated lime will add a nice spark of flavor.

Serves 2 as a main dish

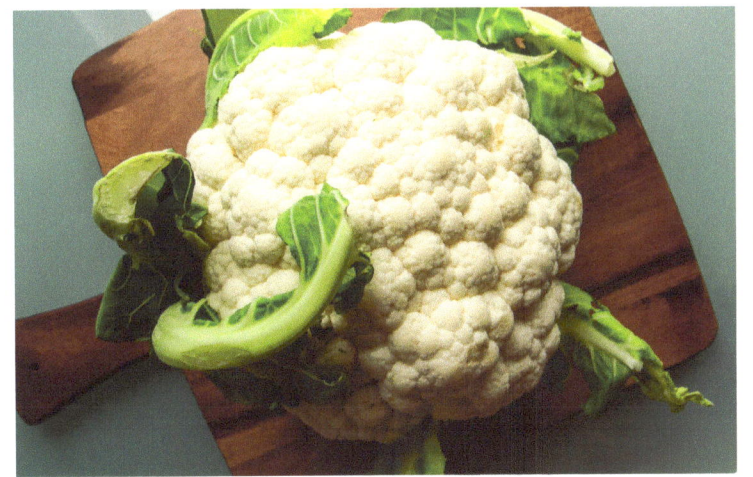
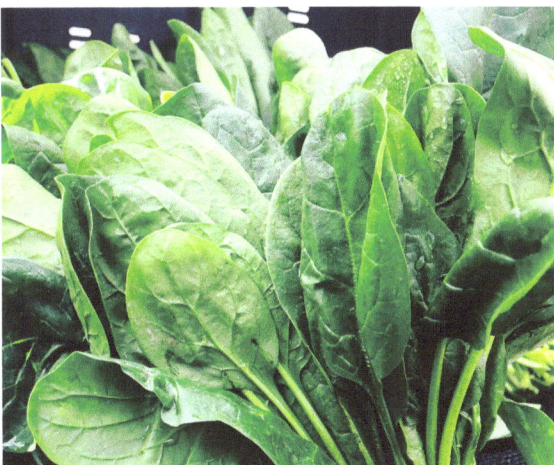
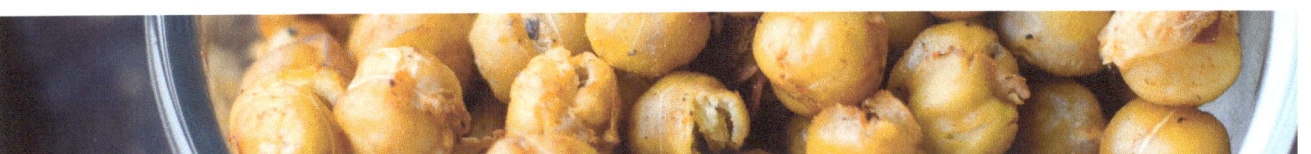

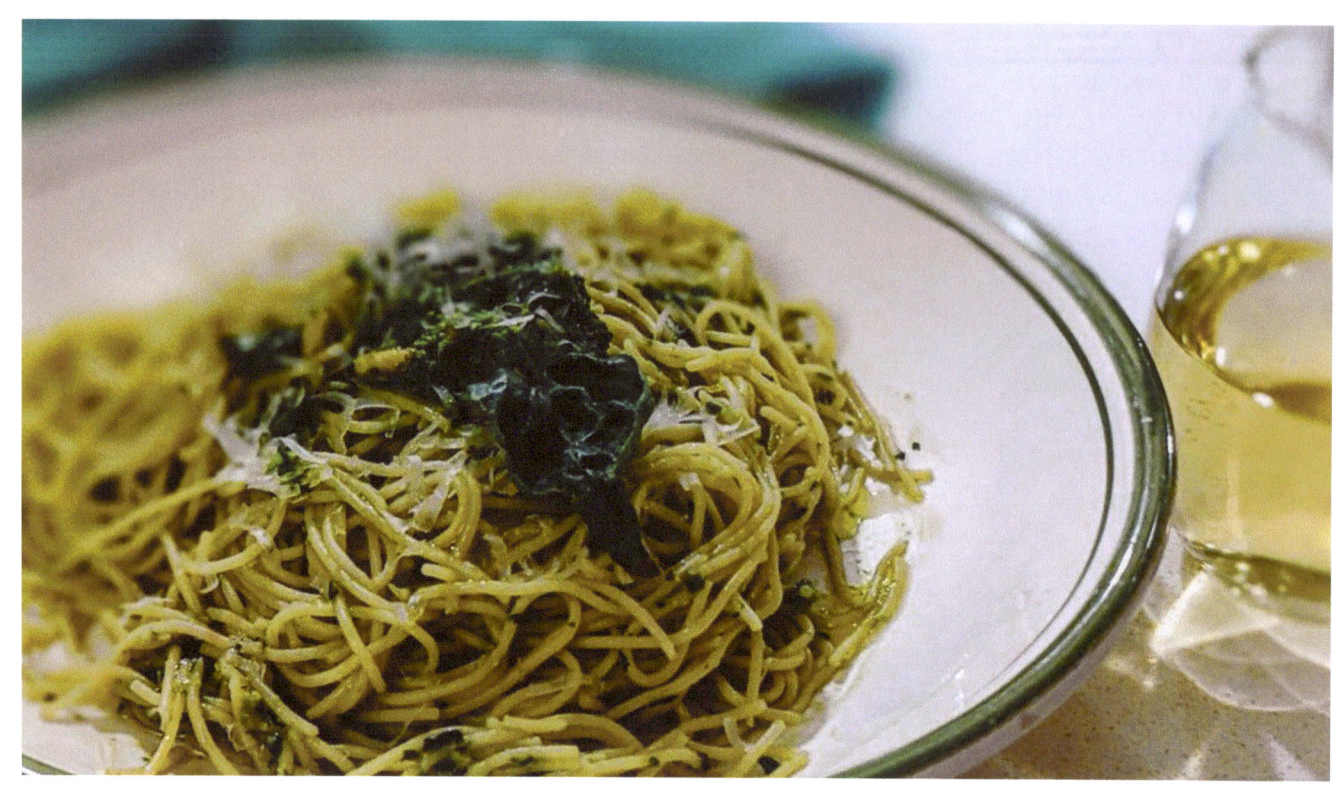

BASIL PESTO WITH YOUR CHOICE OF PASTA

Pesto linguini is my husband's favorite dish. He fell in love with it in Venice (although it originates from Genoa, the capital city of Liguria, Italy), and thus, the dish is a mini-vacation back to Italy. Pesto may sound mundane, but when you can make it with local unique garlic and basil, it takes a simple dish to a whole new level. It is even more special as basil is a bit hard to grow here in Northern Colorado. So, when we can find it, we grab it as quickly as possible! Luckily, EP Greens in Estes Park grows hydroponic basil. There is nothing like the aroma of basil to take you back to a lazy, summer day.

I made this dish with Long Shot Farm's Sicilian Artichoke Garlic. There are multiple garlic growers at the markets, so be on the lookout in late summer. A special varietal finishing olive oil from your favorite olive oil shop magnifies this dish worthy of a mid-week company dinner.

Note: Making pesto is an ordered, magical process. I make this in a mortar and pestle but I have had reasonable results with a very small food processor, and, believe or not, an immersion blender. Just follow the sequence.

Ingredients

- 4 garlic cloves, peeled and roughly chopped
- ½ tsp salt
- 2 handfuls fresh basil
- 2 tbsp roasted pine nuts (**Helpful Tip:** Roast 1 cup pine nuts and freeze for quick use)
- ⅛ cup shredded parmesan (dairy or non-dairy)
- 2 tbsp extra virgin olive oil
- Pasta or gnocchi of choice (the sky is the limit!)

For the Garnish

- Cherry tomatoes, halved
- More parmesan
- A few pine nuts
- 1 sprig of basil
- Extra virgin olive oil

Instructions

Place garlic and salt in mortar and pestle and grind to a smooth paste.
Add the basil ¼ amount at a time until almost smooth.
Add the pine nuts and continue to process to a paste.
Add the parmesan and oil, and stir with a spoon or spatula.
Serve with your pasta or gnocchi of choice.
Garnish with halved tomatoes, additional parmesan, pine nuts, a sprig of basil, and a drizzle of extra virgin olive oil (or use the pesto as a savory topping for soup, potatoes, or tomatoes). Try it with cold pasta for the summer.

Elevate This: Partner the basil pesto with a local pasta such as Pappardelle's Pasta, Pastamore's from Denver, Pastificio's in Boulder, or make your own pasta or gnocchi.

Serves 2 as a topping for pasta

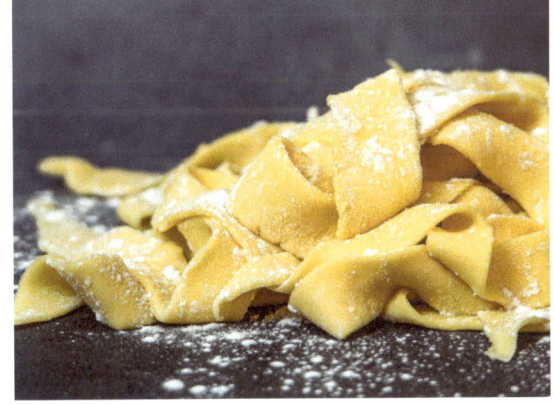
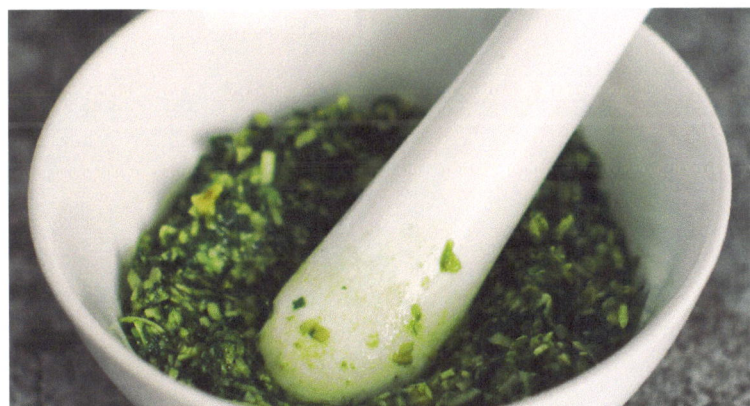
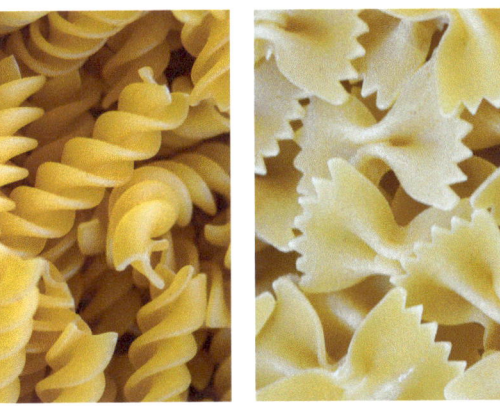
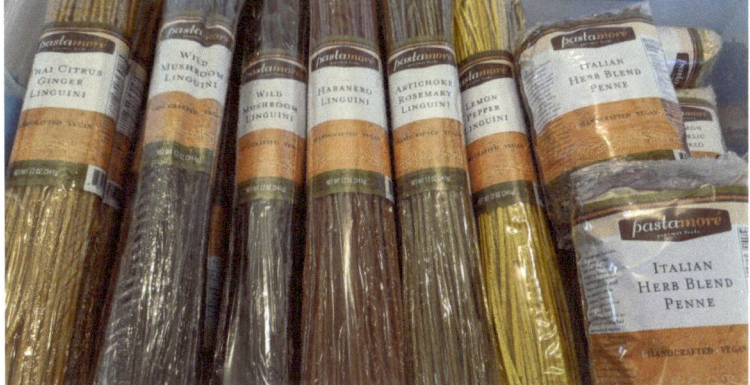

SAFFRON PASTA WITH FRESH TOMATO SAUCE

Pappardelle's saffron pasta makes a beautiful backdrop for the sauce. The fresher or more interesting the color of the tomatoes, the better. For this quick recipe, the tomatoes are not cooked and peeled. Be sure and save the pasta water! Freeze it in jars or cubes. The saffron will add magnificent flavor and color to your next soup!

If you do not have saffron pasta near you, this dish still works with regular pasta. I do highly recommend, though, visiting Pappardelle's online store and have some of their many varieties shipped to your door! You will not be disappointed.

Ingredients
- 8 oz saffron linguini; cooked, liquid reserved
- 1 tbsp oil

For the Sauce
- ½ onion, finely chopped
- 6 garlic cloves, minced
- 2-3 large heirloom tomatoes, cored and diced
- ½ tsp salt
- 1 tbsp fresh oregano, chopped
- 1 tsp basil pesto (tubed or fresh)

For the Garnish
- Toasted breadcrumbs or panko

Instructions
In a large skillet, heat the oil over medium heat.
Add the onions and sauté until soft and golden.
Add the garlic and heat until fragrant, about 30 seconds.
Add the diced tomatoes, chopped oregano, and salt. Sauté for 3-4 minutes.
Add the basil pesto and saffron linguini.
Toss gently and plate in serving bowls.
Garnish with toasted breadcrumbs or panko.

Elevate This: A small side of good quality cured black olives, like Healthy Harvest Black Koutsourelia Olives, or similar, would be perfect.

Serves 2 as a main dish

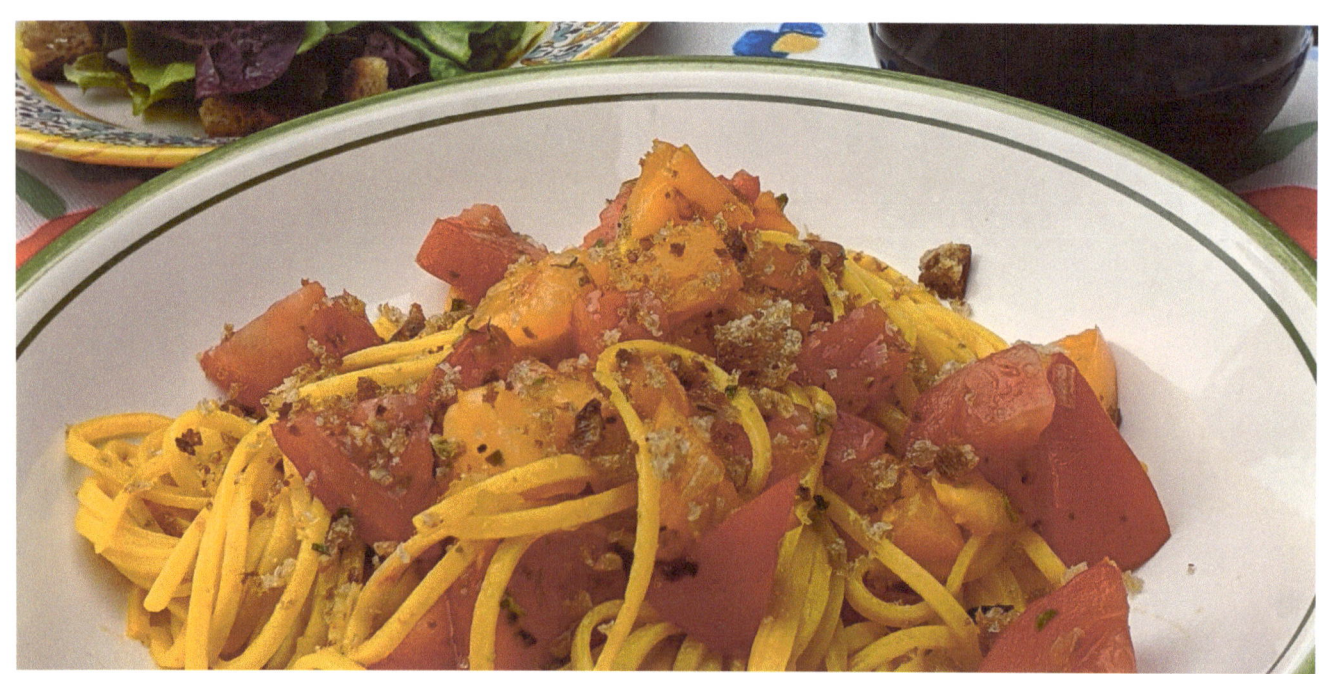

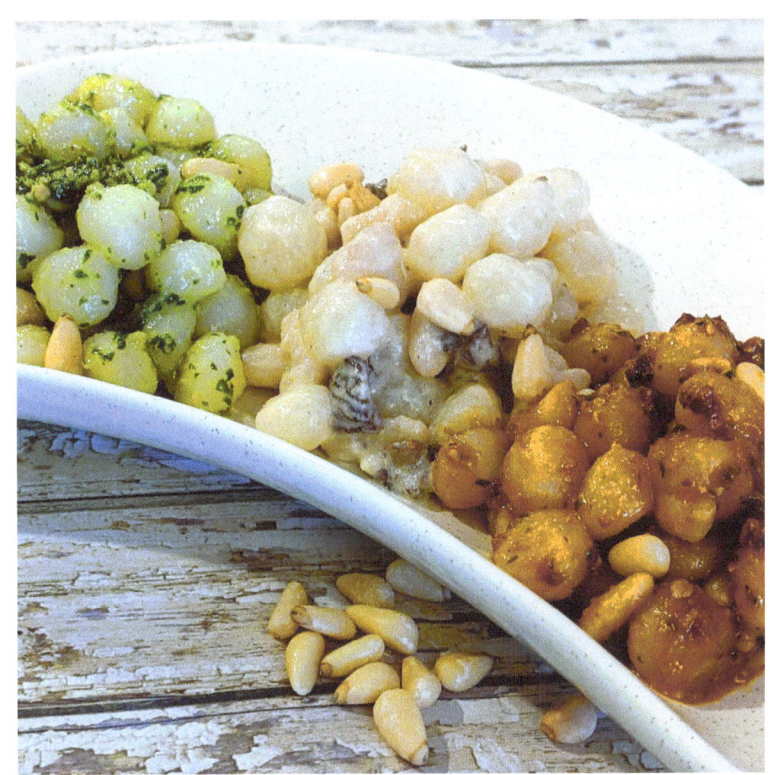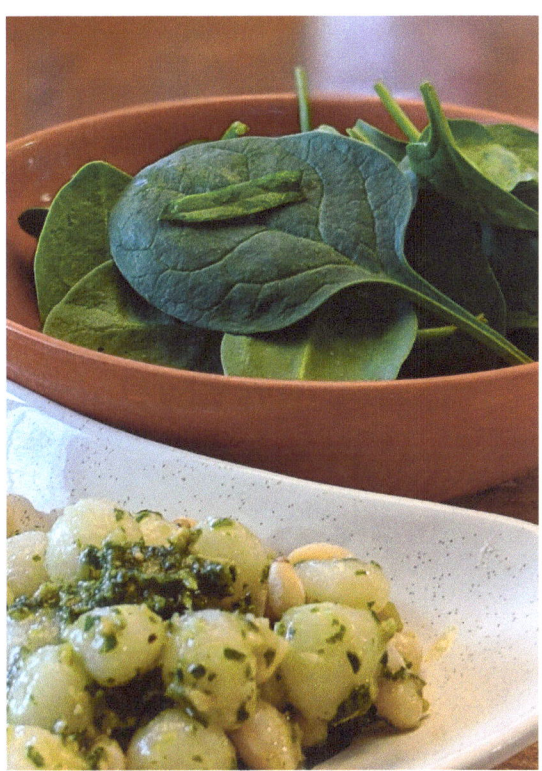

BABY GNOCCHI THREE WAYS

This is not so much a recipe, but is instructions for creatively assembling the delicious food that you are creating. It is entirely possible to think one pasta dish has to have only one sauce. Not so.

This lunch dish came from my many cooking leftovers. You know the drill. Half jars of this, a dab of that. I had three sauces in my fridge: a bit of the Basil Pesto (p. 72), Morel Cream Sauce (p. 37), and a jar of sundried tomato pesto. Inside the pantry was a full bag of baby gnocchi. Rather than choosing which sauce would do with a little gnocchi, I divided the gnocchi into thirds, sauced each with the leftover sauces, sprinkled a few pine nuts, and served on a beautiful dish for lunch. A simple spinach salad completed the ensemble.

Elevate This: *Sprinkle a mixture of nutritional yeast, Italian seasoning, or truffle salt on top. Lay the gnocchi on top of a bit of wilted spinach or swiss chard.*

Serves 1 or more, depending on what you have

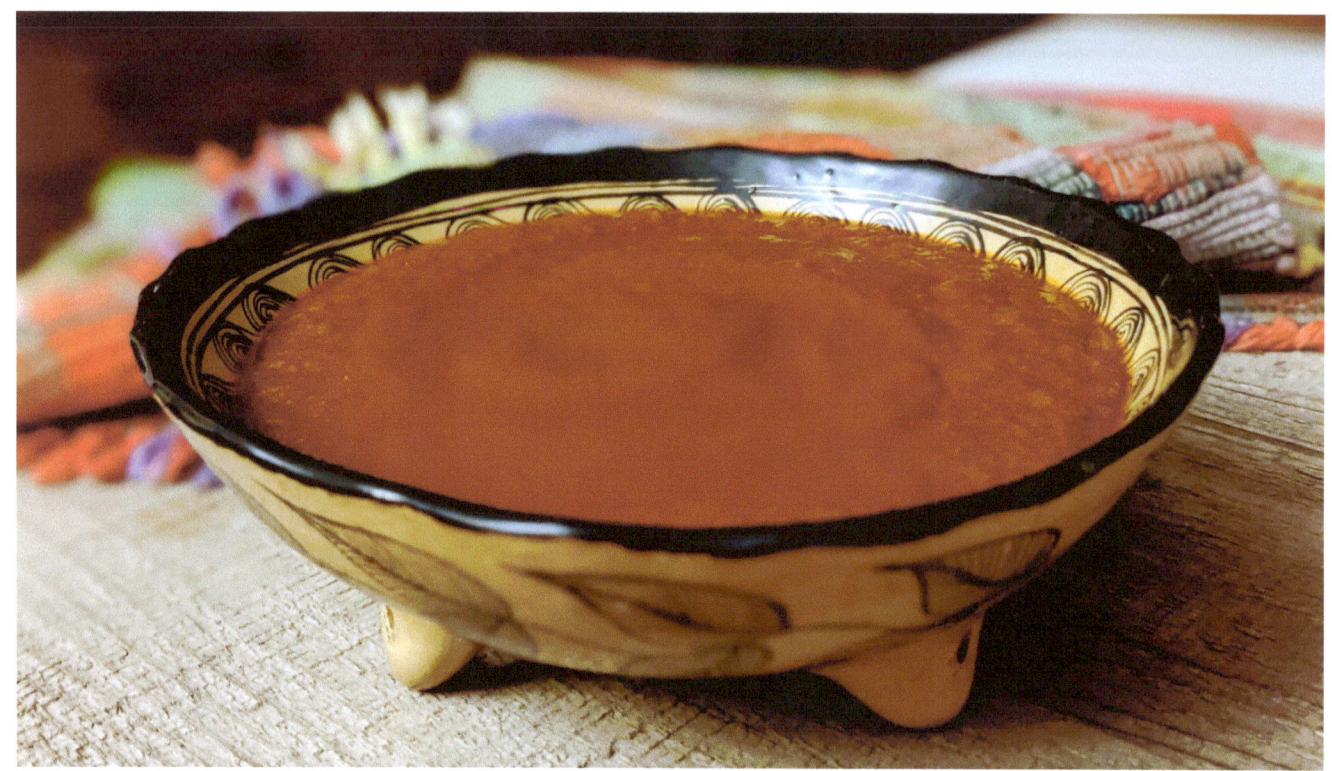

AWARD-WINNING RED CHILI SAUCE

Who doesn't love a smooth, well-rounded, flavorful red chili sauce? This recipe is the base for the beef chili I made for a chili contest in 2018. It won first prize!

Most, or all, of these peppers are available at your local Hispanic market, the international section of your grocery store, or online. The different types of peppers give the chili a depth of smokiness, sweetness, and spice. You can substitute powdered options from a spice shop, but the texture of the sauce may be grainy. Be sure and allow the sauce to blend well in the blender and meld for several hours.

The instructions seem complicated but they are not. Consider the recipe as a series of the following steps:

1. Rehydrate the peppers.
2. Reserve all liquids.
3. Make a sort of mirepoix (sautéing aromatics and spices) as a base.
4. Add final ingredients and blend.
5. Use reserved, flavored liquids for balancing the consistency.

You will find this technique useful for many other projects.

Ingredients

- 2 dried Pasilla peppers
- 2 dried Guajillo peppers
- 3 dried Morito peppers
- 3 dried Ancho peppers
- 3 dried Chipotle peppers (not canned)
- 4 dried New Mexico red chile peppers
- 1 large onion, chopped
- 8 garlic cloves, chopped
- ½ cup water
- 1 tbsp cumin seed
- 1 tbsp cumin powder
- 2 tbsp New Mexico red chile powder
- 1 cup crushed tomatoes
- 2 cups vegetable broth
- 2 cups reserved chile water from soaking
- 2 tbsp oil
- Salt and pepper to taste

Instructions

Place all dried peppers in a bowl and fill with hot water to cover peppers. Place something heavy over the peppers so they stay submerged. (I used my tea kettle). Let rehydrate for at least 20 minutes.

Alternatively, place all the dried peppers in an Instant Pot or pressure cooker. Cover with water and cook on low pressure for 20 minutes. Cool.

As the peppers soak, heat the oil in large Dutch oven or skillet.

Add the onions and sauté until very soft.

Add the garlic and sauté 30 seconds.

Add the cumin seed, cumin powder, and red chile powder, and allow spices to bloom for 1 minute.

Add ½ cup water to deglaze the pan and bring to a simmer. Let cool.

Remove the peppers and save the water. Strain the water if there are any seeds in the water.

Remove stems, seeds, and fibrous membrane holding the seeds from the inside of the peppers. If possible, peel the skin, but this is not always possible.

Place the peppers in a large blender with 2 cups of the reserved pepper-soaked water and blend until very smooth. This may take several minutes. Be patient.

Add the onion mixture and tomatoes to the peppers in the blender, and blend on high until smooth.

Salt and pepper to taste.

At this juncture, you can divide the mixture into several containers and freeze and use for chili or enchiladas.

Alternatively, you can use the chili base with your favorite meat or beans. If using meat such as pork or chuck roast pieces, I prefer to brown the meat, then braise the meat with the sauce at very low temperatures (300°F or less) until the meat is fork tender and shreds. You may add beer or more liquid to make sure there is enough liquid for 3-4 hours of braising.

Check the chili every hour and add more broth or pepper water if necessary. The chili should thicken over time. Skim off any fat if necessary.

Makes 6-8 cups of chili base sauce

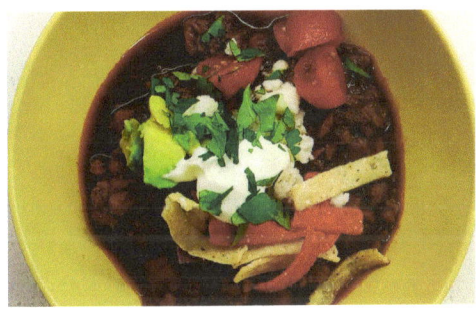

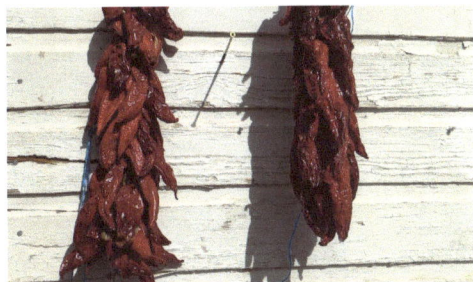

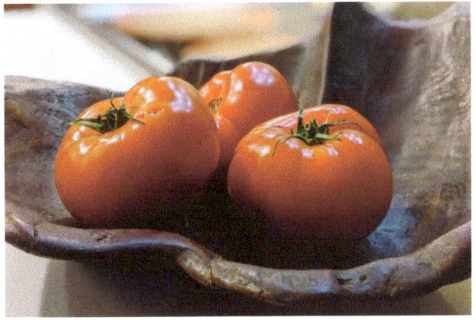

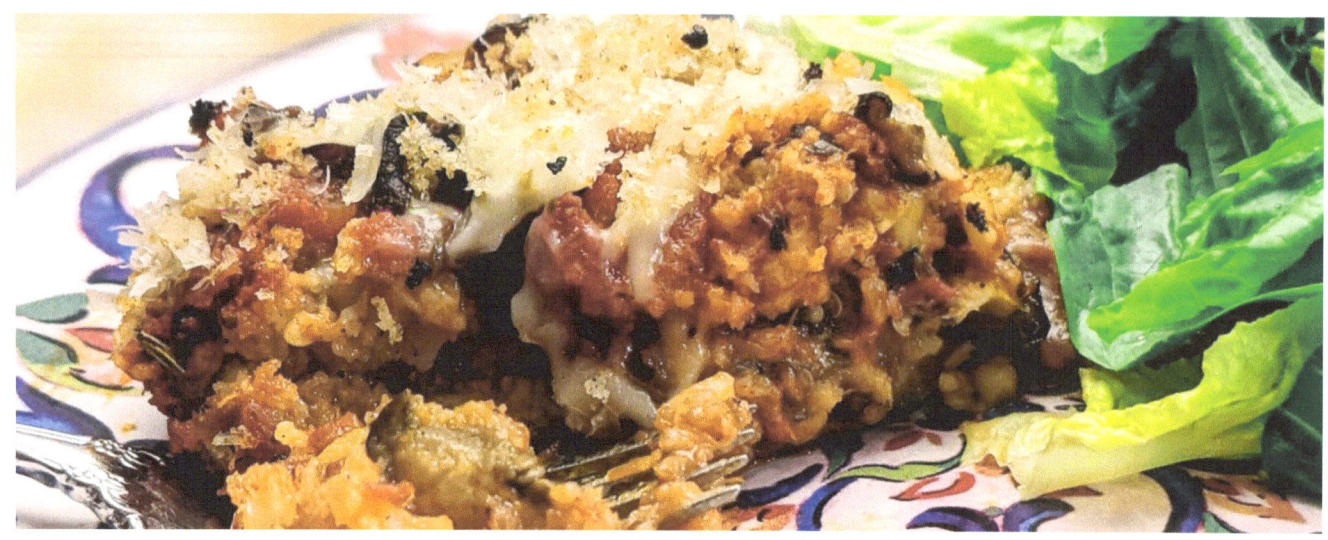

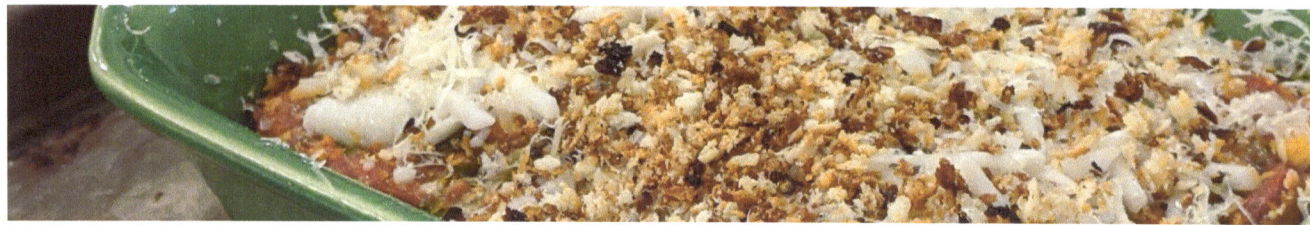

EGGPLANT PARMESAN

Eggplant became my challenge assignment this year. I received a beautiful Italian variety in my FarmFresh CSA and thought, "Oh dear. What do I do?" This plant-based casserole was born.

Over the summer, I began to appreciate the beauty of this vegetable, and the varieties that abound. Personally, when I think of cooking an eggplant, it was always in the style of a ratatouille, grilled, and not much else. Luckily, On the Vine at Richmond Farms also had multiple varieties this year and it was hard to resist giving them a try in different cuisines, including using Japanese eggplant in tacos and white eggplant in rice pilaf.

I will keep working on more cuisines, but in the meantime, I feel comfortable sharing this recipe. The eggplant becomes soft during the baking, the panko crumbs stay crunchy, and the cheese (plant-based as well) melts beautifully in the middle.

Helpful Tip: Take time to drain the eggplant so you won't be disappointed with a soggy dish.

This dish may seem complicated, so let's break it down:

1. Prep the eggplant and your dishes.
2. Roast the mushrooms.
3. Prepare your setup area with the final assembly ingredients.
4. Bread and pan-fry the eggplant quickly.
5. Assemble the casserole.
6. Bake and serve.

Ingredients

For the Eggplant
- 1 Italian eggplant, stem removed and sliced crosswise in ¼-½ slices
- 2 tsp salt
- Oil for pan-frying
- Milk of choice (dairy or non-dairy)
- ½ cup all-purpose flour
- 1 cup of Panko bread crumbs

For the Mushrooms
- 8 ounces shiitake mushrooms, finely chopped, ¼ inch pieces
- 2 garlic cloves, finely minced
- 1 tbsp crushed fennel
- 1 tbsp oil
- A dash of Maggi
- 1 tbsp soy sauce

For the Layers
- 1 jar of Italian marinara or spaghetti sauce
- 1 cup shredded mozzarella (dairy or non-dairy)
- 1 cup grated parmesan (dairy or non-dairy)
- ½ cup feta (dairy or non-dairy)

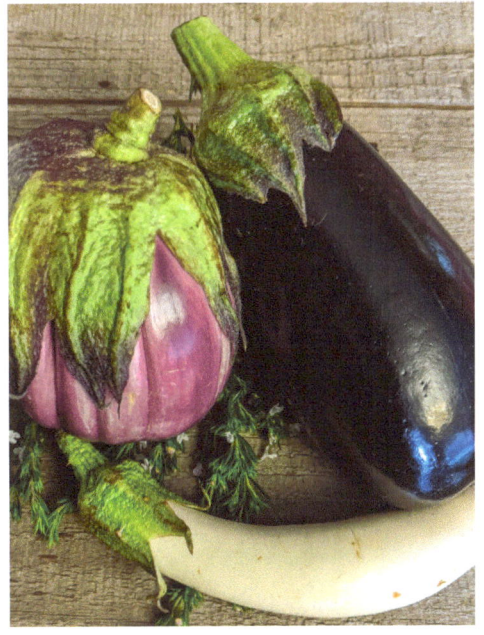

Instructions

Prework
Sprinkle the eggplant slices with the salt. Lay the eggplant slices on a paper towel or clean dish cloth on sheet pan. Allow eggplant to weep for 1-2 hours. Preheat the oven 375°F.

Prepare a sheet pan with foil and non-stick spray. Prepare a 6x8x2 casserole dish with non-stick spray.

Let's Cook
Combine all the mushroom ingredients in a bowl. Spread on the baking sheet and roast for 15-20 minutes, until brown and slightly tender with a fork. Do not roast until crunchy.

Arrange three pie plates or dishes for the dipping method: one for all-purpose flour, one for milk, and one for panko crumbs.

In a skillet, add just enough oil to cover the skillet pan and bring to medium heat.

Dip each eggplant slice into flour, then milk, then bread crumbs. Pan-fry quickly in the skillet. Drain the eggplant slices on a paper towel. Do not overcook, just brown the panko bread crumbs.

Helpful Tip: If there are any leftover crumbs in the skillet, scoop them out and garnish the casserole with the crumbs.

Assemble the Casserole
Arrange a layer of eggplant slices on bottom of pan. Spread a layer of ⅓ of the mushrooms, marinara (or spaghetti) sauce followed by a sprinkling of each type of cheese.

Arrange two more layers of eggplant, alternating the mushrooms, marinara (or spaghetti sauce), and the cheeses.

Note: If using plant-based cheese, add the last layer of cheese 15 minutes after baking.

Bake for 25-30 minutes until golden and cheese is melted, rotating at the 15-minute mark.
If the cheese starts browning too much, cover lightly with foil.

Let sit for 10-15 minutes before serving.

Serves 2-3 as a main dish

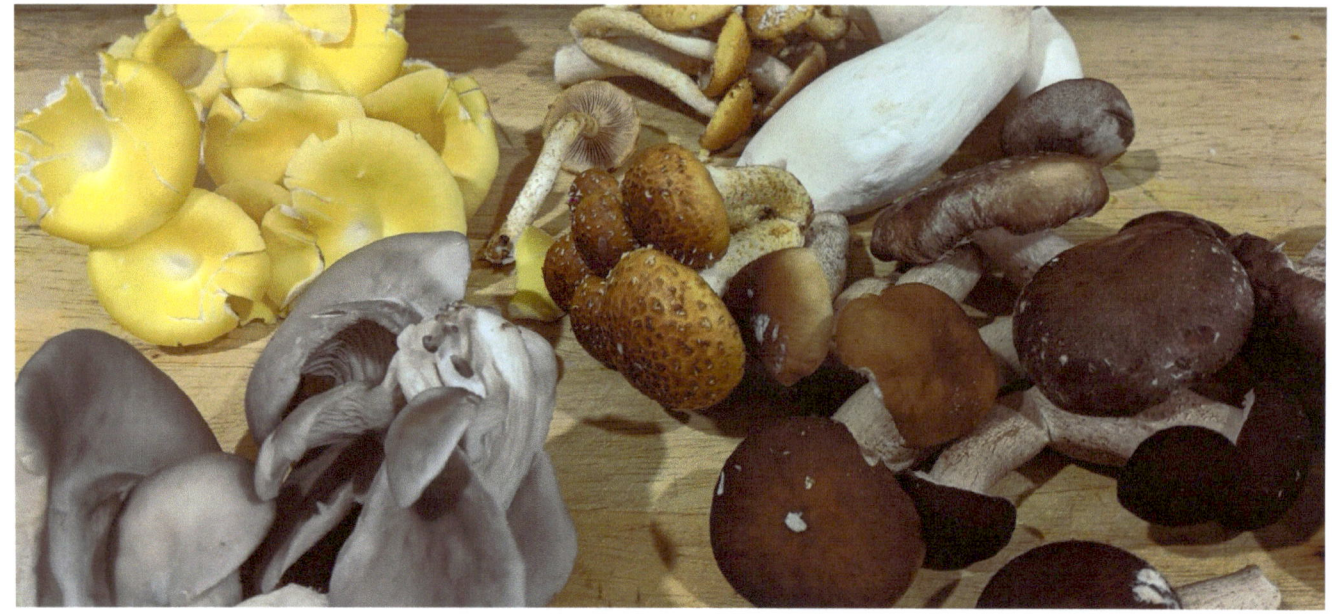
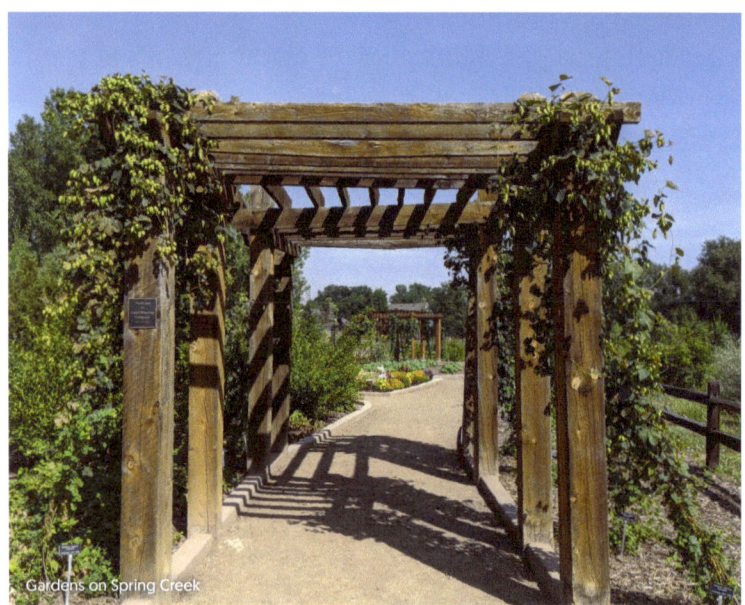
Gardens on Spring Creek
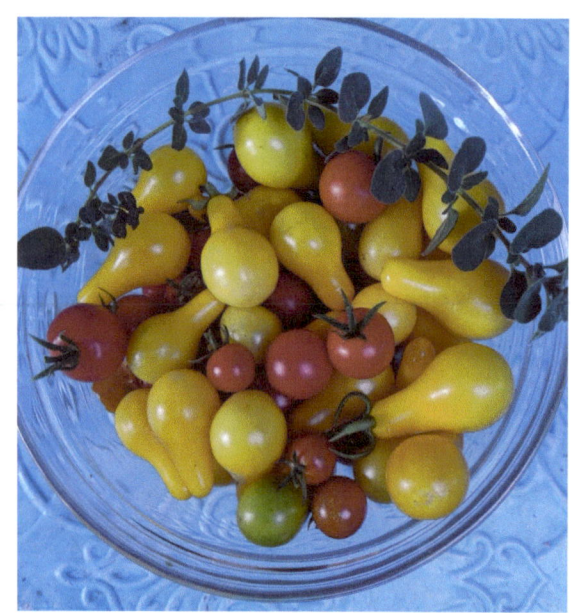
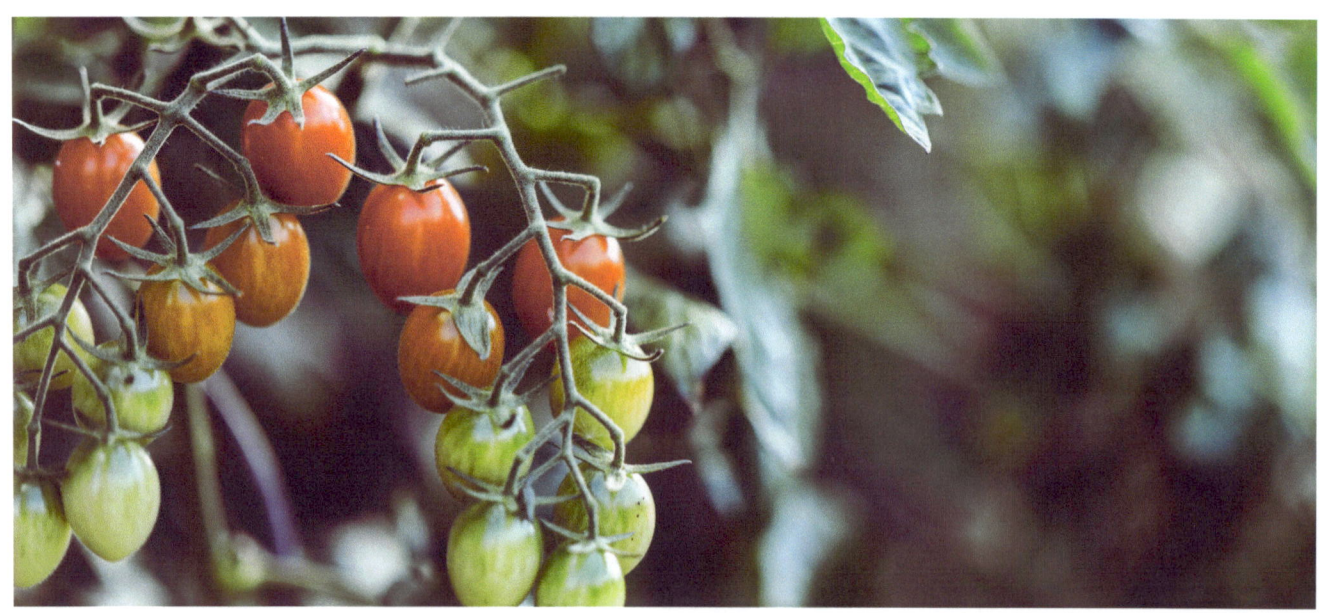

ROASTED TOMATOES & MUSHROOMS IN BRANDY CREAM SAUCE

The 2020 harvest season brought extreme forest fires to our region with smoky, charred days and an extremely early snow slated for the day after Labor Day. One of my favorite farms, On the Vine at Richmond Farms, asked for volunteers to expedite the harvest before the impending freeze. I was placed on the cherry tomato row and picked about 25 pints of various red, yellow, orange and dark purple cherry tomatoes within an hour. It was hot and a bit dizzying. The tomato pickers who gather our cherry tomatoes for the store definitely earn our respect. This is a great recipe to use up those less-than-perfect, slightly shriveled grape tomatoes, and a technique you will want to keep on hand.

Ingredients
- 1 cup grape or cherry tomatoes, halved
- 2 garlic cloves, minced
- 4 ounces mushrooms, sliced
- 1 tbsp olive oil, divided in half
- Salt and pepper to taste

For the Cream Sauce
- 1 tsp olive oil
- ½ shallot, finely minced
- ⅛ cup brandy (or choice liquor)
- 1 tsp tomato paste
- 1 cup milk or cream (dairy or non-dairy)
- 2 tsp cornstarch
- 1 lb gnocchi or 6-8 ounces shaped pasta of choice; boiled, drained, and water reserved

Instructions
Preheat the oven to 400°F. Prepare a sheet pan with foil and non-stick spray.
Combine tomatoes, garlic, ½ tbsp olive oil, and spread on one half of the sheet pan. Salt and pepper to taste. Combine mushrooms with ½ tbsp olive oil. Spread on the other half of the sheet pan. Salt, pepper to taste. Roast tomatoes and mushrooms for 20 minutes, until soft (you may want to remove the mushrooms early). Remove tomatoes from oven, move tomatoes around the bottom of the pan to scrape the caramelization bits from the foil – this adds flavor to the dish.

For the Cream Sauce
Heat the olive oil in a large skillet over medium heat. Sauté the shallots until golden and soft.
Add the tomato paste and stir to coat the shallots. Add the brandy (or liquor of choice) to deglaze the pan. Stir until brandy evaporates and sauce thickens. Turn heat down to low and allow skillet to cool.
Combine milk and cornstarch in bowl and whisk well. Slowly add the milk mixture in ⅓ portions to the skillet. Whisk well after each addition.
Add roasted tomatoes and mushrooms to the skillet. Cook over medium until sauce thickens. Do not boil. Serve over gnocchi or favorite pasta.

Helpful Tip: Add a few tbsp of the pasta water to thin your sauce if it becomes too thick to coat the pasta.

Elevate This: Decorate with some baby arugula or spinach. Use Pastificio Boulder pasta shells made with locally grown ancient grains, or handmade pasta.

Serves 2 as a main dish

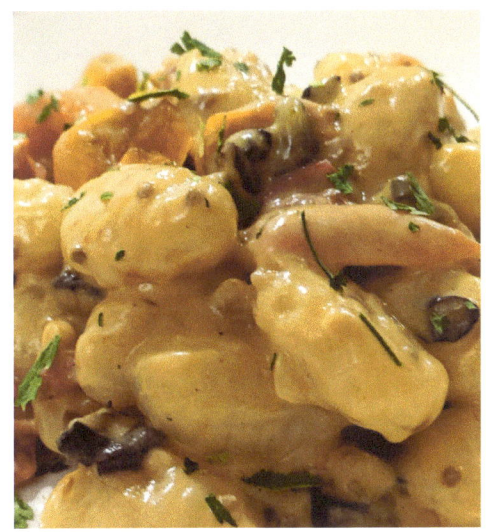

Cherries, Zen and Now

As one drives around Larimer County now, it is hard to believe there was a massive production of cherries 60 years ago. From its humble beginnings in 1915 of 200 acres in cherry orchards, by 1950, Larimer County had over 10,000 acres and almost 155,000 cherry trees in production.

Cherries first came to the Big Thompson valley by William Alexander in 1864 with a small planting of trees on his farm. With the assistance of the Agricultural College's paper, *Fruits for the Farmer* in 1893, the farming area quickly became a hotbed of cash crops such as apples, raspberries, and plums. In 1904, Buena Vista Orchard planted the newly bred cherry tree that could withstand the chill of winter and thrive in arid summers and the area boomed.

During the late 1920s the Spring Glade orchard was the largest cherry orchard west of the Mississippi producing more than $1 million worth of cherries per year. Cherry picking was hot, dusty, sticky work and the pitting preparation for the canning companies was labor-intensive work. Research states that the cherry industry through the 1960s offered summer work to almost every man, woman, and child in the area.

A series of droughts, a shortage of canning supplies during World War II, and later freezes that extensively damaged the trees, decimated the industry and began its decline. By 1960, the Loveland farmers could not compete with cherry growers in California and Michigan. Loveland still celebrates its cherry legacy with an annual Cherry Pie Festival in July.

Sour cherries are still grown in many backyards in Northern Colorado. Today, varietals are being developed that are a bit hardier. The bright red fruit sparkling in the sun and dangling in triad clumps are a beautiful thing to behold on a bike ride or walk. Northern Colorado cold patterns are iffy, so there is the possibility of losing beautiful Spring cherry blossoms to a late snow.

Fortunately, the Colorado Western Slope farmers are planting Montmorency sour, Bing, and Ranier cherries for our enjoyment. Thanks to family growers near Palisade and Paonia, if my cherry tree loses flowers to a freeze, there will hopefully be beautiful Colorado options at our local farmers market in July. The fresh sour cherry season is short, but the cherries freeze beautifully for future use in pies, tarts, crumbles, jams, cordials, and liqueurs.

I love sour cherries and could eat the sweetened jam or filling with a spoon. Dessert recipes abound for sour cherries, so I opted for an interesting recipe for a savory and tart side dish.

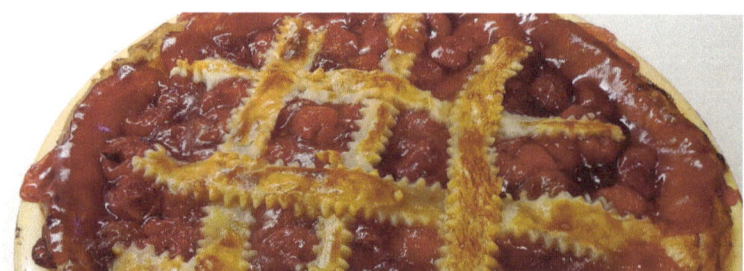
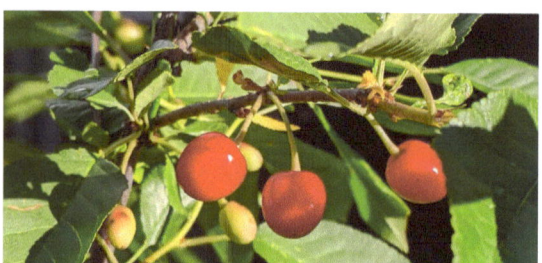
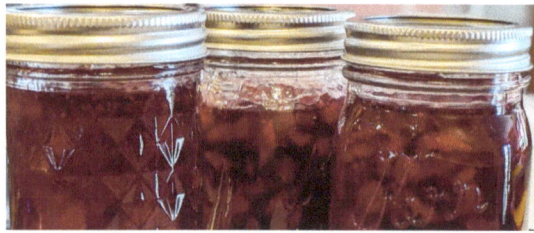
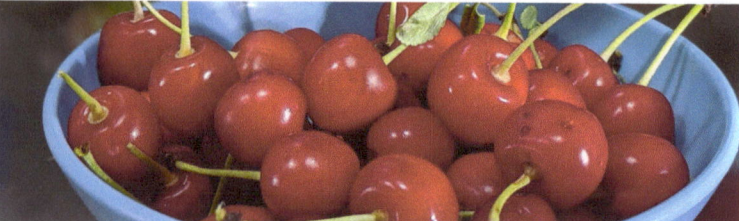

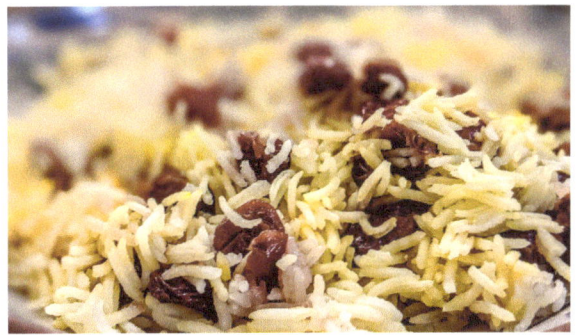
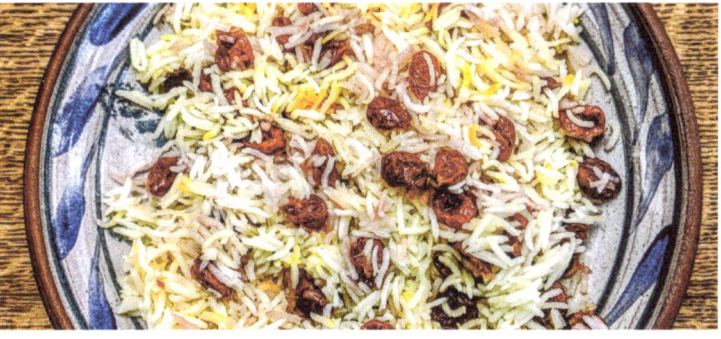
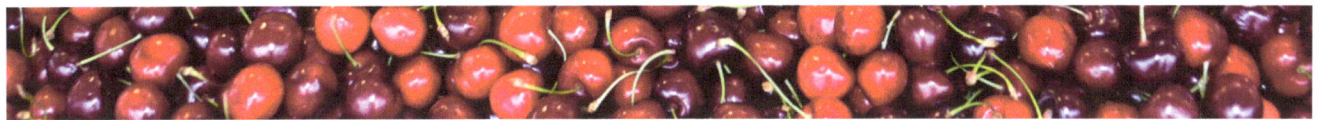

ALBALOO POLO

(Sour Cherry Rice) Sometimes less is more. Thinking outside the box for an unusual sour cherry dish, I discovered this Persian dish of rice, sour cherry sauce, butter (dairy or non-dairy), and saffron. Albaloo Polo is four simple ingredients, and highlights the Colorado sour cherry season for a sweet and savory dish. If you don't want to make the fruit sauce, use a jar of sour cherry jam.

Ingredients

For the Sour Cherry Sauce
- 2 cup sour cherries, pitted
- 2 cup sugar
- 1 tbsp powdered clear gel or cornstarch, mixed in 1 tbsp water

For the Rice
- 4-5 saffron threads (optional, but highly recommended)
- 1 tbsp hot water
- 1 cup uncooked white rice (I used long grain, but medium grain basmati or jasmine will work)
- 1 ¾ cup water
- 1 tsp salt
- 1 cup sour cherry sauce above or 1 cup sour cherry jam
- 4 tbsp butter (dairy or non-dairy), cut into 12 small pieces

Instructions

For the Sour Cherry Sauce
Bring sour cherries to soft boil over medium heat. Cook 5 minutes to remove moisture. Slowly add sugar. Cook until mixture begins to thicken (~190°F). With a small sieve, sprinkle powdered clear gel or cornstarch mixture over sour cherries. Stir to dissolve until the sauce becomes clear red. Remove from heat and cool. Once cooled, remove 1 cup of sauce and strain with a strainer. Keep the remaining cherry sauce for other uses, such as desserts, or on a crêpe.
Place saffron in 1 tbsp hot water, steep for 5 minutes.

For the Rice
Add rice, water and salt to sauce pan and cook for 7 min. Rinse rice with cold water and place in a separate bowl. Return ⅓ of the rice to the sauce pan. Poke 4 holes in rice and add 1 piece of butter (dairy or non-dairy) to each hole. Cover with ½ the cherry sauce. Cover the cherry sauce with ⅓ of the rice. Repeat the hole and butter process. Cover with remaining cherry sauce. Top the cherry sauce with remaining rice and last 4 pieces of butter. Sprinkle the saffron water on top. Cover with a lid and cook on medium low for 20 minutes. Fluff and serve.

Elevate This: Add sliced almonds or an herb. Practice and play, but allow the cherries to remain center stage.

Serves 4 as a side dish

Peach Perfect

Peaches, peaches, peaches. There are South Carolina peaches, Georgia peaches, Texas Hill Country peaches. and California peaches. The piece de resistance of the peach family, in my humble opinion, is the Palisade Peach, found in Colorado.

What makes a Palisade peach so incredibly special? Palisade is situated on Colorado's Western Slope or Grand Valley. The warm days and cool nights help the sugars develop. The area grows several types of peaches including freestone, cling, and semi-cling. The peach I most love is called a "yellow melting flesh" peach, a freestone variety. The skin is soft, meaning you can almost use your fingers to pull the peach—skin and all—off the stone.

The pericarp, or skin, is distinct. A perfectly ripe Palisade peach is a beautiful peachy color with accents of light rose. The flesh is a beautiful yellow-orange. The endocarp (area closest to the stone) on a true Palisade peach, is a deep garnet or slight bronze color. Hence, as pictured in the Rustic Peach Crumble, you may see a bit of ruby or garnet in your dish. Having tasted all other peaches, the juiciness of a Palisade peach is unparalleled – always sweet with nectar dripping down to your elbows. Ah, one of the most enjoyable annual eating experiences.

How do you know you are getting a Palisade peach? You know you are getting a Palisade if you research the name and the grower has a Palisade address, or better yet, follow the grower and growing season directly on social media. Just because a seller labels a peach "Colorado," does not mean the peach is from the Palisade area.

Cling and semi-cling harvests begin in late June and freestones begin in late July. It is a very short season. Once the peaches are gone, they are gone. They are not kept in cold storage for winter distribution. If you want to enjoy a Palisade peach off season, buy a box and freeze them in small batches. I peel the peaches, remove the pit, cut the peaches into slices, soak briefly in lemon juice to prevent browning, and freeze them in Glad Press'N Seal. Then they will be ready to be enjoyed as a topping on your yogurt or ice cream, or in a crumble.

You will find backyard peach trees on the Front Range that are lovely and offer excellent peaches, but we all appreciate the efforts of the Palisade peach community in bringing their bounty from across the Rockies to the Front Range late summer farmers markets.

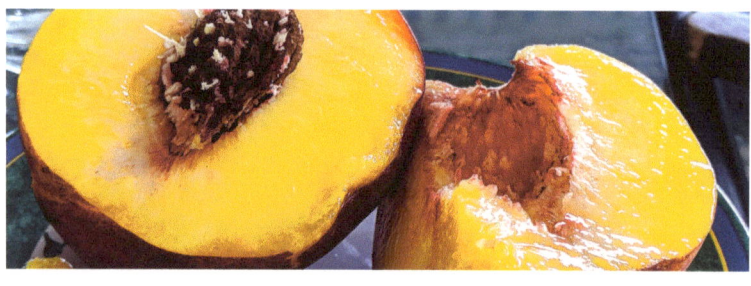
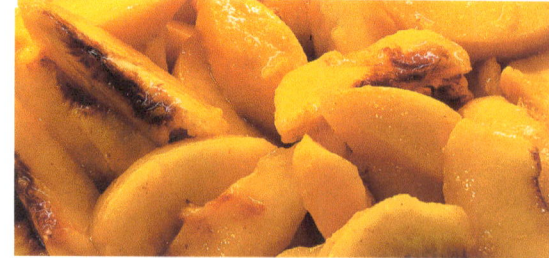
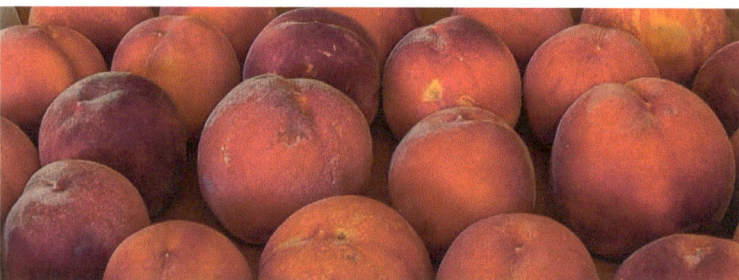
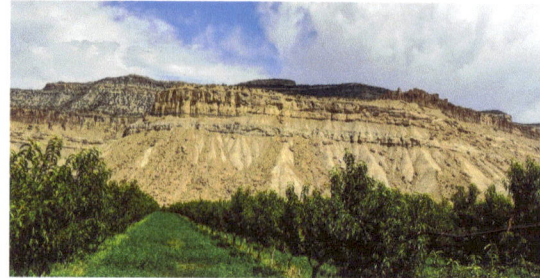

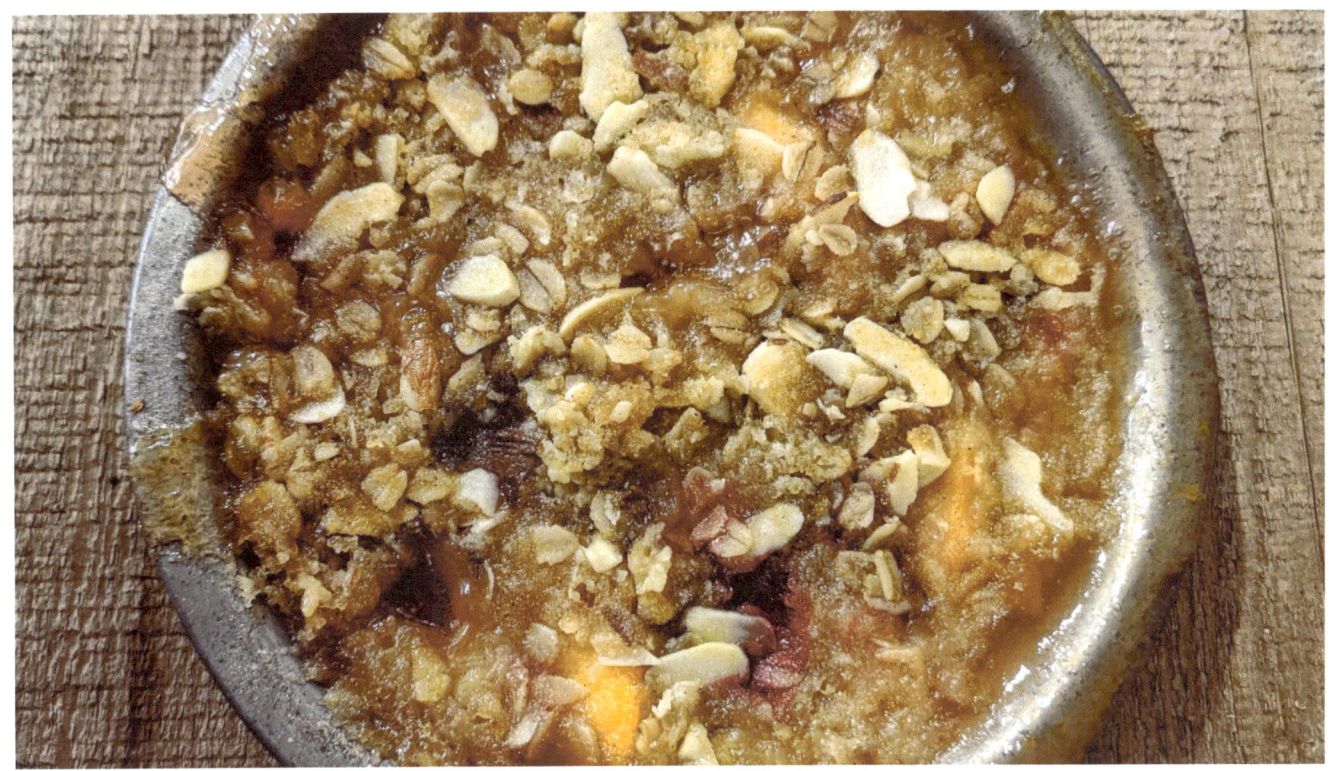

RUSTIC PEACH CRUMBLE

This crumble comes together quickly, fulfills my sweet tooth, and treats special guests without a lot of kitchen fuss. I use this recipe in the spring with rhubarb instead of peaches, and I substitute with cherries in the summer.

Ingredients
- 3 large Palisade peaches; peeled, pitted, and sliced
- 1 tsp lemon juice
- 2 tbsp cornstarch
- 4 tbsp cold butter (dairy or non-dairy), cut into ¼-inch pieces
- ⅓ cup all-purpose flour
- ¼ cup brown sugar
- ¼ cup old-fashioned oatmeal (not 1-minute oatmeal)
- ¼ cup sliced almonds
- ½ tsp cinnamon

Instructions
Preheat oven at 375°F and spray an 8-inch pie plate with non-stick spray.
Combine peaches, lemon juice and cornstarch in a bowl until cornstarch dissolves. Pour into prepared pie pan.
In a bowl, combine the butter (dairy or non-dairy) and flour with your fingers. Press the butter pieces throughout the flour. It is okay if there are little chunks of butter, they need to melt to make the crust.
Add the remaining ingredients to the flour mixture. Arrange the flour mixture on top of the peaches.
Place the pie pan on a baking sheet (in case it boils over). Bake for 20-30 minutes until bubbly.
Cool a bit before scooping.

Elevate This: Add a few raspberries or blueberries to the peaches, especially if you don't have enough peaches to cover the pie pan.

Serves 3-4 as a dessert

Tomatoes, Corn and Melons, Oh My!

Almost every region of the country has its own tomato, corn, and melon season. Ours starts in August. The long, warm days and cool nights make for spectacularly sweet heirloom garden tomatoes, Rocky Ford™ melons, yellow watermelons, and corn. All will continue to produce until mid-September when the days begin to shorten, cool down rapidly, and we must say goodbye to these treats until the following year.

Private and community gardens have an endless variety too, including cherry, grape, yellow pear-shaped, Heirloom Cherokees and more. Tomatoes in farmers market bins are like the brilliant modern artwork of Wassily Kandinsky. Smashes of bright orange, gold, yellow, green, cherry red, maroon, purple, and almost black. They are almost too beautiful to cut – but, do!

Colorado's own special variety of corn is Olathe Corn. The Olathe, Colorado area in the southern Front Range used to grow beets and barley, but switched to a sweet corn variety that thrived in the climate. Sweet, crunchy, soft, and firm – all in one bite. Our local growers, including On the Vine at Richmond Farms, Miller Farms, and FarmFresh CSA—among others—grow many single and bi-color varieties such as Spring Treat, Providence, Serendipity, and Honey Select.

Rocky Ford™ melons have been around since the 1890s, shipped to all areas of the country, and served at the finest restaurants in New York City. Rocky Ford melons are grown on the lower east Front Range in Rocky Ford, Colorado, near the Arkansas River. In the early years, George Swink convinced his neighbors to build the first irrigation system in the valley, forever transforming the area into a top crop-producing region. A sweet, short season luxury is to cut off the peel, seed, and try not to eat the whole melon in one standing.

How to Peel and Cut a Cantaloupe:

1. Wash the melon and pat dry.
2. Cut off both ends.
3. Stabilize the cut side of the melon on a cutting board.
4. With a sharp knife, cut strips of peel down the sides from top to bottom.
5. When all peel is removed, cut the melon in half, remove the seeds, and cut into wedges or chunks.

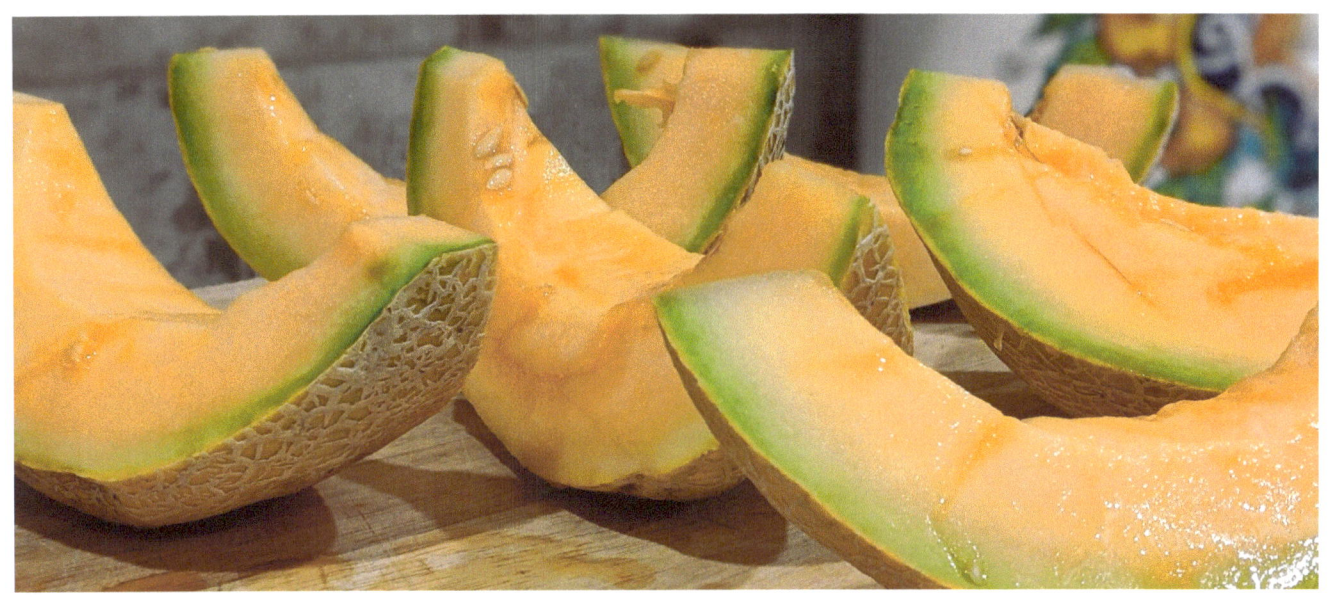
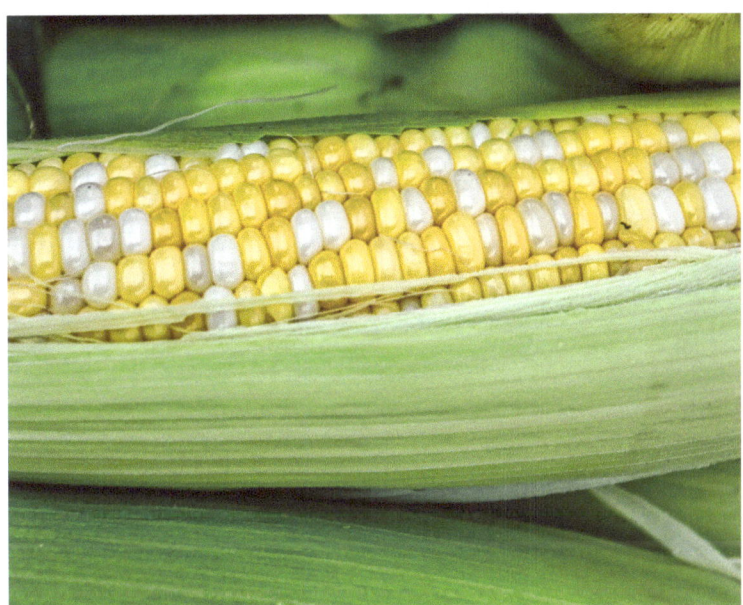
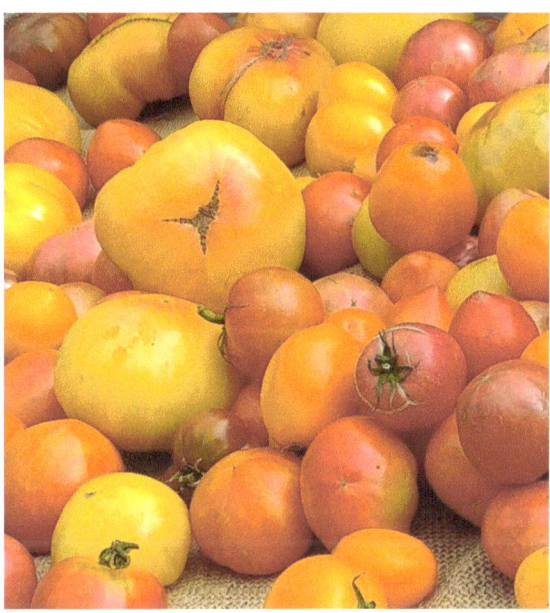
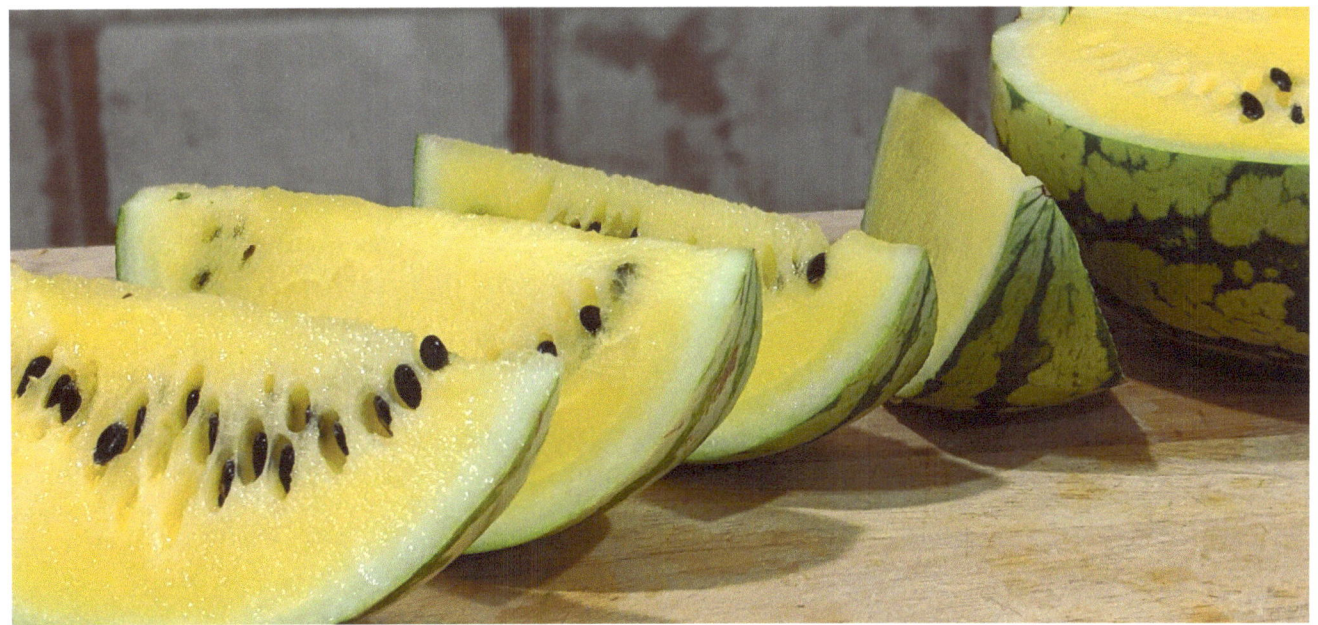

Honey Bee FAQs

Backyard beekeeping is popular in Northern Colorado. As beekeepers in an arid, elevated, cold climate, our beekeeping coincides with the short growing season. The bees begin to emerge in March. We work diligently to create a healthy, sustainable environment for them. The strongest honey flow is from June to late August. As the tree and garden flowers wane, our work begins to feed and treat them for parasites, and get them ready for winter by October.

Why should I buy local honey? Raw honey has antibacterial, antiviral, and antifungal properties, and promotes digestive health. Raw, local honey also contains a blend of local pollen, which can strengthen a person's immune system, and reduce pollen allergy symptoms. Local honey is not processed, heated or combined with any other liquid sugar products. Most importantly, research has shown you get more than four times the amount of antioxidants in local, versus processed, mass produced honey.

What are the anatomical parts of a bee? Each honey bee has six legs, pair of compound eyes, wings, nectar pouch and abdomen.

What is that yellow stuff I see on a bee's legs? Pollen.

What percent of our food is pollinated by bees? $\frac{1}{3}$ of our global food supply.

How much honey does one bee "make?" $\frac{1}{12}$ of a teaspoon in its lifetime.

How far do bees fly for pollen and nectar? As a rule of thumb, the foraging area around a beehive extends for two miles, although bees have been observed foraging two and three times this distance from the hive.

At what temperature do bees stop flying? Bee behavior is affected by temperature. They rarely work when the temperature is below 57°F or above 100°F. They cannot fly when the temperature is below 55°F. On very hot days, bees cluster outside unshaded hives and do not work. This is called bearding.

How long does a bee live? In warm weather, approximately 42 days. In cold weather, 4-6 months.

How long does a Queen bee live? About 2-3 years. The hive either replaces her, or the beekeeper manually replaces her with a new queen. Yes, I have had to kill a poorly-laying queen. They definitely take one for the team.

Is it true most bees are female? Yes. The queen lays mostly female eggs. Females do all the work.

So, what kind of work do they do? During their lifetime, they serve as nurse bees taking care of eggs to capped brood, housecleaners (they are fastidious and even carry out and fly out their dead!) and foragers to the end of life. They also guard the hive and fight off predators.

How many eggs does a Queen lay? She lays about 1,000 eggs per day. That is enough to create a rotation of future worker generations.

Do bees hibernate in the winter? No. Worker bees rotate in and out of the bee huddle, much like penguins do to survive the cold. They keep the hive temperature around a balmy 95°F.

Why do bees swarm? Short answer, bees swarm for additional space and to reproduce in the spring and early summer.

What is the biggest difference between a bee and a wasp? While honey bees can attack when provoked, wasps are naturally more aggressive predators. Honey bees are hairy, while wasps usually have smooth and shiny skin.

Is it true we are losing honey bees? Yes. At the time of this writing, beekeepers are losing approximately 40% of their hives. Bees are harmed by the use of neonicotinoid pesticides, parasites known as Varroa mites, colony collapse disorder, and they are losing areas to forage. We can manage the pesticides, treat hives for mites, and plant for pollinators!

What is the deadliest home pesticide for foraging bees? Sevin dust. Although any product with neonicotinoids is extremely harmful. There is ongoing research on many home and agricultural pesticides and bee health.

I see more and more backyard beekeepers. How can I help the bees in my area?

- Reduce your lawn footprint.
- Plant pollinator-friendly flowers and trees.
- Limit pesticides.
- Know who to call if you see a swarm (for example, your local swarm hotline).

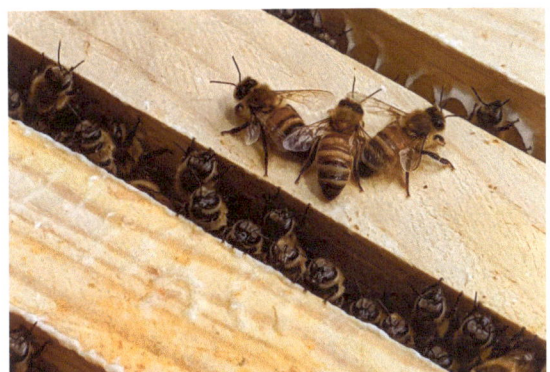
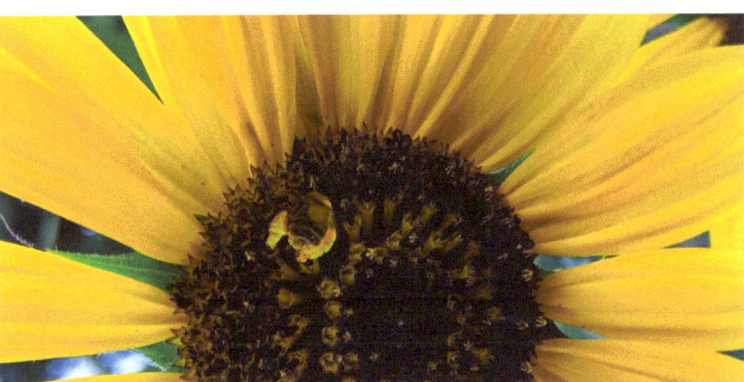
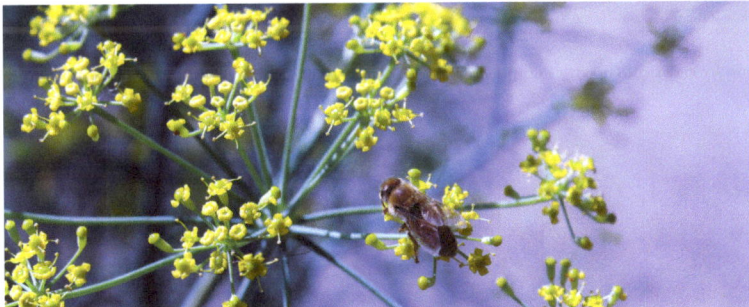
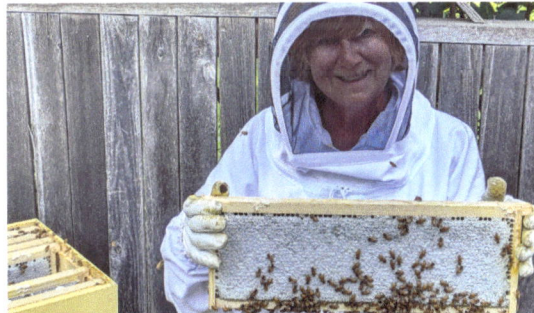
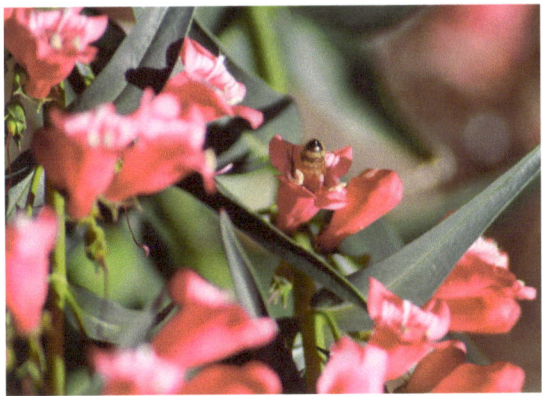
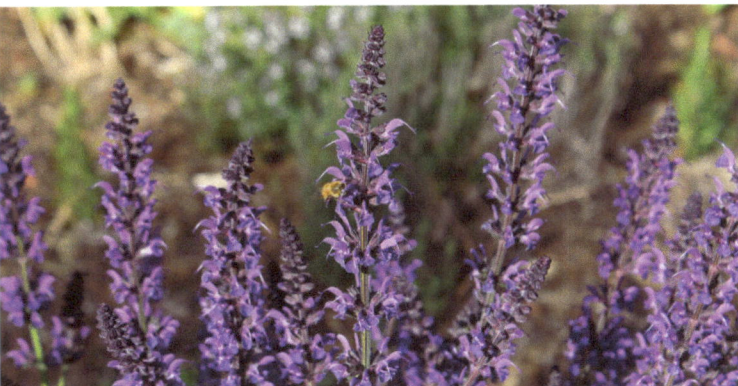

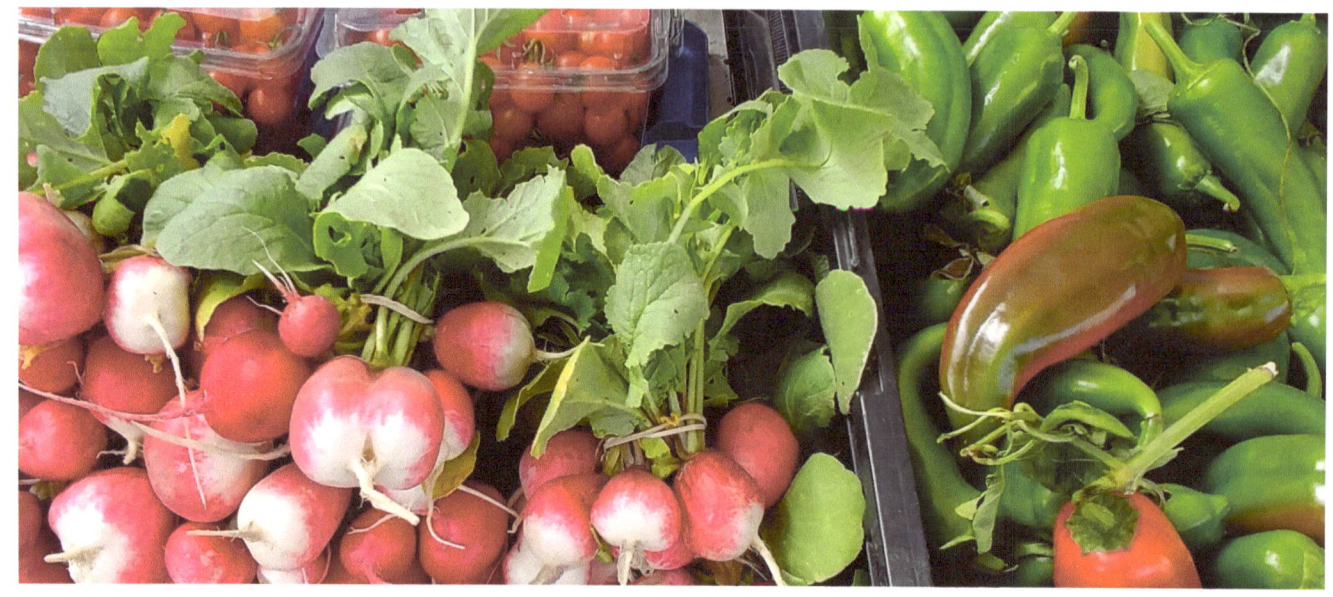
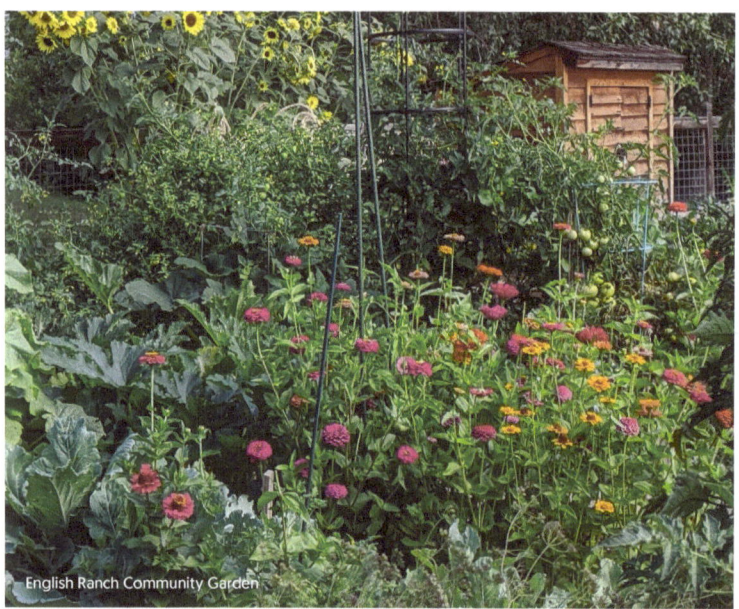
English Ranch Community Garden
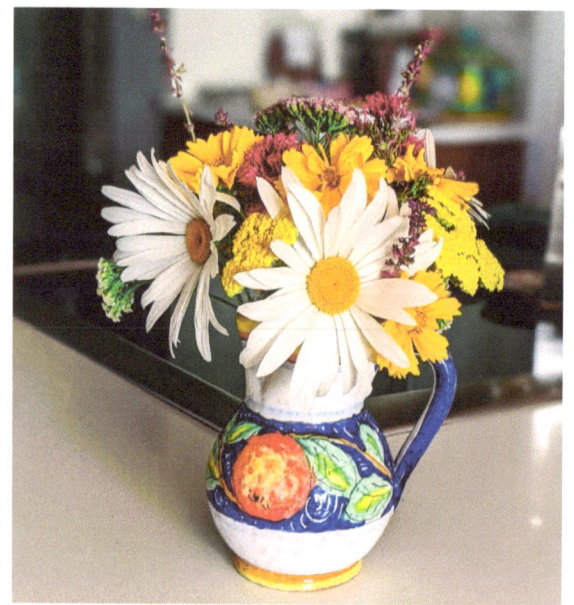
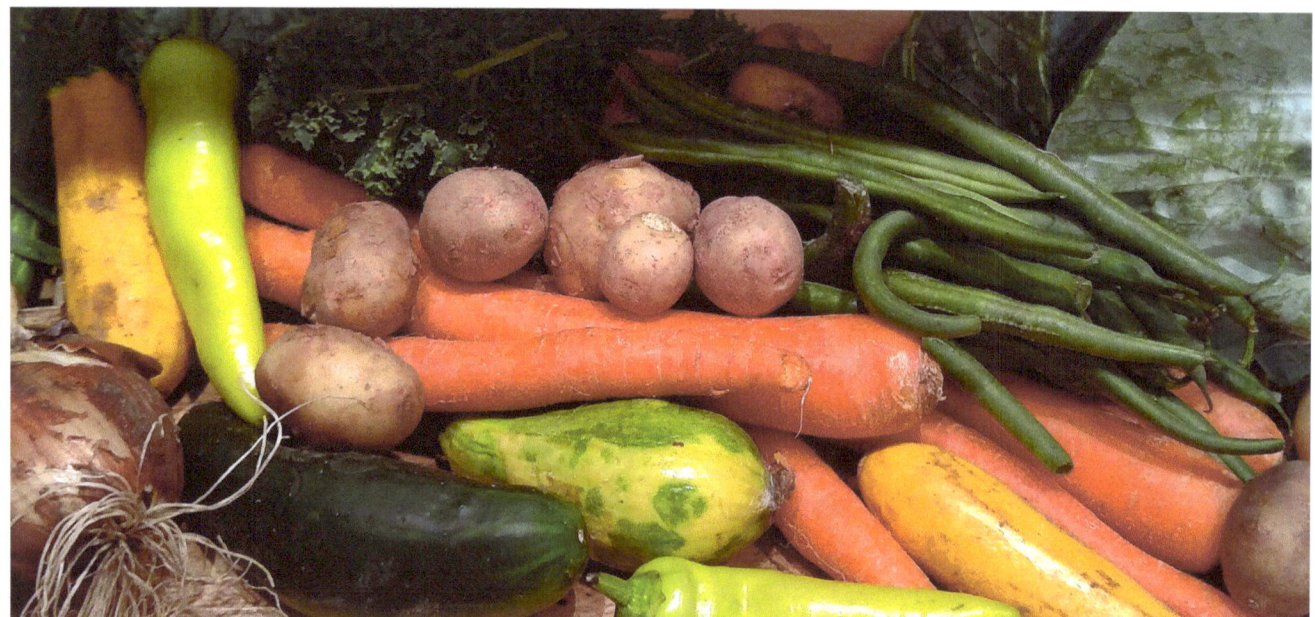

AUTUMN

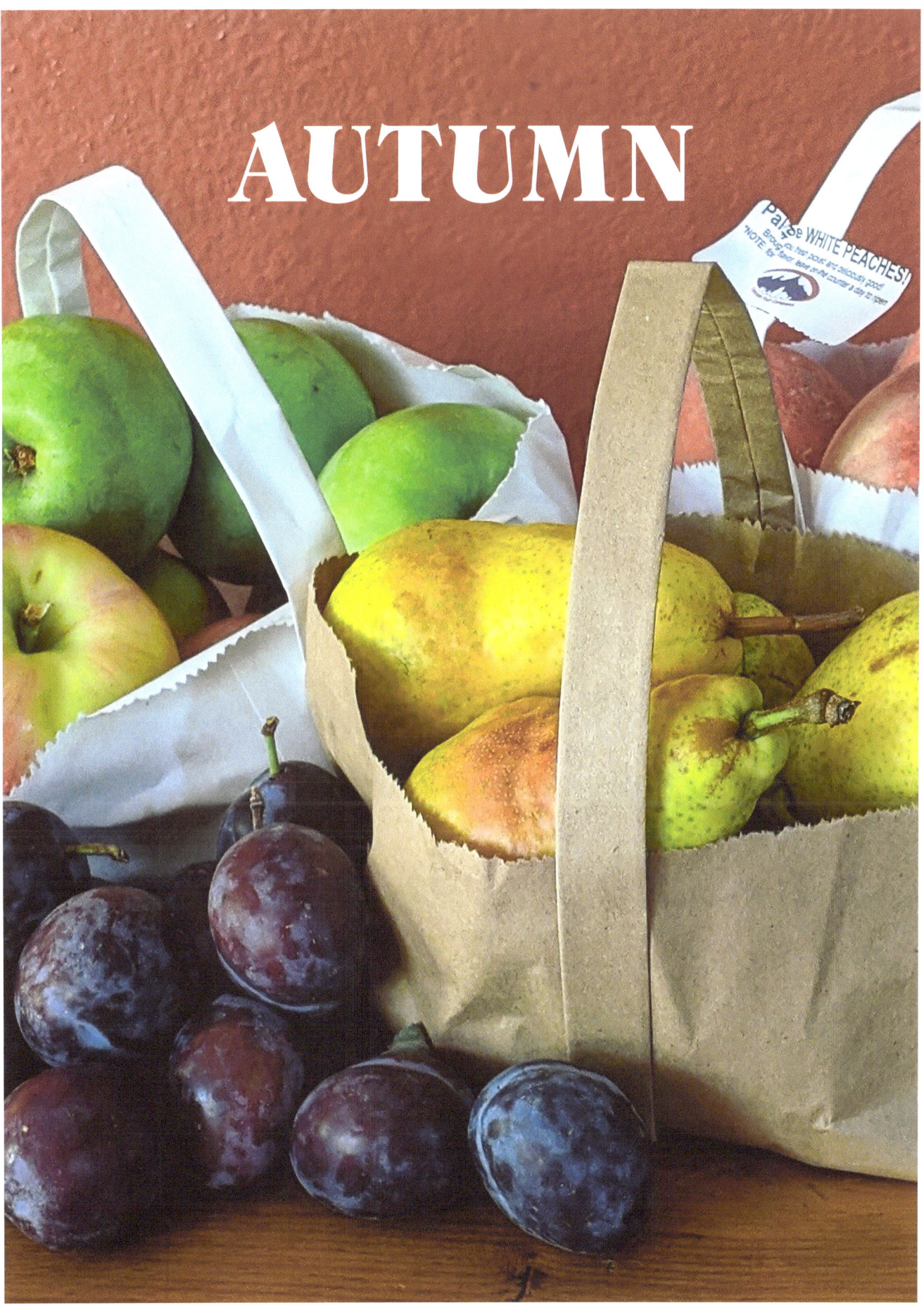

The days are waning. Shadows are long. The aspens and cottonwoods up the Poudre River are beginning to turn.

Geese are clumping and flying in formations to various watering holes and resting spots around town, their plaintiff honking overhead. Bees are foraging the last of the purple asters, summer sunflowers and autumn crocuses, and we are getting the hives ready for the first snow — which could be anytime from Labor Day to Halloween.

It's the golden hour, and the world puts its autumn glow onto Horsetooth Mountain, over the Front Range foothills, for the final few moments of day.

The evening is here. What shall we make for supper?

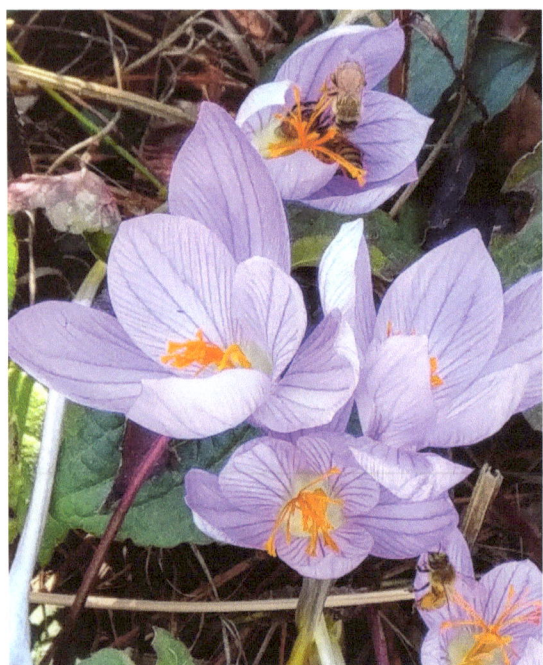
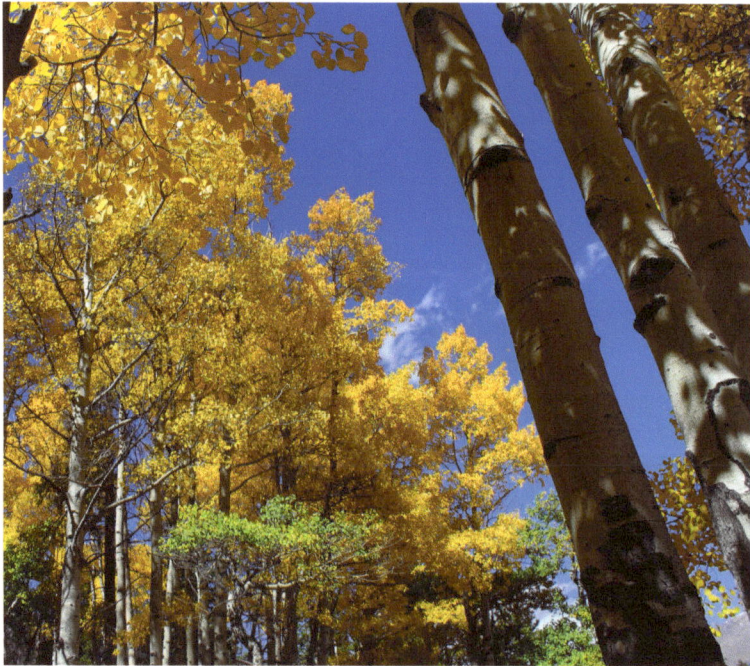
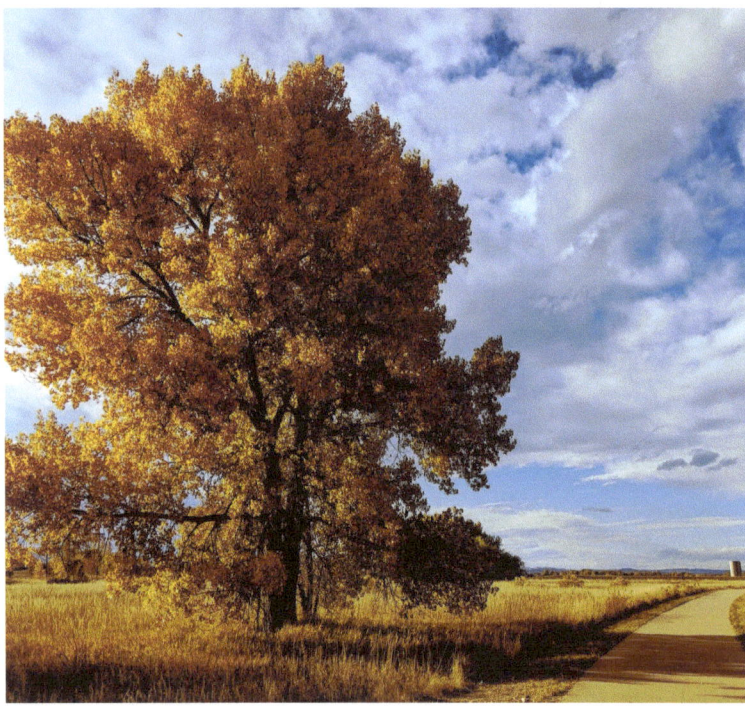
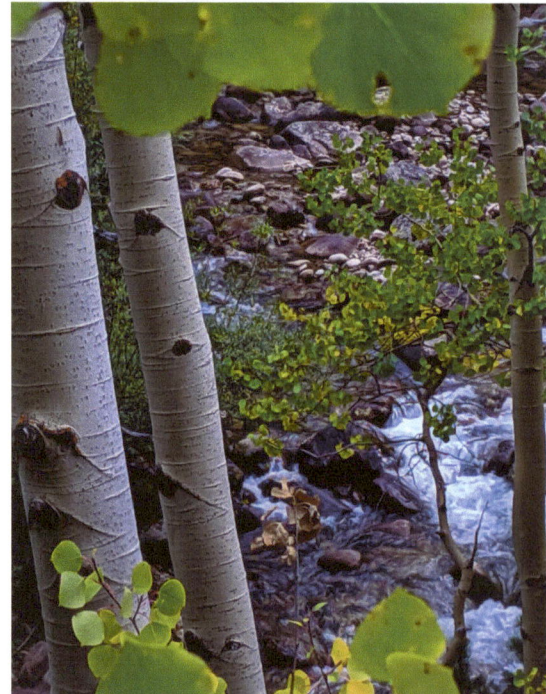

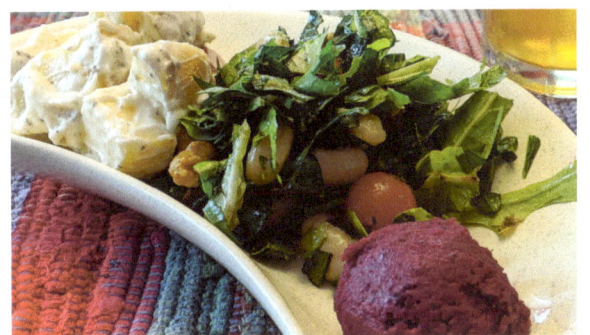
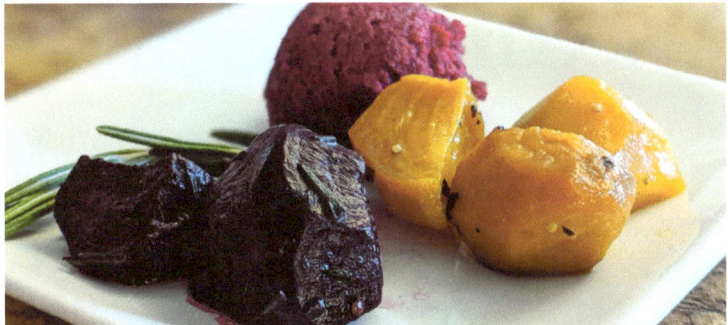
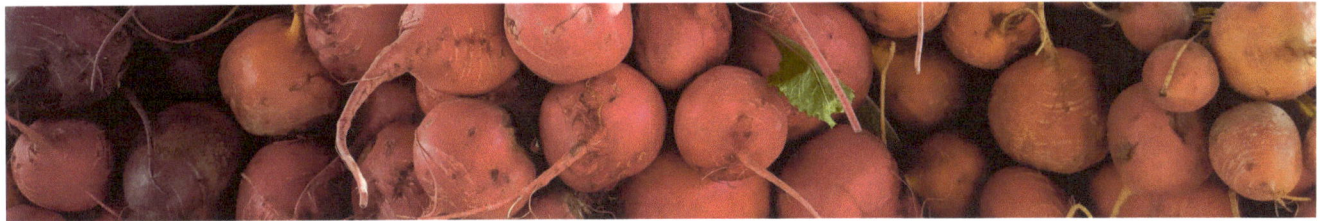

A TASTING OF BEETS THREE WAYS

Beets, beets, and more beets. I am the only one in my household who eats beets, so I thought I would get creative. This is really an idea page more than anything.

Consider a veg as something you can steam, boil, mash, smoke, bake, roast, preserve, pan sear, sauté, or marinade. You can even pair it with fruit or grain or marry it with another vegetable. The nice thing is, if you just have one of a certain veg, you can blend it with a second veg into something wonderful and enough for a serving or two.

A: Mash a steamed or boiled beet with a steamed or boiled purple potato. I tested puréeing beets with white beans, white potatoes, sweet potatoes, and purple potatoes. I preferred the purple potatoes, but experiment for yourself. Have some fun and mash away with a food processor for best results.

B: Smoke or roast yellow beets with a nice smoked pepper (I like Durango smoked pepper from a local spice shop) and finish with a flavored finishing salt. There are so many salts to choose from. The sky is the limit. Peel and cut the beets into ½ inch or so bites. Toss in oil and salt and pepper. Smoke at 220°F until fork tender. Or roast in the oven at 400°F until fork tender.

C: Pressure cook red beets for 20 minutes. Let cool. Peel. Quarter. Marinade in ¼ cup olive oil, 2 tsp balsamic vinegar, and some chopped rosemary. Be creative! Use different olive oil varieties and think interesting vinegars, such as sour cherry, lemongrass mint, or any of the other fun infused balsamic vinegars on the market.

Helpful Tip: When serving mashed food, use an ice cream or cookie scoop. The rounded form creates a lovely presentation on which to garnish or separate the dish from something else on the plate.

It's About Garlic

Most of us grew up on one variety of garlic – white, soft neck from the grocery store. That's it. I had no idea until we moved to Colorado there were so many other varieties!

Across Northern Colorado, there are multiple farmers growing as many as 18 varieties of heirloom garlic, including Long Shot Farm in Longmont. Long Shot sells their garlic in the fall after harvest at the local county farmers markets. But, a trip to their farm stand is a lovely drive along county roads and vista views that are particularly beautiful after the first snow in September or October.

There are hard neck and soft neck varieties, in variations of red, blue, and purple. Some of my favorites are Music, Early Red Italian, Spanish Roja, and Oregon Blue.

I think a box of a dozen garlic varieties would make a superb gift for the experiential home chef, don't you?

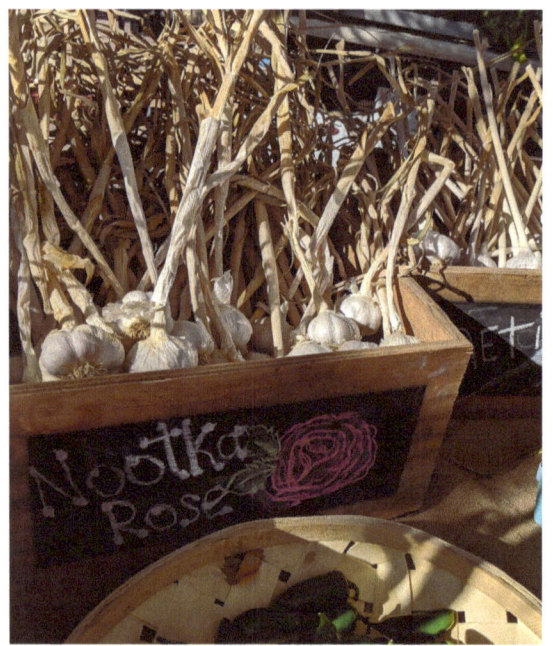
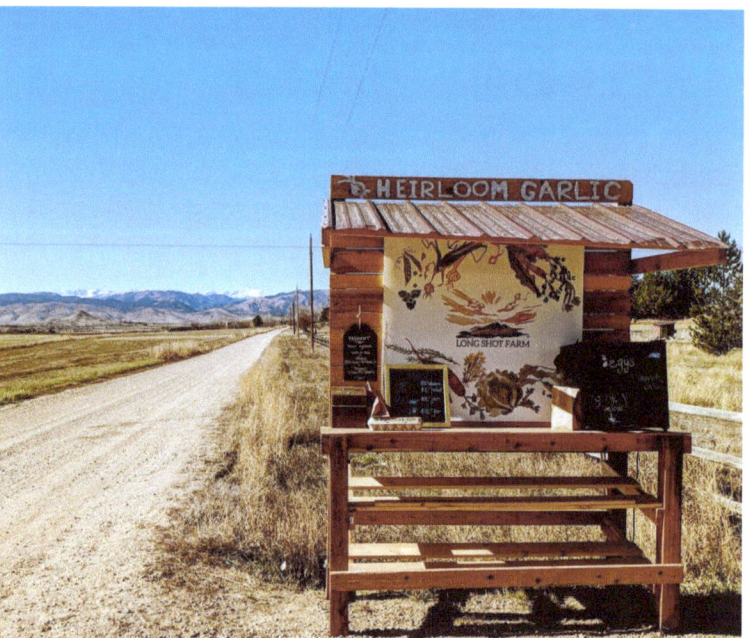
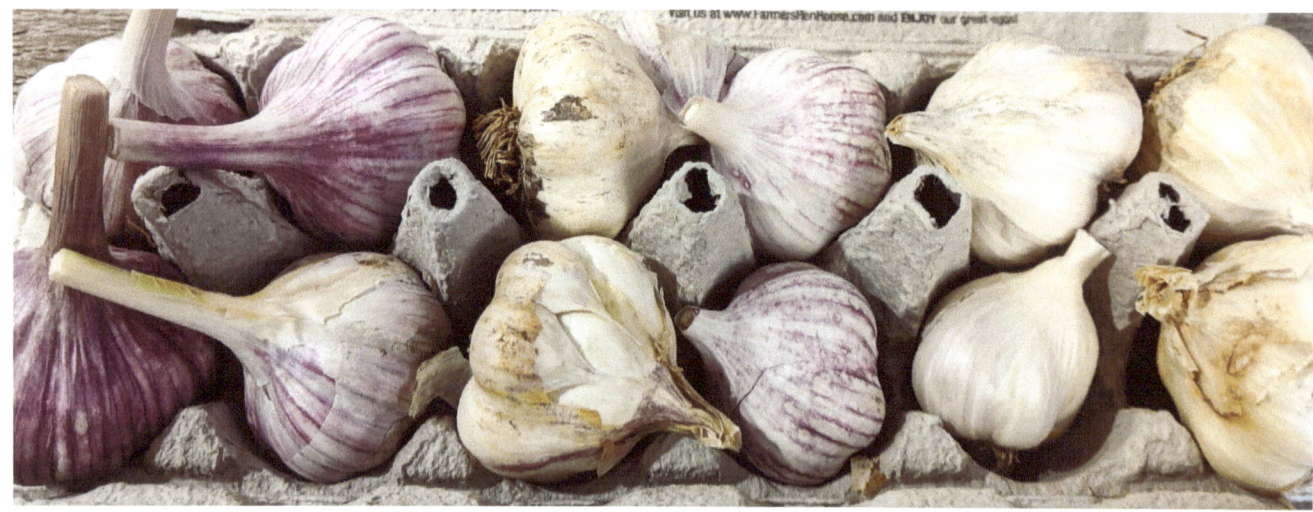

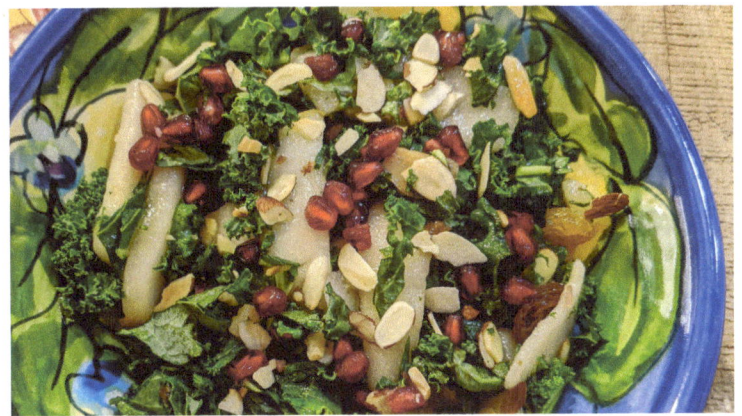
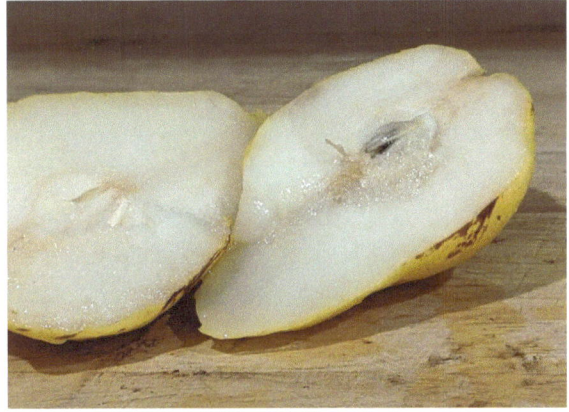
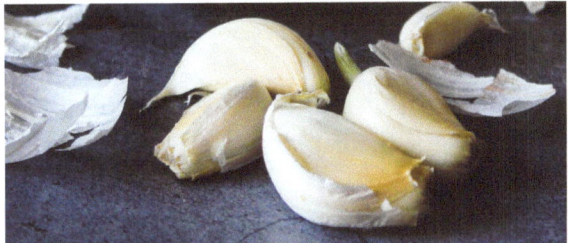
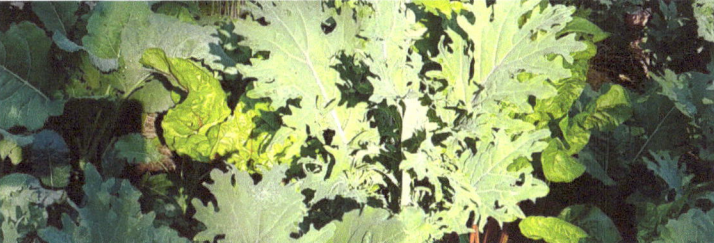

KALE, PEAR, CANDIED GARLIC, ALMOND AND HONEY SALAD

Fall signals in early polytunnel or hoop crops, such as kale, and the last of the pears from the Western slope. A touch of recently harvested, local honey transitions this dish into what my husband calls, "a dessert green salad." The candied local garlic and poms give a touch of hot and touch of tart. If you don't like the sweetness, just cut back on the honey.

Ingredients

For the Salad
- ½ lb kale; stem-stripped, roughly chopped, and massaged
- 1 pear, sliced and seeded
- ¼ cup pomegranate seeds
- ¼ cup toasted almonds

For the Dressing
- 6 garlic cloves, peeled and thickly sliced
- ¼ cup Madeira, Masala, or red wine
- 1 tbsp sugar
- ½ tsp sea salt
- 2 tbsp local honey
- ¼ cup golden raisins

Instructions

For the Dressing
Place the garlic in a small saucepan. Cover with water and boil five minutes. Add the Madeira, sugar and sea salt, and reduce to a thin syrup. Add the honey and raisins and cook until the syrup thickens, but is not gooey. Keep warm. If it gets too thick, then add a little water to thin it out.

Assemble
Combine all the salad ingredients in a bowl. Add the warm dressing, toss, and serve.

Elevate This: Experiment with finishing salts and peppers. Honey pecans or chopped dates will be a nice addition as well.

Serves 2-3 as a salad dish

Apple Me This

Ginger Gold. Florina. Pixie Crunch. Wynoochie Early. The names by themselves exude the elegance, history, glamour, fun, and taste of heritage apples. You may not find all of these varieties in your local grocery store. Nor will you find the gloriously elegant and versatile Kandil Sinap (a Turkish or possibly Crimean apple) that was discovered in the 1800s and is now available in Colorado. You will only find these locally at Masonville Apple Orchards.

Masonville Orchards started in 1988 in the Masonville Valley, near Stove Prairie, a few miles southwest of Fort Collins. The valley provides the right mix of soil, elevation, cool overnight temperatures, and warm days for apples to blossom and mature. Spring can be a little tricky with a late frost, but the orchards have been in production for over 30 years.

Walt Rosenberg, owner and orchardist, had a deep passion for orchards. Growing up in Kentucky on a farm, Walt was exposed to all aspects of farming life including tobacco, cattle, and orchards. After completing a successful life as an engineer, he journeyed back to his love of orchards, selecting the Masonville Valley as his starting point for the first of what would become multiple orchards in Northern Colorado. It may not be an exaggeration that Walt brought heritage apples back to Colorado. He built a wonderful legacy with Masonville Orchards that all of us can enjoy.

Having little experience with apple orchards growing up, I was particularly intrigued by what a fresh, heritage apple looked, smelled, and tasted like. What is a good eating apple, a pie apple, a cider apple or a multi-purpose apple? What does an apple taste like right off a tree? We can get multiple varieties in stores, but nothing like what is offered through our area orchards, like Adam's Apple U-Pick Orchards.

In 2019, Walt gave me and my friend Shari a tour through the Cobb Lake orchard, and provided an opportunity for us to experience the glory of apples first-hand. Walt was kind enough to give us a lengthy introduction to heritage apples and show us the literal fruits of his labor.

The Cobb Lake orchard is situated on the east side of I-25 along Cobb Lake, with a magnificent view of the mountains. On a clear day, one gets a view of beautiful red, green, and gold apples, rows of irrigated, heavily-laden trees weighted with fruit, a length of pasture, the lake and the mountains. We walked through the orchard as Walt described his work and the different varietals, with each apple becoming more beautiful and luscious than the last.

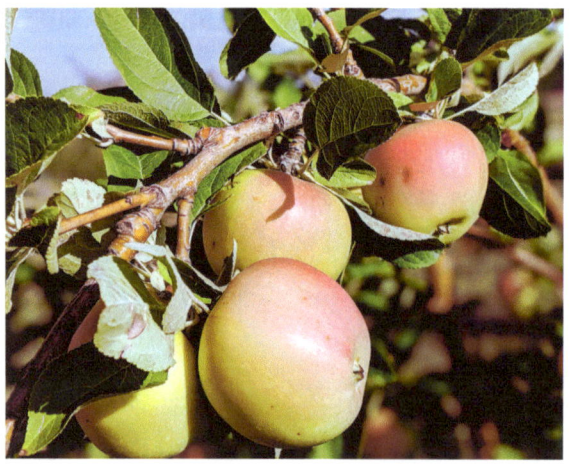
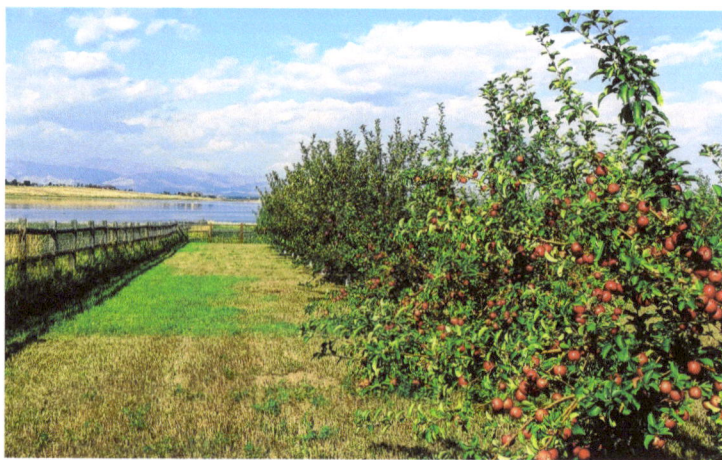

Ten Things I Have Learned About Local Orchards and Apples:

1. Fort Collins orchards offer over 200 varieties of apples, pears, and plums, many of which most of us have never heard.
2. There are at least five criteria that chain stores need to accept apples in their distribution system including size, shape and color, storage, ability to ship, and of course price. The margin for grocery stores is very tight, so hand-crafted, historical, and perhaps, magical, slightly misshapen apples may not quite fit criteria.
3. Sweetness is a factor in the cold storage process. The sweeter the apple, the harder it may be to keep cold for long periods of time.
4. Consumers generally like perfect, large, and inexpensive fruits and vegetables. Hence, the cute little crispy sweet Pixie Crunch, that packs a punch of taste within a fruit about the size of racquetball, may take a while to make it into your grocery store.
5. Washington State provides us with the most accessible apples through huge distribution chains. Not a bad thing. Though in my humble opinion, local orchards provide us with the best tasting experience.
6. Apples have distinctive characteristics, sort of like wine. Fruity, tart, mouthfeel, crunchy or a bit tender.
7. A fresh red apple has oxidized spots on it while on the tree, which makes it look like it has a fungus. Polish it a bit with a wipe and it will suddenly become a Snow-White awesome, picture-perfect apple.
8. The Red Delicious apple became the crown jewel of America's apples, and potentially our "standard" for an eating apple.
9. Orchardists are in it for the long haul. It takes as many as eight years for an orchardist to harvest the first crop of apples.
10. Colorado was one of the most prolific apple-growing areas in the 1800s. Then came the Great Depression, science, and new varietals that didn't grow well here. Thanks to Walt and the new, up-and-coming growers, apples are making a comeback to the Front Range.

What I find most inspiring is the love Walt had for the care of the orchards and the quality level for his customers. Customers from as far away as California requested his apples. His orchards have transitioned to new owners who have the same love for the mystique and beauty of local heritage apples. His apples will live on in the new orchards and backyards of those in who are purchasing scionwood for grafting, and continuing the tradition of apple-growing in our area. Northern Colorado owes him a debt of gratitude for bringing apples back to our area – thank you, Walt.

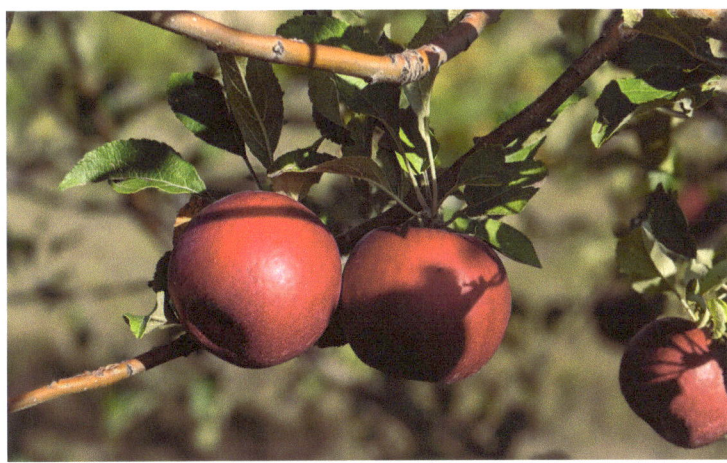
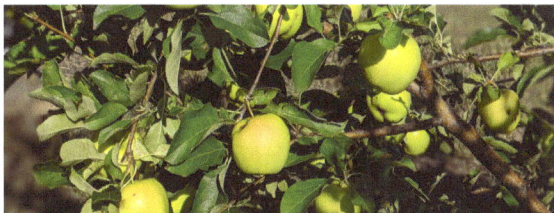
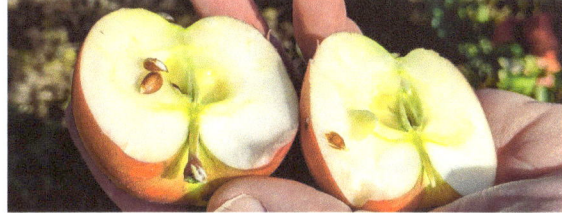

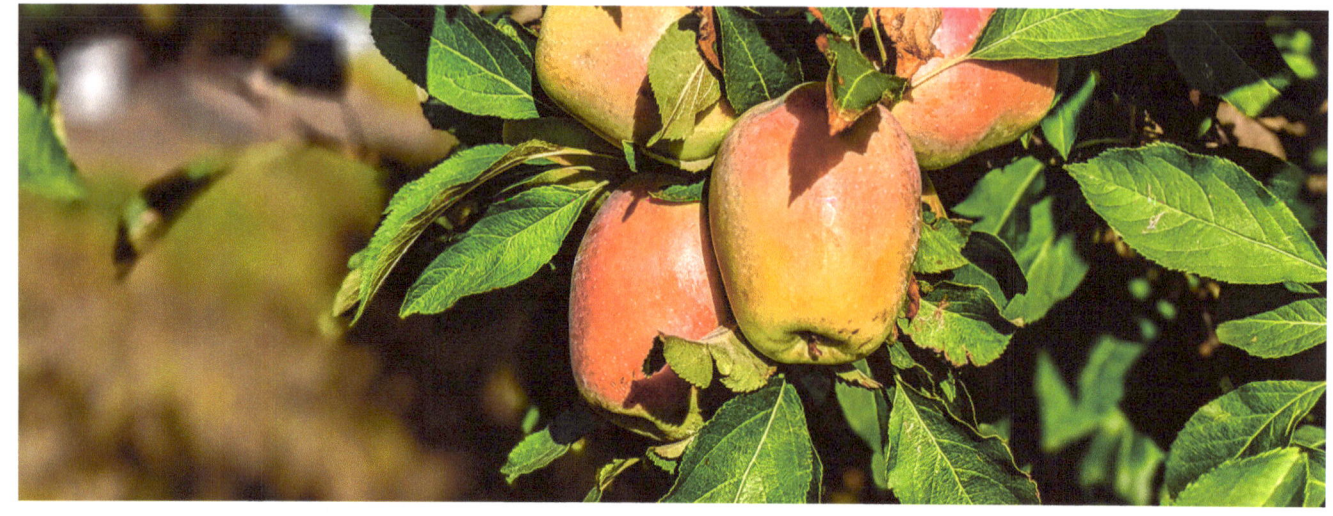
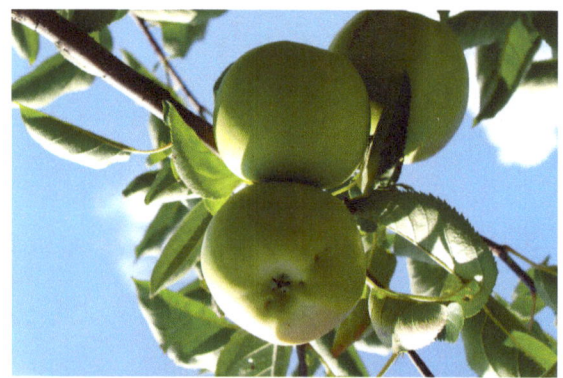
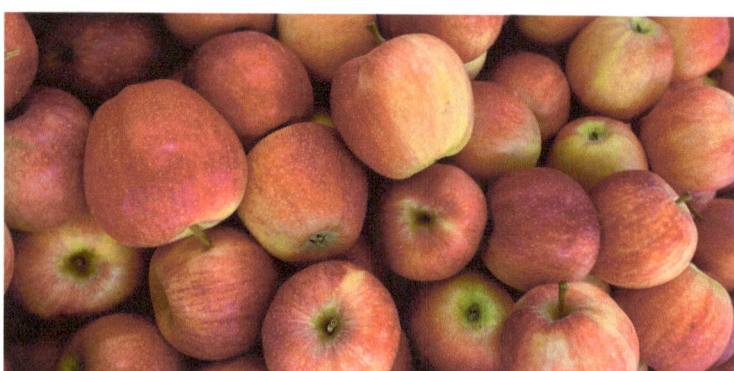
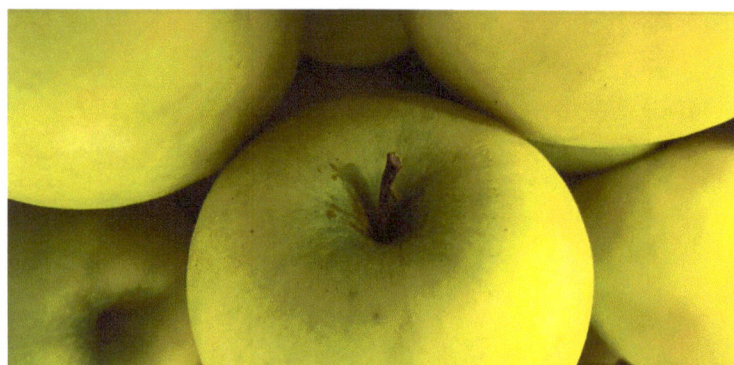
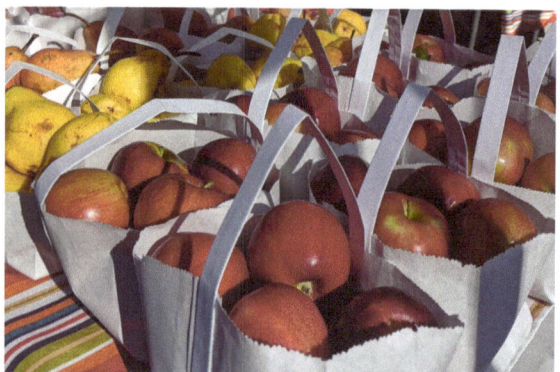
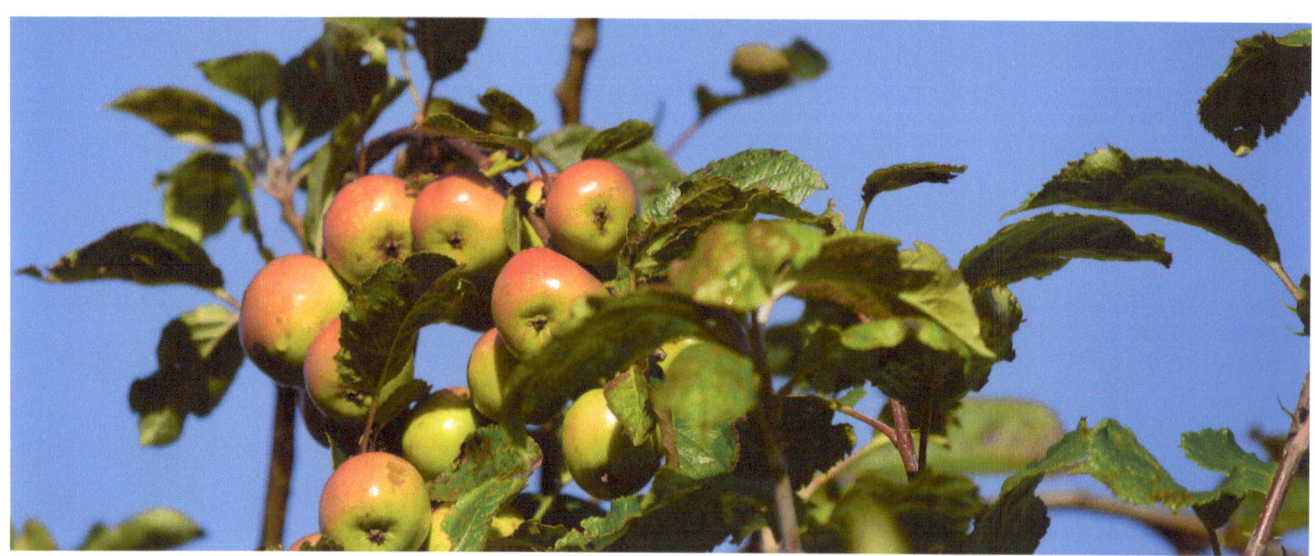

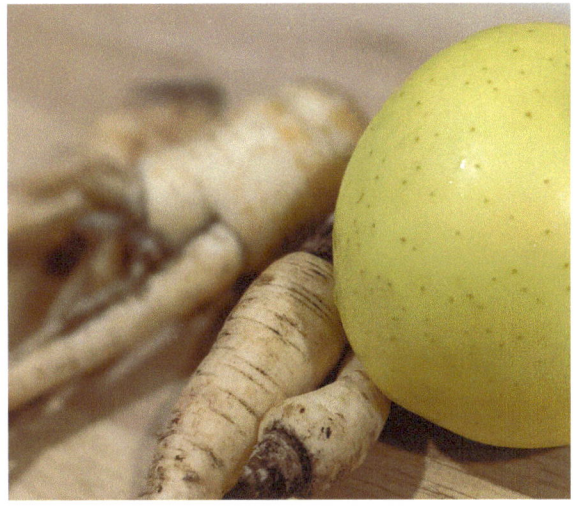
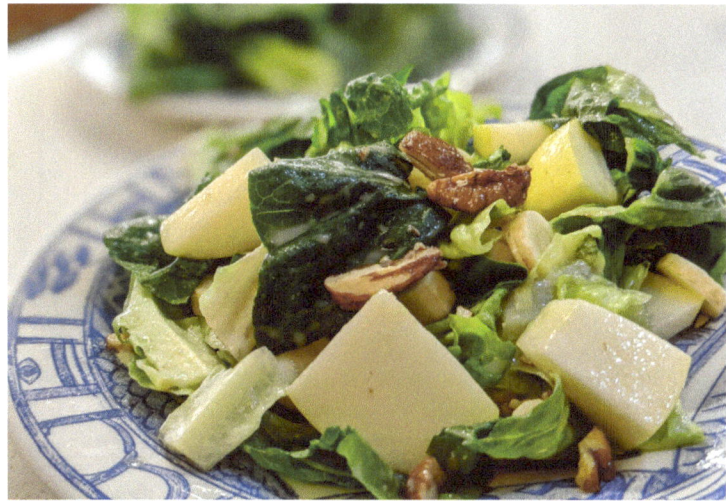
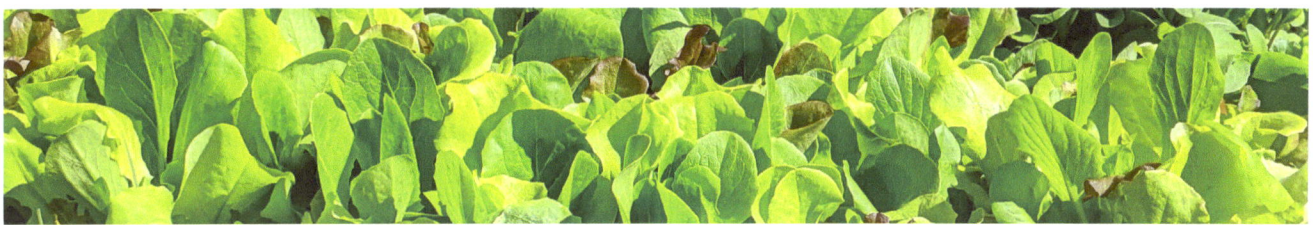

APPLE PARSNIP SALAD

Think of parsnips as white carrots. Slightly sweet. Crunchy. Moist. This salad blends the tartness of the green apple with the sweetness of the parsnip and maple dressing. A medium parsnip will work well, as large ones tend to be a bit fibrous.

Ingredients

For the Salad
- 1 Granny Smith apple; cored, sliced, cut slices in half
- 1 medium parsnip, peeled and cut into ¼ inch rounds
- About 3 cups of beautiful leafy green lettuce

For the Dressing
- 1 tbsp mayonnaise (regular or vegan)
- 1 tbsp oil
- 2 tsp apple cider vinegar
- 2 tsp maple syrup (more if you want sweeter)
- ½ tsp sea salt

For the Garnish
- Pecans, walnuts, or almonds

Instructions

Place the apple, parsnip, and lettuce in a bowl.
In a separate small bowl, whisk the salad dressing ingredients together until creamy.
Toss the greens with the dressing.
Garnish with your nut of choice and serve.

Elevate This: A bit of purple lettuce will add a splash of color. Thinly sliced candied ginger will give the salad an extra pop.

Serves 2-3 as a salad dish

Keep Squash and Carry On

I know your pain. Pumpkins and winter squash are the harbingers of autumn. They photograph beautifully and decorate holiday tables. We mound them in bowls and let our children and grandchildren wander through the corn patches and later, choose a wonderful, shapely, orange globe with the perfect stem and curling vine tendril. Now what? Which are edible, and which are decorative? What do I do once I impulse buy four acorn squash, three pumpkins, two butternuts, and a gorgeous delicata? Which are edible and how do I process?

First, a pumpkin is a type of squash in the Cucurbitaceae family. Most skins are tough but the newer varieties, such as delicata and sweet dumpling, have thinner skins which can be eaten when cooked. All are edible, but smaller winter squash tend to be sweeter than larger, Cinderella-style pumpkins.

Squash has quite a fascinating history. A wild vine in Central America, the Norte Chico people began to cultivate it for food, baskets, and utensils. This was especially important as the Central American people wiped out a great majority of their large animal sources which carried the seeds in the wild. Squash is part of the Central American Three Sisters of farming – squash, beans, and corn. The corn provided support for the beans, while the squash kept the weeds down and kept the water from evaporating. These food groups are also the basis for Southern succotash.

Winter squash now crosses all cuisine lines. Beyond the basic roasted cubes and squash casserole, winter squash can be used to fill Italian ravioli, Indian dosas, and French crêpes, elevate Mushroom Parmentier, and yes, make cupcakes. You can make flatbreads and soups, fritters, and beautiful sweet and savory salads.

Curing and Storing Squash

Winter squash store well, particularly here in Colorado. Feel free to cure it first. Curing winter squash requires about 10-14 days of simply letting the squash sit in a warm place with good air circulation and not letting the squash get wet. I'm pretty sure squash at the winter farmers market is cured – but always ask.

Curing Winter Squash: Set it on an elevated rack or mesh frame (a cake cooling rack would work) and let the air circulate.

Storing Winter Squash: Store at 50-55°F with a relative humidity of 50 to 70 percent. Higher humidity can result in rot. Store cured squash on a shelf or rack, not on the floor. Keep the skins of cured squash dry to prevent the growth of fungi and bacteria.

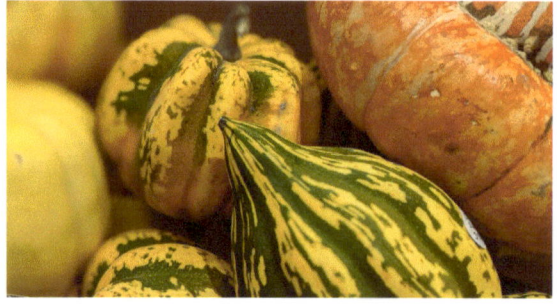
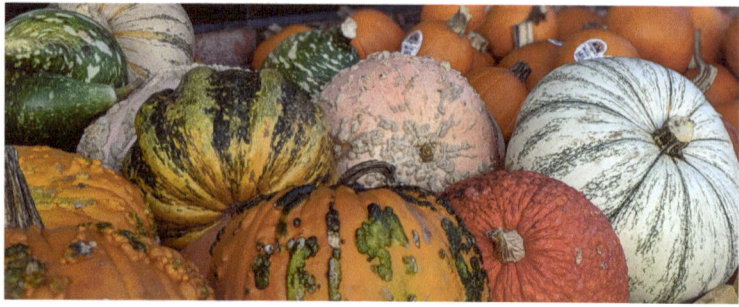

Prepping and Cooking Hard-skinned Squash (Mostly Pumpkins)

Pressure Cooking: If your pressure cooker or Instant Pot is large enough, you can pressure cook a three-pound pie pumpkin, whole. Yes, whole. My suggestion is to read and follow the instructions for your specific device but, in general follow these instructions:
Place the pumpkin in a steamer basket in the electric pressure cooker, adding enough water to come to the bottom edge of the basket.
Pressure cook on high for about 15 minutes. Your pumpkin flesh will be a little wetter as it is a steam cooking process, so be aware of that in your dish.
Peel, purée your pumpkin flesh, and freeze in portions in the freezer.
If your purée is too wet, heat the purée over the stovetop on medium low heat to cook off some of the moisture. Cool and package to freeze.
Note: You can also pressure cook the sections of the pumpkin that have been cut and seeded, but reduce pressure cooking time to 5 minutes.

Roasting: I won't lie, cutting a hard-skinned squash (i.e. pumpkin) can be challenging. You need a very sharp knife, a cutting board, leverage, and instructions. The general instructions include:
If your pumpkin is not completely flat on the bottom, slice off the bottom to create a flat base.
Place the pumpkin on its flat bottom. Beginning along the side of the stem (not on the stem), cut down through the pumpkin flesh to the bottom of the pumpkin. Repeat the process on the remaining three sides. Remove the seeds. ***Helpful Tip:*** This is also how to cut a bell pepper!
You may either roast the pieces as is; or remove the flesh from the skin, cube, season, then roast.
Roast in the oven at 400°F for 15-30 minutes (depending on the size of the pieces) until the pumpkin is easily pierced with a fork.

Smoking: A friend of mine smoked quartered pumpkin pieces, skin on, and they were divine. She skinned and puréed the flesh and it took a pumpkin dish to a whole new level. A little cream or cashew milk. Some cumin or spice mix. Dish elevated.
To smoke, follow the cutting instructions above and place on prepared smoker pans. Smoke at 225°F until you can easily pierce the flesh with a paring knife or fork.
Cool. Skin. Purée. Package.

Prepping and Cooking Thin-skinned Squash

Most thin-skinned squash are smaller, and thus, easier to handle. A good sharp chef knife and a smaller knife to remove the seeds is recommended.
Since the squash are smaller, cuter, colorful, and more decorative looking, they open up different possibilities for roasting or stuffing.
After cutting the squash in half, scoop out the seeds and discard them. Before baking, stuff the squash with a stuffing of your choice, or simply sprinkle it with oil and spices.
Bake at 350°F until fork tender.
Alternatively, cut the smaller squash in half, and depending on the shape, cut in rings, half-moons, or whatever shape the squash seems to give you.
I have provided multiple recipes for you in the Autumn and Winter sections – several pumpkin dishes, plus one recipe each with acorn, delicata, and sweet dumpling squash. Their original shapes determined the shape of the dish and outcome.
Of course, you can always prep and purée a smaller squash, but I personally would leave that process to the larger varieties.

Practice and Play. Keep squash and carry on.

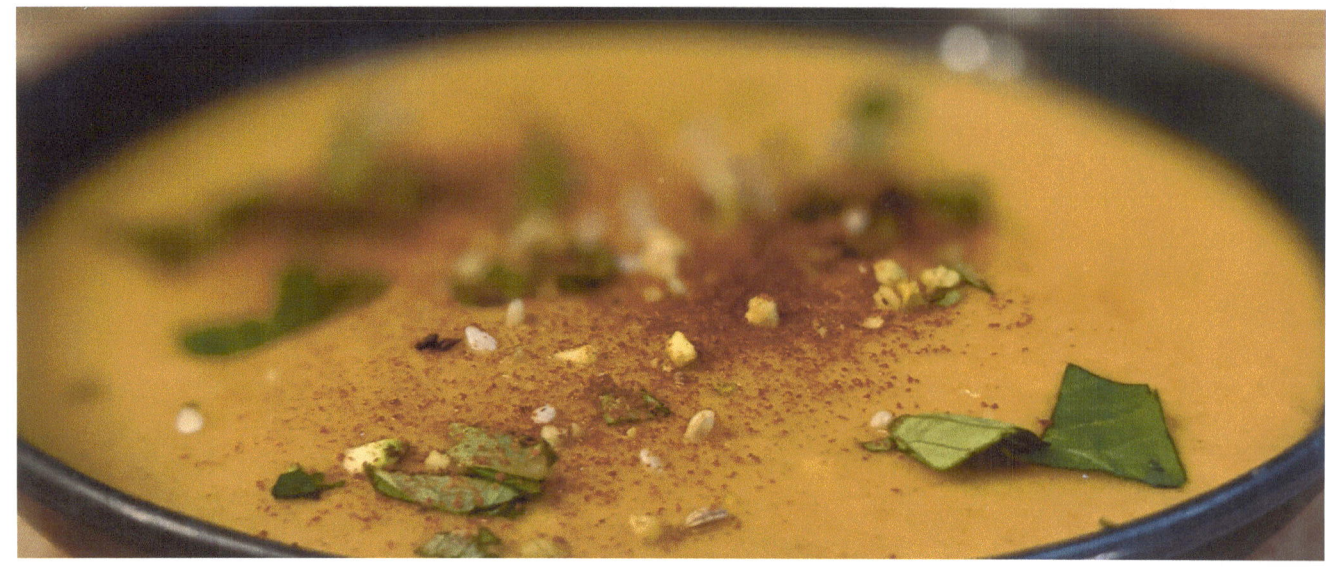

PUMPKIN PEANUT SOUP

Honestly, I have not always been a pumpkin girl. But Cheryl, a friend of mine, grows them in her garden and has given me many packages of pumpkin purée to change my perspective. Another friend gave me some peanut soup to try, and voilà, we have a pumpkin peanut soup and multiple pumpkin recipes in this book. This soup is elegant enough for a holiday first course.

Ingredients
- 8 garlic cloves, peeled and roughly chopped
- One 4-inch piece of ginger, peeled and roughly chopped
- 2-3 tbsp oil
- 1 cup pumpkin purée
- ¼ cup cashew cream or half and half
- 2 tbsp peanut butter
- ½ cup vegetable broth
- ¼ cup aquafaba (optional, but thickens without adding fat or flour)
- 1-2 tsp cumin to taste
- 1-2 tsp bittersweet or hot smoked paprika to taste
- 1-2 tsp white pepper to taste
- 1 tsp asafetida (optional, but adds depth of flavor)

For the Garnish
- Chopped cilantro
- Paprika
- Dukkah

Instructions

Place the garlic, ginger and oil in a small food processor or immersion blender and blend until creamy and smooth. Reserve 1 tbsp and refrigerate the excess ginger garlic cream sauce to be used for any future recipes (this sauce is delicious and you will want to add it to many dishes).

Add 1 tbsp of the above ginger garlic cream to the remaining ingredients in a saucepan and stir well. Warm soup to desired consistency.

Garnish with chopped cilantro, paprika, and dukkah, and serve.

Elevate This: Bits of crushed croutons, a few roasted mushrooms, or a dab of Microgreen Pesto (p. 129) will add texture and another layer of flavor.

Serves 2-3 as a soup dish

KOHLRABI BEAN BARLEY SOUP

Kohlrabi is not a new veg. It can be found in many grocery stores, three or four tucked neatly by the beets. Sometimes we give them a brief nod, skirt our eyes over to the carrots, and walk by, not knowing what to do with them. Then, you get one in your CSA, and it's time to figure it out.

This soup has a transparent, soup base. The color of the saffron just shines through. I used the pasta water from the Saffron Pasta (p. 74), but feel free to use a pinch (3-4 threads) in water.

The vegetables are to be cooked but not mushy. Don't leave out the Marmite. Marmite is a go-to umami that will bring depth to a dish without having to use mushrooms or tomatoes. An additional nod to the area's barley industry, and you have a wonderful autumn soup.

Note: *Cook barley until al dente – it will continue to soften as it cools. Spread on a cookie sheet and freeze for future meals. This broth is also a nice sipping broth for a nippy, fall day.*

Ingredients

For the Broth
- 1 quart saffron water or 5-6 saffron threads steeped in 4 cups of water
- 2 sage leaves, whole
- 1 sprig rosemary
- 1 sprig of thyme
- 1 tsp Marmite

For the Vegetables
- 3 small potatoes, steamed
- 3 carrots, cubed or rounds, microwaved for 3 minutes
- 1 kohlrabi; peeled, cubed, and microwaved for 4-5 minutes
- 1 cup cooked flageolet or cannellini beans (canned is okay)
- 1 cup cooked barley or grain of choice

Instructions

Steep the broth ingredients for 15-20 minutes over low heat. Remove herb stems and leaves.

Add the cooked vegetables and cook on low heat for 10 minutes.

Place grains into a bowl and pour the soup over the grains, then serve.

Elevate This: Top with a touch of Microgreen Pesto or Microgreen Pistou (p. 129).

Serves 2 as a soup dish

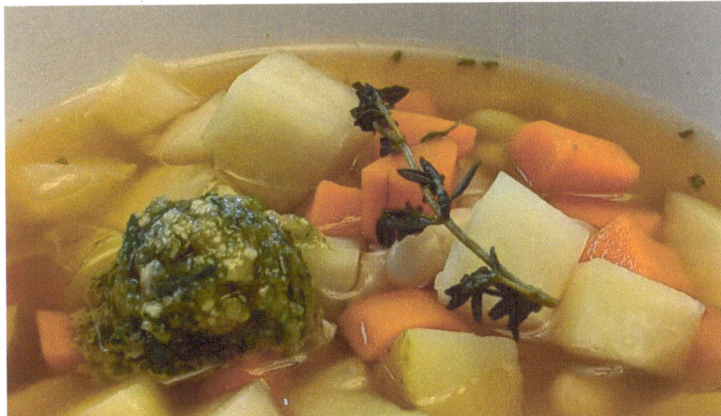
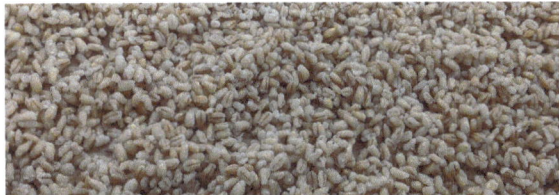
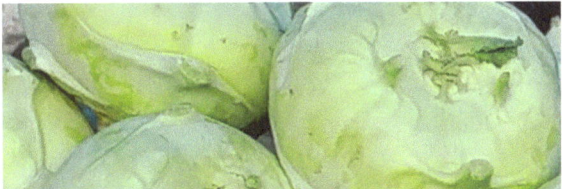

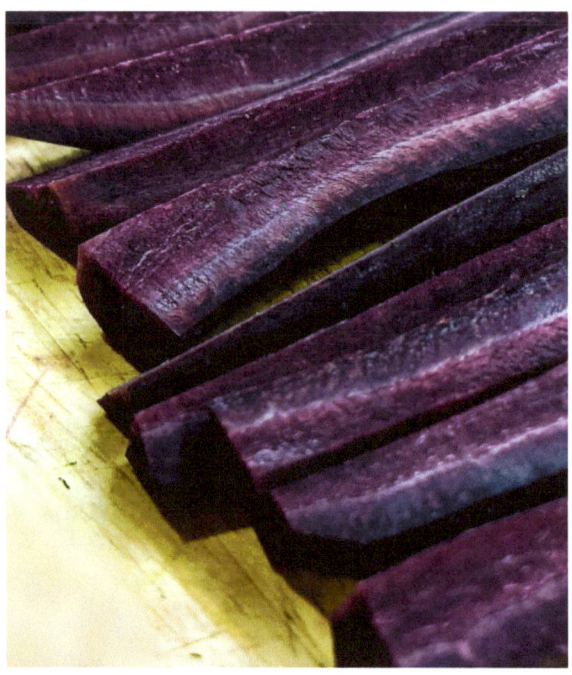
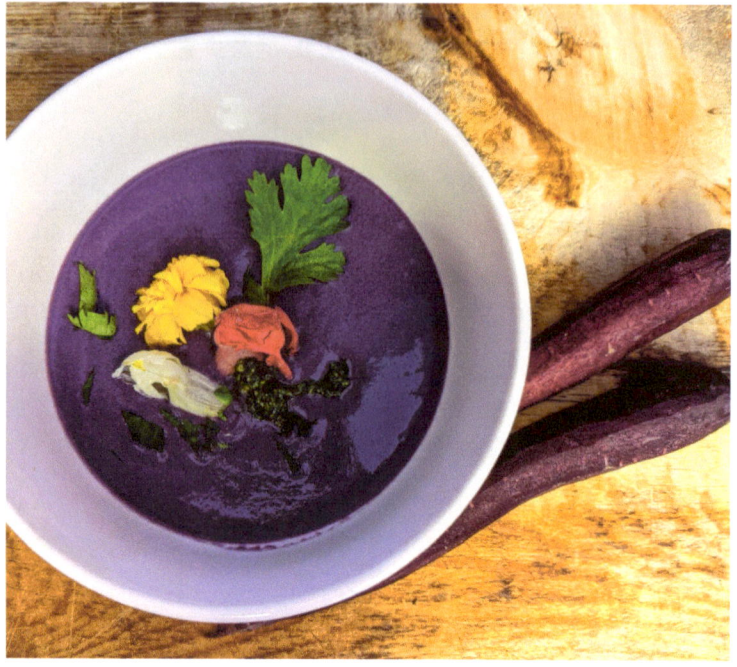

PURPLE CARROT SOUP TWO WAYS

Hoffman Farms is a family-owned and operated farm specializing in vegetables. It is owned and operated by Hanmei and Derrick Hoffman. They are proud to call Colorado their home, and their children are the 6th generation of Hoffmans born in Northern Colorado. The couple farms multiple locations in Weld County, from north of Greeley to Ft. Lupton, and currently grows over 60 varieties that they sell direct to consumer.

Derrick is a third generation farmer and a direct descendant of Germans from Russian immigrants who moved here to work in the sugar beets of Northern Colorado in the 1900s. His family grew barley, corn, pinto beans and alfalfa. After a career in managing technology systems, he returned to the farm. Alongside his wife Hanmei—a third generation farmer from the Fuzhou province in southern China—he rapidly expanded the farm and its multitude of vegetable varieties. An example of one variety is the featured Delicata Squash with Apricots, Poms, and Pecans (p. 144).

The purple carrots I bought at their vendor stall were the darkest, most complete shade of eggplant purple (#431C52 on color charts) from foot to stem. I roasted them as a trial run and then thought it might be a mind-bender to enjoy a dark purple soup. Voilà! You have two options to choose from – one with a slight Asian twist, and one more traditional savory variety.

Aquafaba, literally "bean water," was coined in December 2014 by musician Joël Roessel, who discovered you can whip the liquid leftover from a can of chickpeas into a meringue. Drain the chickpeas, reserve the liquid, and freeze in freezer cubes until needed. The aquafaba will thicken the soup without thickeners or cream.

PURPLE CARROT COCONUT SOUP

Ingredients
- 2 garlic cloves
- ½ tsp salt
- 1 tbsp oil
- ½ cup aquafaba
- 1 tsp lemon
- 4-5 purple carrots, peeled and steamed until fork tender
- ½ cup coconut milk
- Milk of choice to thicken the soup (I used cashew almond milk)
- Salt and pepper to taste

For the Garnish
- Cilantro
- Microgreen Pesto or Microgreen Pistou (p. 129)

Instructions
Purée the first five ingredients in a blender or hand immersion blender until garlic is completely puréed. A small food processor works well, it just will take more time to purée completely.
Add carrots and coconut milk and purée until smooth. Add your milk of choice to thin the soup to your desired consistency.
Salt and pepper to taste.
Let sit for 10 minutes to allow the color to enhance. Garnish with cilantro and Microgreen Pesto or Pistou.

Elevate This: Try the soup with an addition of some Thai green curry spice mixture – just a touch.

Serves 2 as a soup dish

PURPLE CARROT SAVORY SOUP

Instructions
Follow the ingredients and instructions above, but instead of coconut milk, substitute chicken broth or vegan chicken broth.

Serve either version warm or at room temperature, with a sprinkling of cilantro and a dab of spicy Microgreen Pesto or Microgreen Pistou (p. 129).

Elevate This: I intentionally did not add any spices so you could practice and play with a delicious, simple base of a soup. A bit of cumin, Aleppo pepper, or the slightest dash of berbere might complement the gentleness of the soup without overpowering the sweet carrot. Sometimes, less is more.

Serves 2 as a soup dish

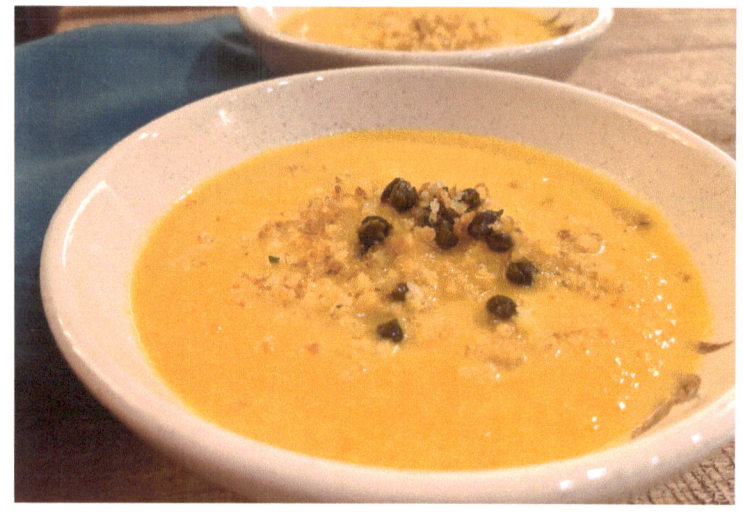
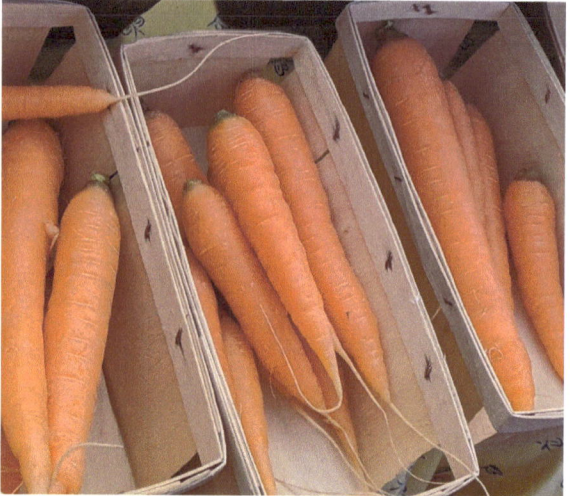
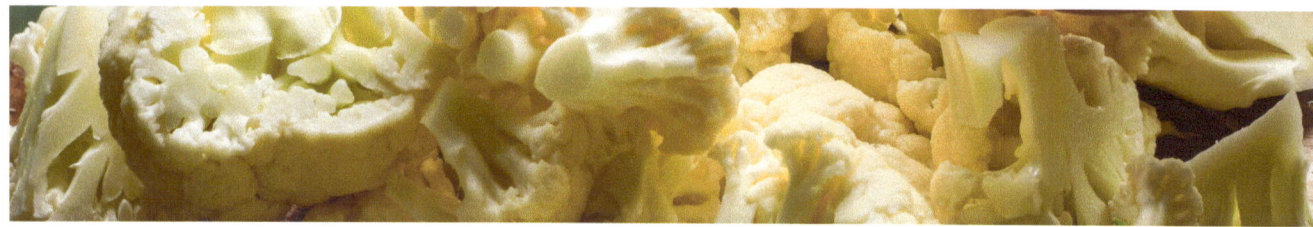

CREAM OF CAULIFLOWER AND CARROT SOUP

This simple soup is a great way to use one off, lonely, leftover veggies in your fridge veg box; in this case some cauliflower and a carrot. Add your milk of choice and you will create a tasty, effortless autumn soup.

Ingredients
- ¼ pound of cauliflower
- 2 carrots until soft
- Milk or cream (dairy or non-dairy) in the amount of the consistency you prefer
- Salt and pepper to taste

For the Garnish
- Toasted, seasoned breadcrumbs or panko crumbs

Instructions
Steam the cauliflower and carrots until soft.
Purée in a blender, adding the milk or cream (dairy or non-dairy) to the consistency you prefer.
Salt and pepper to taste.
Garnish with toasted, seasoned breadcrumbs or panko crumbs.

Elevate This: Rinse 1 tbsp capers. Pat dry. Place them in a bowl with 2 tsp oil. Microwave on high for 2 minutes, or until crispy, not burnt. Garnish with the Crispy Capers found in the *Elevations* section (p. 168).

Serves 2 as a soup dish

PUMPKIN FLATBREADS

Roasted pumpkin chunks and purée freeze beautifully. These flatbreads can be made with pretty much any root or winter vine vegetable. Think butternut squash, orange and purple sweet potatoes, and sweet white yams. Also, avocados! This flatbread can be your go-to wrap when you have only one of something staring at you in the pantry, but need to serve 2-3 people.

Ingredients
- 1 cup cooked fresh pumpkin
- 1 cup flour, plus enough flour to make a stiff dough
- Dash of sea salt

Instructions
In a food processor, purée the pumpkin and salt.
In thirds, slowly add 1 cup flour, processing well after each addition.
Keep adding 2 tbsp of flour until you have a stiff dough in the processor. It should not be sticky. The dough will pull away from the sides of the processor. Process for about 4-5 minutes, adding 1 tbsp of flour if the dough becomes sticky.
You should be able to pull the dough out without getting sticky fingers. Once the dough is firm, pull the dough out.
Place on a board and knead for about 30 seconds to check the consistency. If still sticky, add a little more flour and knead, or place back in the processor to knead.

Flatten the dough into a 4-inch circle, place on a plate, cover and refrigerate for 30 minutes to an hour. Remove from refrigerator. Cut dough into 4 pieces. Roll each piece into a ball, then, with a rolling pin, roll into an 8-inch circle.
Heat a large cast iron or non stick skillet on medium heat (high heat will burn the flatbread).
Place flatbread in skillet and allow one side to cook. The flatbread will puff up. Flip to cook the other side. Repeat process for the remaining three dough balls.

These are delicious just by themselves, or you can fill them with whatever you have leftover in the fridge. The layers of flavor filling for this recipe project were Toum (p. 130), purple potatoes, a few final slices of eggplant sautéed in Greek seasoning and bread crumbs, the last of the halved grape tomatoes with mojo spices and olive oil, lentils, microgreens, Microgreen Gremolata (p. 129), and a drizzle of harissa.

Elevate This: Add turmeric for more color. For a dinner party, make smaller flatbreads (street taco size) of different colors. Add ground spices like cayenne, Aleppo pepper, or a touch of berbere.

Makes 4 flatbreads. Serves 2-4 as a side dish

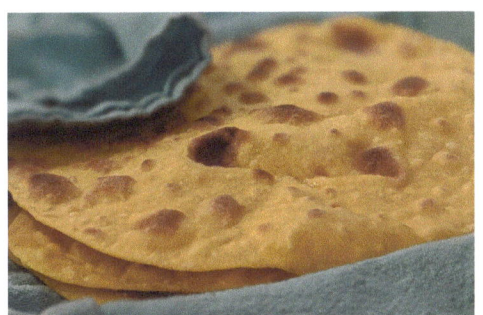
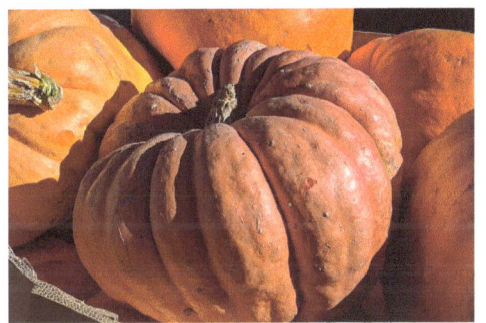
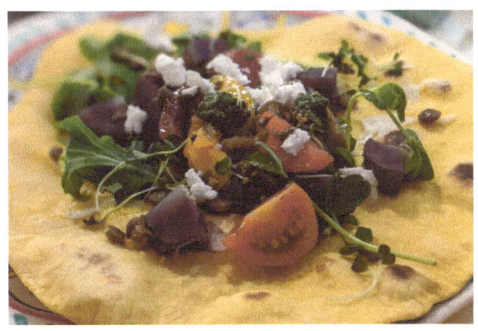
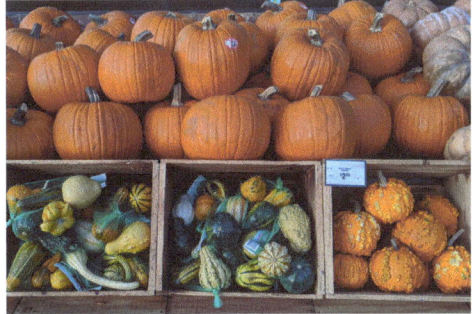

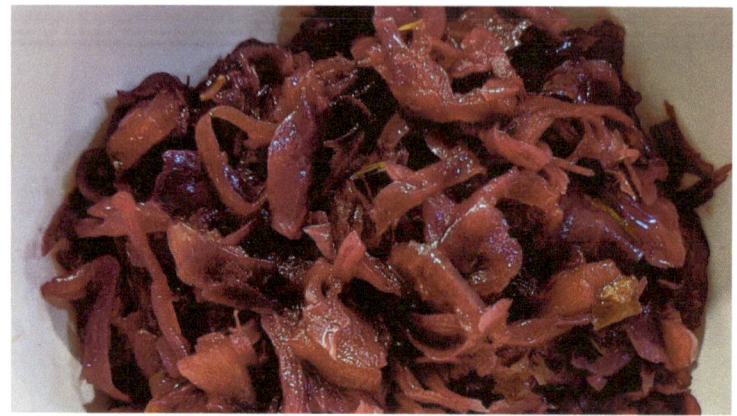
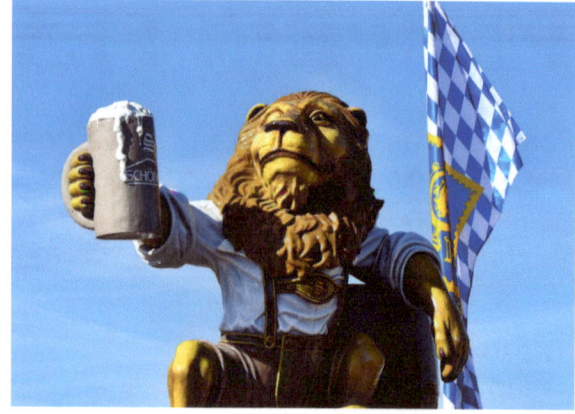
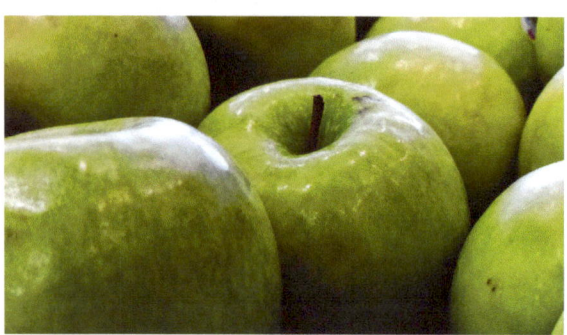
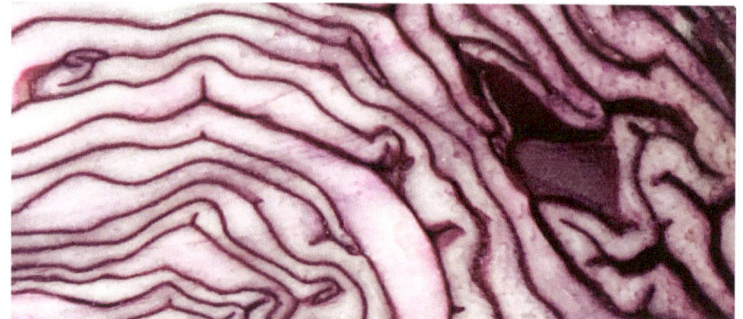

TRADITIONAL GERMAN ROTKOHL

(Sweet/Sour Red Cabbage) *Fort Collins is in what is called the Napa Valley of beers, and starting in late September, we have our fair share of Oktoberfest events! This recipe is a share from my friend, Tracy. She made this wonderful dish for our annual Oktoberfest party several years ago and it received rave reviews, so why change anything? I adjusted the proportions to serve 3-4 people.*

This Rotkohl is the traditional accompaniment for a Sunday roast, rouladen, sauerbraten and potatoes, spaetzle, or knoedel. Some kartoffelkloesse, spaetzle, or even lentils, will make great additions to your plate. During the 2-hour simmering, you can be doing other things, like unloading the dishwasher, reading emails, or enjoying a nice cup of tea in the autumn sun. You can also use purple cabbage for sauerkraut as well. Just follow the recipe for Super Simple Sauerkraut in this cookbook (p. 110).

Ingredients
- ¼ cup butter (dairy or non-dairy)
- ½ large yellow onion, finely diced
- 1 large Granny Smith semi-tart apple, peeled, cored and diced
- 1 lb pound red cabbage, very thinly sliced (I used ½ of a medium head)
- ¼ cup vegetable broth
- 2 tbsp sour cherry preserves or jam
- 2 tbsp red wine vinegar (up to 2 tbsp additional red wine vinegar to jazz up the flavor)
- 1 tbsp white sugar
- 1 tbsp brown sugar

For the Herb Seasoning
- 1 bay leaf
- 3 whole cloves
- 3 juniper berries (yes, it's necessary, but the bag or jar will last you 10 years, so… buy it!)
- 1 tbsp fennel seeds, whole, slightly crushed in a mortar
- 1 tbsp caraway seeds, whole, slightly crushed in a mortar
- ½ tsp salt
- Dash of Accent (10 grains is enough to pop flavor)

Instructions
Melt the butter (dairy or non-dairy) in a Dutch oven over medium heat.

Add the onions and apples, and cook for 7-10 minutes until just beginning to brown. Lower heat and add a bit of water if necessary, to avoid burning.

Add the cabbage and cook for 5 minutes.

Add the broth, cherry preserves (or jam), red wine vinegar, white and brown sugars, bay leaf, cloves, juniper berries, fennel seeds, caraway seeds, salt, and a dash of Accent.

Bring to a boil, reduce the heat to low, cover, and simmer for 2 hours, stirring occasionally. Add more broth if needed. Add more salt, sugar and vinegar to taste after it's cooked about 1.5 hours.

Tracy's Helpful Tips
- I used a heavy Le Creuset style Dutch oven—which allows the dish to braise nicely on a stove top—but you can also use a deep skillet with a lid.
- It improves if cooked for 2 hours.
- At 1.5 hours, adjust flavors if necessary. Sweet and sour is a personal preference. It if is flat in flavor, add more red wine vinegar or more brown sugar, salt, and 1 tbsp jam or preserves to sweeten it up.
- It takes more vinegar and brown sugar than you'd expect, and it helps to add these in increments as it cooks. I always finish the dish by adding another bit of red wine vinegar once the heat is off.

Serves 4 as a side dish

SUPER SIMPLE SAUERKRAUT

My grandmother made sauerkraut, but I never really paid attention to the process. The canned version we get in the store is more than likely just brined but not truly fermented cabbage. Fort Collins folks are focused on fermenting. From beer and kombucha, kefir to sauerkraut, you can find something fermenting somewhere in our area. This is my husband Mike's recipe.

This recipe works for any size batch as you will be weighing ingredients and calculating the salt requirements. You will need a fermentation vessel—big enough to hold the cabbage—and a kitchen scale.

Ingredients
- Cabbage (the fresher the better, because it will have more moisture)
- Salt (kosher or pickling, *not* iodized)

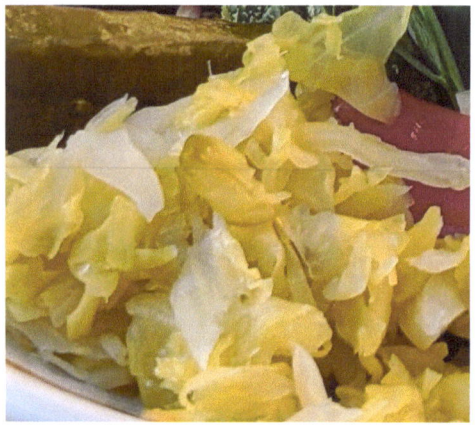

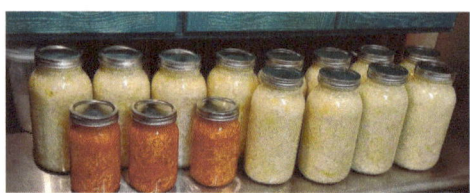

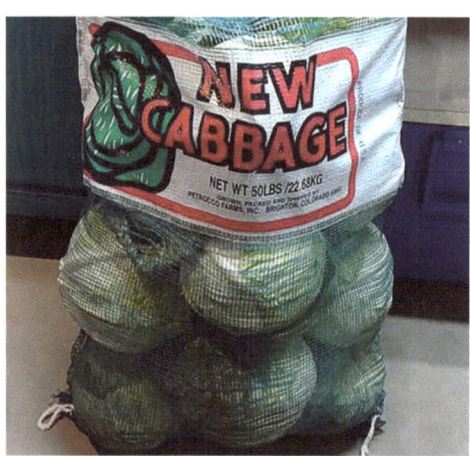

Instructions
Rinse the cabbage and/or remove the outer layer. Cut the core out of the cabbage head and discard. Weigh the cabbage, then measure out 2% of that weight in salt.
Shred or chop the cabbage.
Mix the cabbage and salt in layers in the fermentation vessel. After a while, the salt will draw out the water from the cabbage.
Repeat the mixing until the liquid covers the cabbage. Be patient, it may take 60 minutes or more.
Place something on top of the mixture to hold the cabbage below the surface of the liquid. This could be a plate, a bag of marbles, or similar. The important thing is to avoid oxidization from the cabbage rising above the liquid.
If absolutely necessary, a 2% saline solution can be added to cover the cabbage. To make a 2% solution, weigh the water, then measure out 2% of that weight in salt and mix with water until dissolved.
Cover the mix with a lid that will allow the CO_2 from fermentation to escape.
Let the vessel sit for a couple of weeks – not too hot, not too cold, not opened. A Fort Collins basement works great, as many are around 65°F.
Then the saurkraut is ready for packaging, canning, and, of course, eating.

Elevate This: You may add your choice of other grated vegetables such as carrots, carrots, or daikon radish for a bit of bite. A few caraway or fennel seeds add a nice touch.

Serves 2 as a side dish

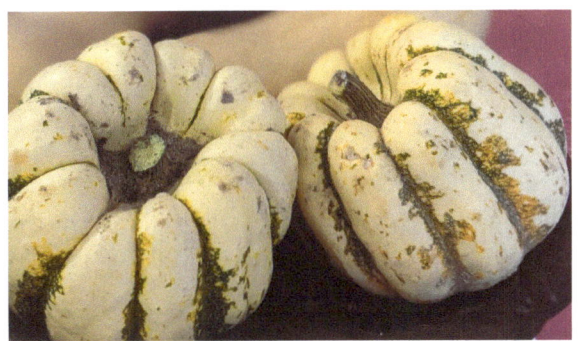 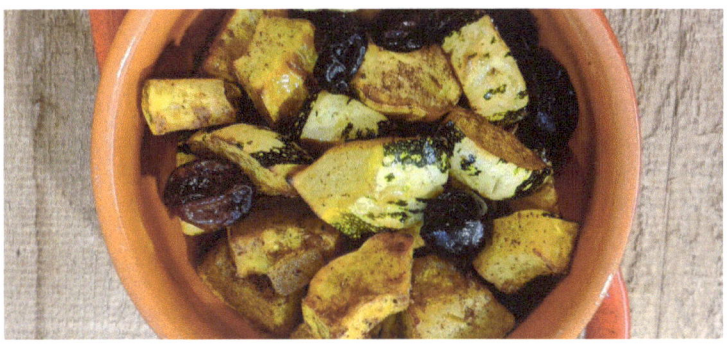

SWEET DUMPLING SQUASH WITH RAS EL HANOUT, CANDIED GINGER AND DRIED FRUIT

Fall squash is not your basic acorn squash anymore. There are many cute, stubby varieties that can almost be a personal squash meal. The sweet dumpling variety is no exception. The skin is the softest of the winter squash, the interior is beautiful yellow orange.

I wanted to experience another method of roasting these little gems, this time with Ras El Hanout spices, a North African spice mixture which usually consists of over 12 spices. Common ingredients include cardamom, cumin, clove, cinnamon, nutmeg, mace, allspice, dry ginger, chile peppers, coriander seed, peppercorn, sweet and hot paprika, fenugreek, and dry turmeric.

Our area has so many spice shops – I suggest popping in and buying the spice mix, unless you want to make it yourself. Many of my friends and cooking students prefer to have the pre-mixed spices to speed things up and reduce the cost. I have all the individual spices, but the efficiency of ready-made spice mixes was hard to resist. Ras El Hanout can also be ordered online and many grocery stores are carrying it now in the international spice sections. Don't leave out the candied ginger, as it creates a super nice "bite" and balance to the Ras El Hanout.

Ingredients
- 1 Sweet Dumpling Squash; cut into rings, remove the seeds, then cut into 1-inch pieces along the dimples of the squash
- 2 tsp Ras El Hanout spice mixture
- 2 tbsp water
- 1 tbsp oil
- Two 2-inch pieces of candied ginger, minced or thinly sliced thin
- Dried fruit of choice, soaked in water for 15 minutes

Instructions
Preheat oven to 375°F.
Prepare sheet pan with foil and non-stick spray.
Add the water to the pan.
Place the squash, ginger and fruit and oil in a bowl. Sprinkle with the spice mixture and coat the squash with the spice mixture.
Arrange squash on the tray and cover tightly with foil. Bake for 15 minutes or until squash is fork tender. Uncover the pan and bake another 15 minutes until the water evaporates and a glaze forms on the squash. Place in a serving dish and enjoy.

Elevate This: Top with mint or cilantro, a bit more candied ginger, and perhaps crushed fennel seeds.

Serves 2-3 as a side dish

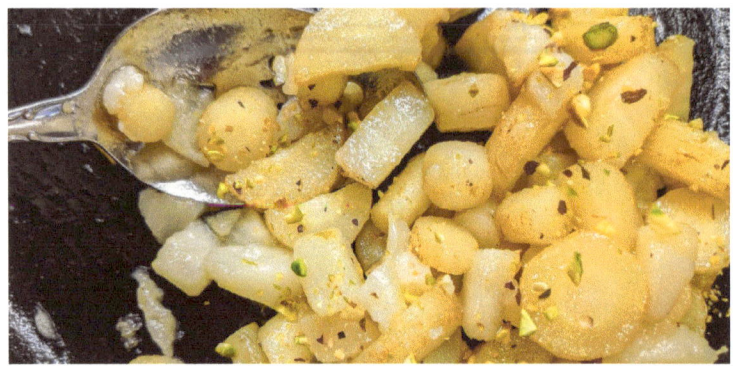
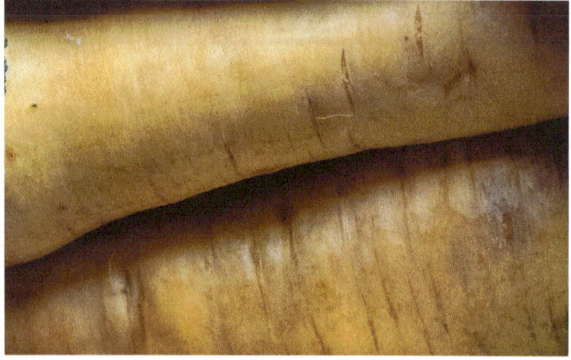
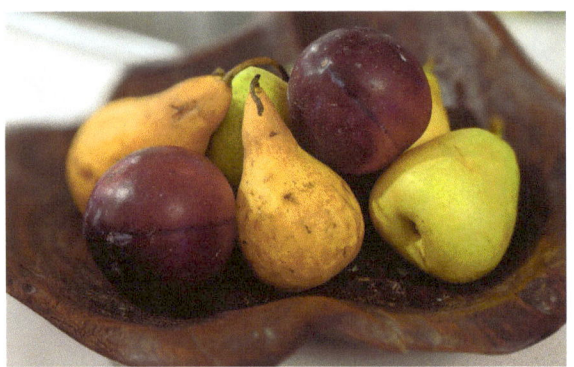
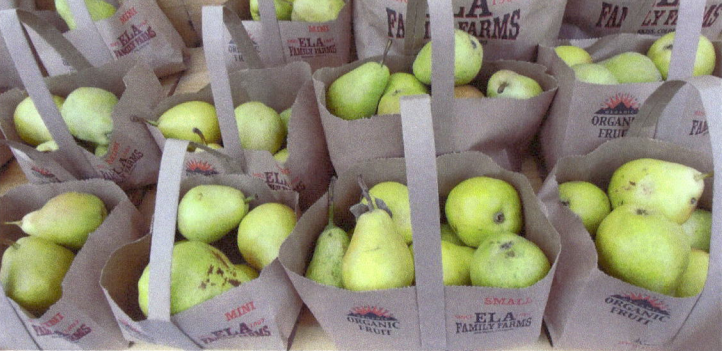

PARSNIPS AND PEARS

Fruits and veg marry well in this dish. Simple ingredients. Complementary textures. The sweetness of the parsnips and sweetness/tartness of the pear. I used a cast iron skillet for this recipe, but the technique does well in stainless steel pans as well. A simple dish, perfect for a holiday meal or family get-together.

Ingredients
- 4 medium parsnips, peeled and cut in ¼ inch slices
- 1 pear, pealed, cored and cut into ½ inch pieces
- ½ cup water
- 1 tbsp oil
- 2 tbsp local honey
- 2 tbsp pistachios, chopped and roasted

Instructions
Add the water and oil to large cast iron skillet. Add the parsnips. Bring to a boil then reduce heat. Cover and simmer for 15 minutes, or until fork tender. Increase the heat and boil off the water.
The parsnips will begin to brown in the remaining oil. Add the pear pieces and stir until both the parsnips and pears begin to brown.
Remove from heat.
Drizzle with honey and pistachios.

Elevate This: Add an interesting infused honey such as lavender or thyme, a dash of nutmeg, or cinnamon. Consider a sprinkle of Aleppo pepper, or use maple syrup instead of honey.

Serves 2-3 as a side dish

SMOKED GARLIC

Minced, chopped, sliced, whole, and puréed garlic are all awesome. Smoked garlic is an excellent elevation tool to pull together ingredients in making a great dish. The fresher the garlic, the better – my favorite sources are Aspen Moon Farm and On the Vine at Richmond Farms.

Ingredients
- Whole garlic heads
- Olive oil
- Salt and pepper to taste

Instructions
Set your smoker at 225°F.
Prepare a sheet pan with aluminum foil and non-stick cooking spray.
Cut about ½ inch off the top of the head of the garlic so the garlic cloves are exposed.
Drizzle olive oil on the open garlic cloves or paint it on with a silicone pastry brush. Salt and pepper to taste.
Smoke with your favorite wood for 1 hour or until soft.
If you don't have a smoker, mix the olive oil with 1 tsp liquid smoke or dry mesquite smoking powder, wrap lightly in foil (leave a little airspace), and roast in the oven at 400°F for 30 minutes, or until soft.
Cool and store in an airtight container in refrigerator.

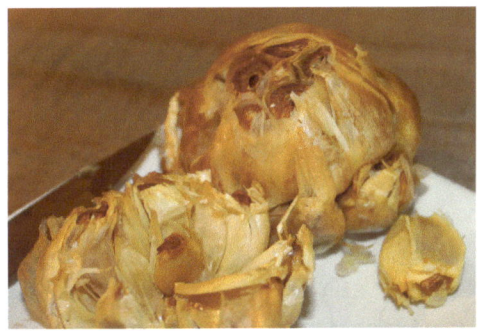

What to Do with Smoked Garlic: Hand mash garlic cloves as needed. Spread on crostinis with a bit of olive and sundried tomatoes or use as a sandwich or panini spread. Mash with avocados to elevate your guacamole, or purée with canned lima beans for a different take on traditional bean dip. Make an easy tapas dish with the recipe below!

PATATAS Y GARBANZOS EN PIMENTÓN

(Potatoes and Chickpeas in Paprika)

Ingredients
- 5-6 smoked garlic cloves (prepared as above recipe)
- 1 can of chickpeas, drained (remember aquafaba trick, p. 104)
- 6-7 baby Dutch yellow potatoes, steamed and quartered
- 1 tsp hot smoked or bittersweet paprika
- 1 tbsp oil
- 1 tsp lemon juice
- ½ tsp salt

For the Garnish
- Chopped parsley

Instructions
Place a few smoked garlic cloves into a hand immersion blender with the oil, salt and lemon juice. Place all the ingredients in a bowl and toss well. Sprinkle a bit more of your paprika of choice and garnish with chopped parsley.

Serves 3-4 as a side dish

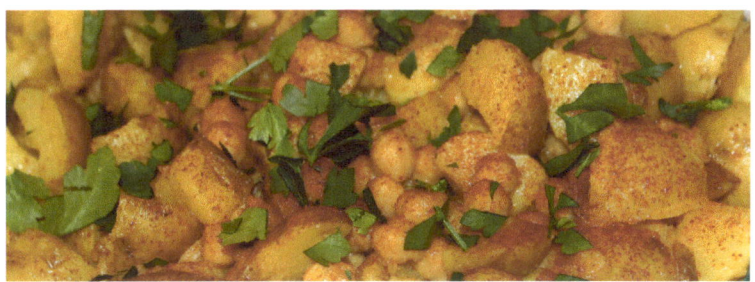

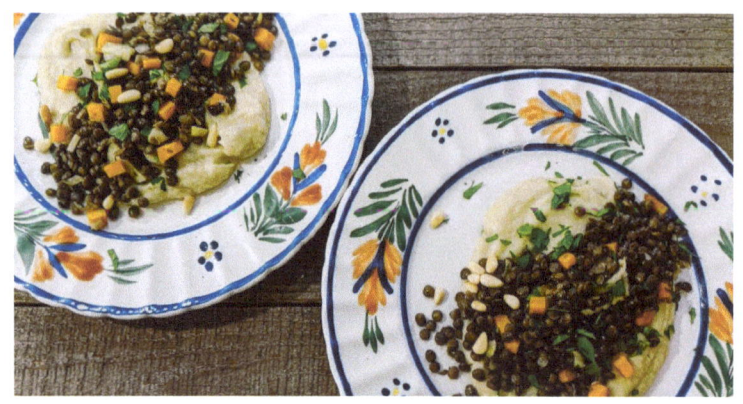
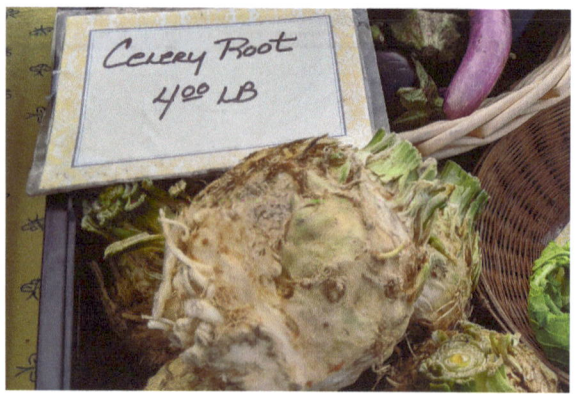

LENTILS WITH CELERIAC TRUFFLE PURÉE

It is entirely possible you might get a celeriac in your CSA, or perhaps you feel adventurous and want to try a new vegetable. This purée can be used as a base for the lentils, or experiment with a soup or chowder.

Ingredients

For the Celeriac Purée
- 1 celeriac; peeled, cut into chunks, steamed in Instant Pot for 10 min.
- 1 tbsp oil
- 1 leek (white part only), thinly sliced
- 1 tsp salt
- 1 garlic clove, minced
- ½ cup milk (dairy or non-dairy)
- ⅛ cup nutritional yeast
- 1 tsp truffle oil or ½ tsp truffle salt

For the Lentils
- 1 cup French lentils, rinsed and picked over
- 1 bay leaf
- 2 sprigs of thyme
- 1 tbsp oil
- 1 carrot; peeled, diced, microwaved for 5 minutes, drained
- 1 leek (white part only), thinly sliced
- ½ bulb fennel bulb, thinly sliced
- 1 tsp dry savory
- Salt and pepper to taste

For the Garnish
- Chopped parsley, toasted pine nuts, and/or fennel frond sprig

Instructions

For the Celeriac Purée
Heat oil over medium heat in a small skillet. Add leek, garlic and salt and sauté until soft.

Add the celeriac chunks, leek and garlic mixture to a blender. Add the milk and nutritional yeast and blend until smooth. Stir in truffle oil or salt to taste. Set aside.

For the Lentils
Place the lentils in a sauce pan and cover with water. Add the bay leaf and thyme and cook for 20 minutes or until al dente. Do not allow to burst.

Remove from heat, let cool and drain. Remove bay leaf. In the same skillet as above, heat the oil on medium heat. Add the leek and fennel. Sauté until golden soft. Turn heat to low and add the lentils, carrots and savory. Salt and pepper to taste.

Serve
Attractively smear the purée on the plate, and add the lentils on top. Garnish with chopped parsley, toasted pine nuts, and/or a sprig of fennel frond.

Elevate This: Sprinkle the dish with a bit of fennel pollen. The Sage Roasted Shiitakes (p. 145) will make a nice addition to this dish.

Serves 2 as a main dish

INDIAN CABBAGE WITH TURMERIC AND PEAS

Late fall cabbage is heavenly. It is big and juicy, and perfect for sauerkraut. If not making kraut, a large cabbage means you need lots of options to use it up. So many other cuisines use cabbage beyond the usual postulation of Germans, Czechs, Russians, Polish, and other Slavic countries. Think kimchi and colcannon (one of my favorites for St. Patrick's Day celebrations!) This sturdy vegetable can be eaten fresh, fried, stuffed, baked, roasted, fermented, sautéed, and souped. I happened upon this dish in one of my cookbooks and loved it. You can marry it with a side of chickpeas and potatoes, naan, or lentil soup. A few tweaks from my kitchen – here we go!

Ingredients
- 1 tbsp oil or ghee
- ½ medium onion, minced
- ½ tsp whole cumin seeds
- ¼ tsp asafetida (optional, but it adds oomph to the dish)
- 1 whole red, dried Thai or Cayenne chile, broken into 2-3 pieces
- ½ tsp Garam Masala
- 2 bay leaves
- 4 cups roughly chopped or thinly sliced cabbage (your choice)
- Splash of water
- ½ cup frozen green peas
- Salt and pepper to taste

For the Garnish
- Chopped cilantro

Instructions
Heat the oil or ghee in large skillet or wok.
Add the onion and sauté until soft.
Add the next 4 spice ingredients and allow the spices to bloom for 30 seconds.
Add the bay leaves and cabbage and toss to coat with spice mixture.
Add a splash of water to deglaze the pan a bit, cover and simmer for 5 minutes.
Stir in the frozen peas and cook peas until done, about 5 minutes.
Remove bay leaves.
Salt and pepper to taste.
Garnish with chopped cilantro and serve.

Elevate This: Add ginger or garlic paste while sautéing the onions. Sprinkle Nigella seeds for crunch and décor. Add grated carrot or purple cabbage for added color.

Serves 2 as a main dish

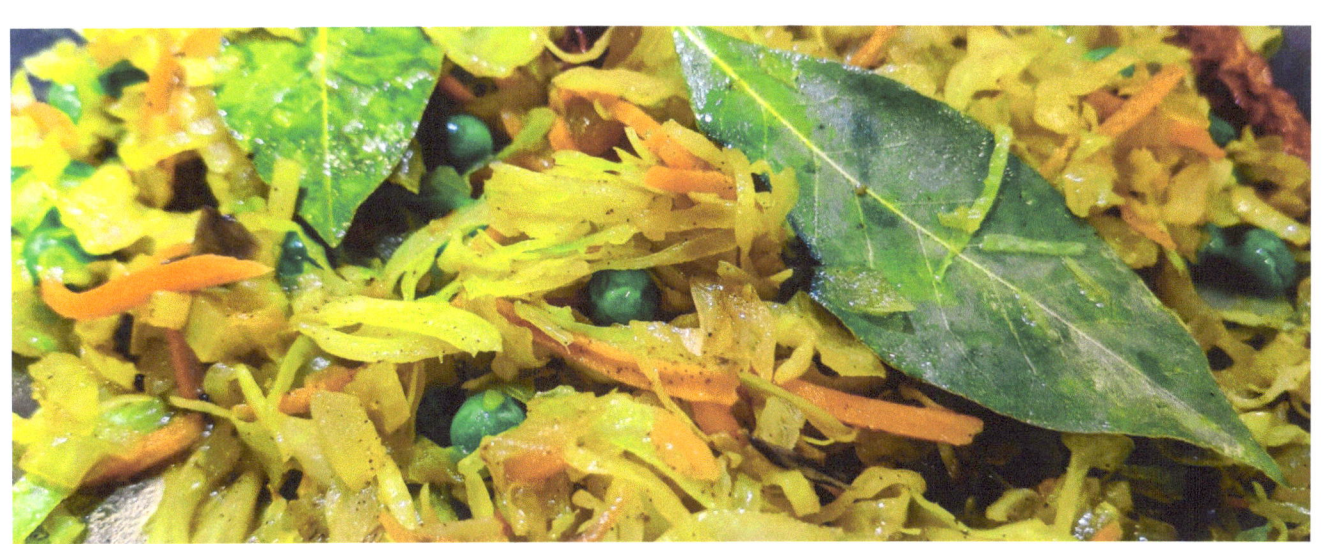

Aspen Moon Farm

Aspen Moon Farm in Boulder County is a USDA Certified Organic and Demeter Certified Biodynamic farm. This means their produce is truly 100% natural and bee-friendly. Starting in 2009 with one acre in cultivation, Aspen Moon Farm now has 25 acres in production.

The team—made of family members, farm crew, and interns—practices a variety of sustainable agriculture, including biodynamic composting, cover cropping, and crop rotation. Crops are carefully tended and hand-harvested if necessary, so customers get the freshest and most nutritious produce possible. Crops include a wide range of seasonal vegetables, organic flowers, berries, heritage grains and beans—such as White Sonora, Blue Emmer, and Rouge De Bordeaux—and starter plants for the spring garden.

I happened upon Aspen Moon Farm at the Longmont Saturday Farmers Market around holiday time. At that time, I was researching heritage grains and beans. Aspen Moon Farm had neatly packaged lovely Red Italian Heirloom Cornmeal. I've always thought, if it is Italian, it must be good. So off I went back to my kitchen armed with local heirloom cornmeal to make polenta and cornbread. The flecks of red cornmeal created a beautiful contrast to the yellow cornmeal, and this polenta was perfectly flaky and "toothy."

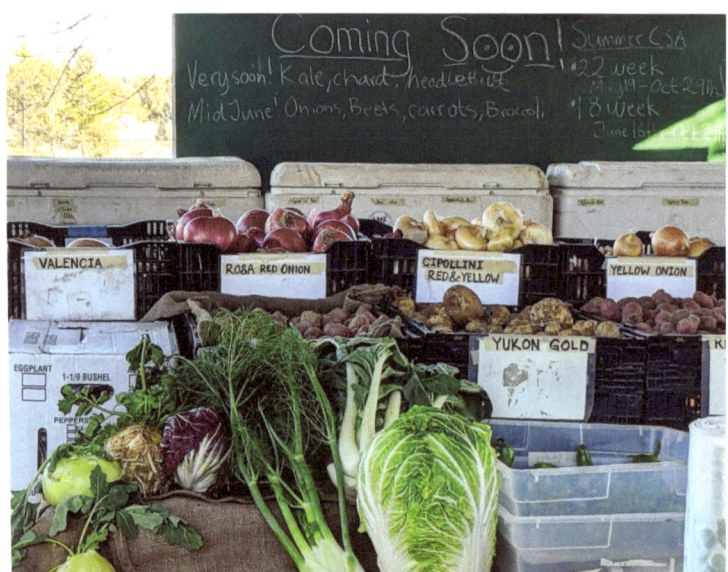
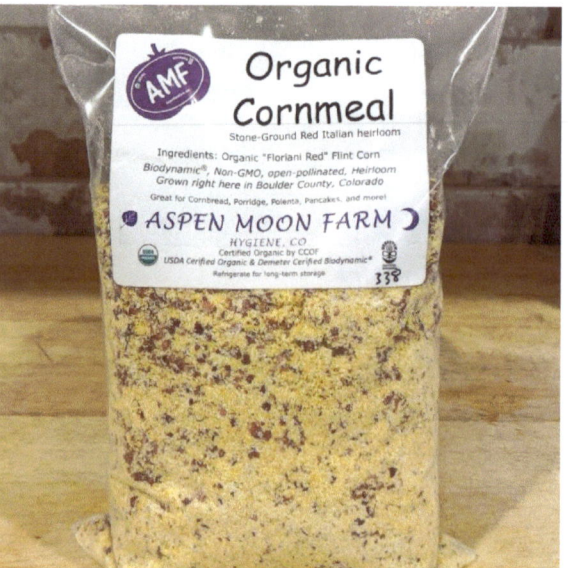
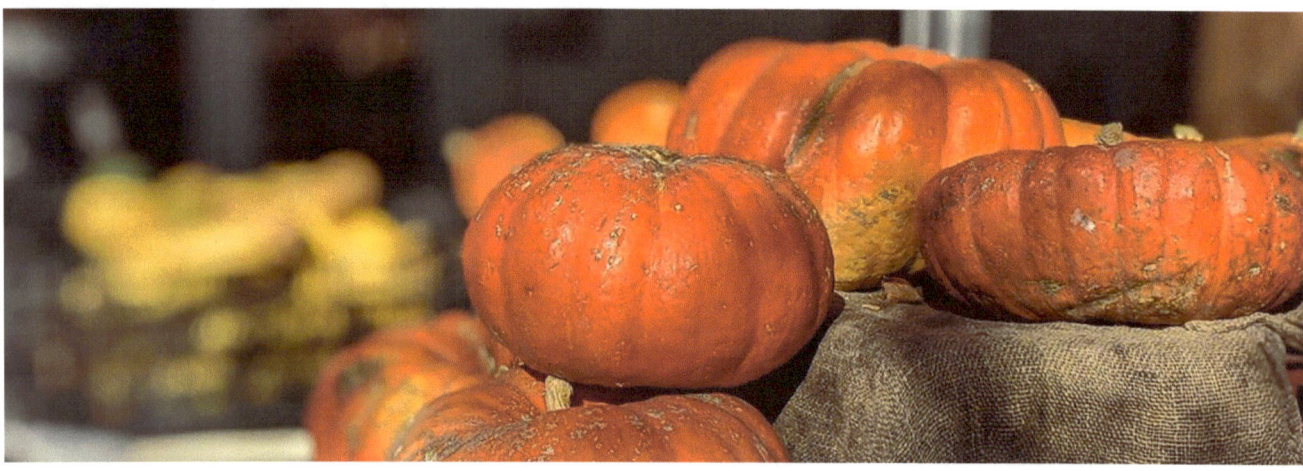

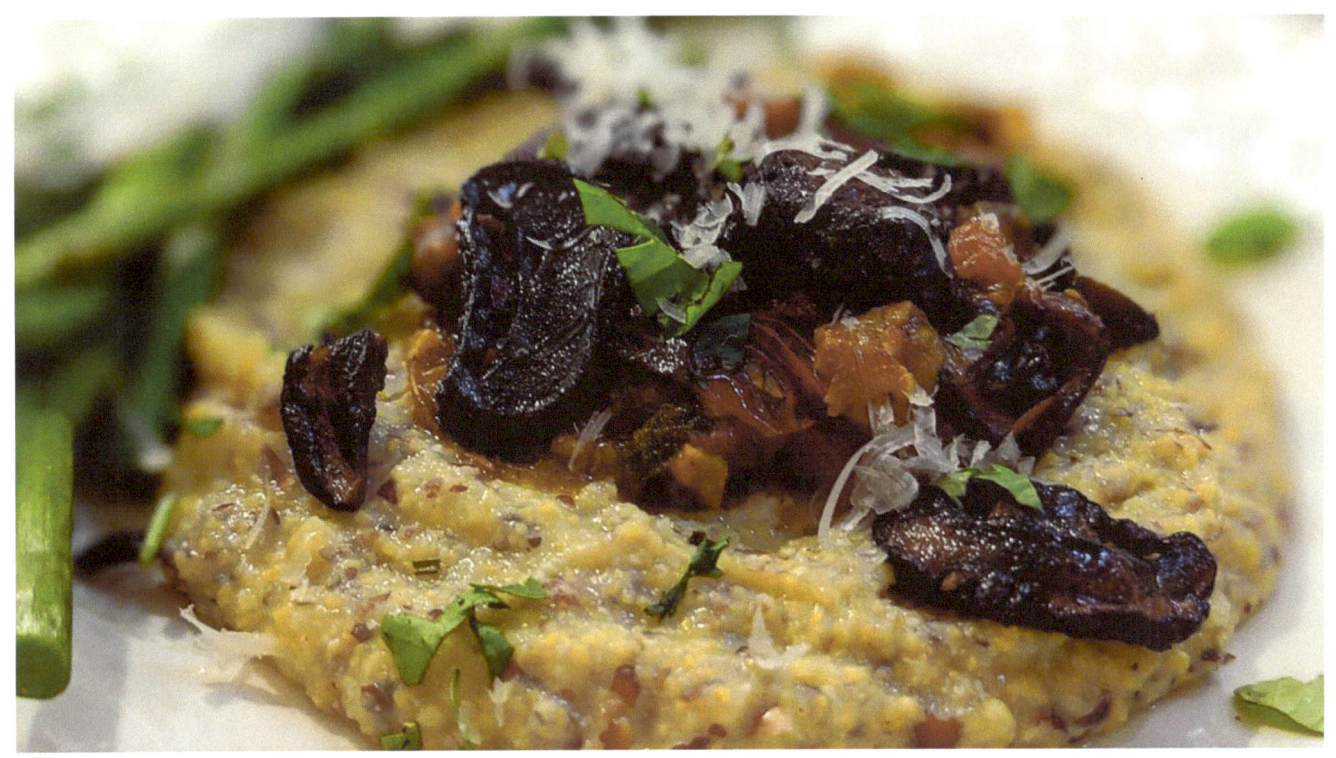

ASPEN MOON FARM POLENTA WITH ROASTED GRAPE TOMATOES

Ingredients

For the Polenta
- 1 cup Aspen Moon Farm Organic Cornmeal
- 3 cups water
- 1 tbsp grated parmesan (dairy or non-dairy)
- 1 tbsp milk (dairy or non-dairy)

For the Tomato Sauce
- 16 multicolored grape tomatoes, halved
- 1 garlic clove, minced
- 1 tbsp olive oil
- 2 sage leaves
- Salt and pepper to taste
- 1 tbsp dry vermouth
- 1 tbsp milk (dairy or non-dairy)

For the Garnish
- Additional grated parmesan (dairy or non-dairy)

Instructions

For the Polenta
Bring water to boil in a large saucepan. Slowly add the cornmeal while stirring. Lower heat to medium low and stir until mixture thickens.
Add the parmesan and milk (dairy or non-dairy). Salt and pepper to taste.

For the Tomato Sauce
Preheat oven to 400°F. Line a baking sheet with foil. Mix tomatoes, oil, garlic and sage in a bowl. Spread the mixture onto the foil. Roast 20 minutes until soft. Push tomatoes to the side and pour dry vermouth on the baking sheet. Roast again for 5 minutes. Push the tomatoes back in the middle to soak up the juices. Add the milk. Roast again for 5 minutes.

Serve
Spread the polenta on a plate or bowl. Top with tomato sauce and garnish with additional grated parmesan.

Elevate This: Top with vegan bacon or crispy, smoked mushrooms (as pictured).

Serves 2 as a main course

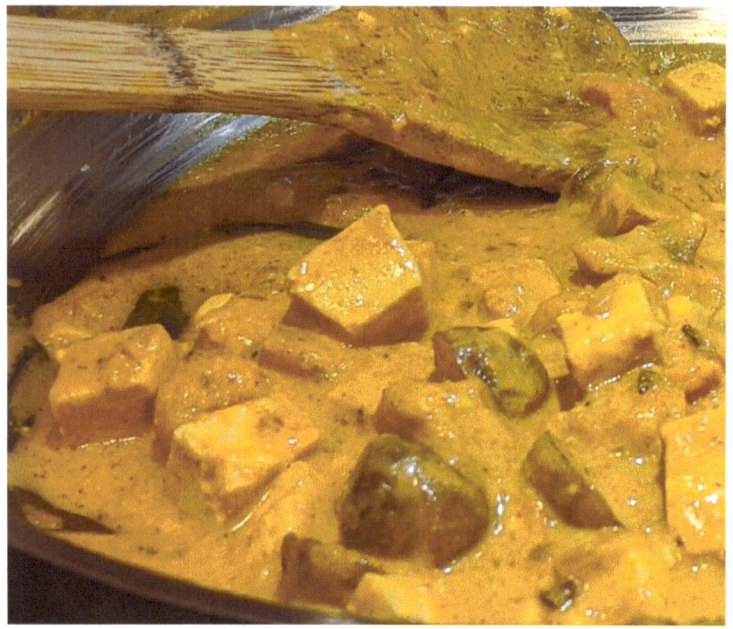
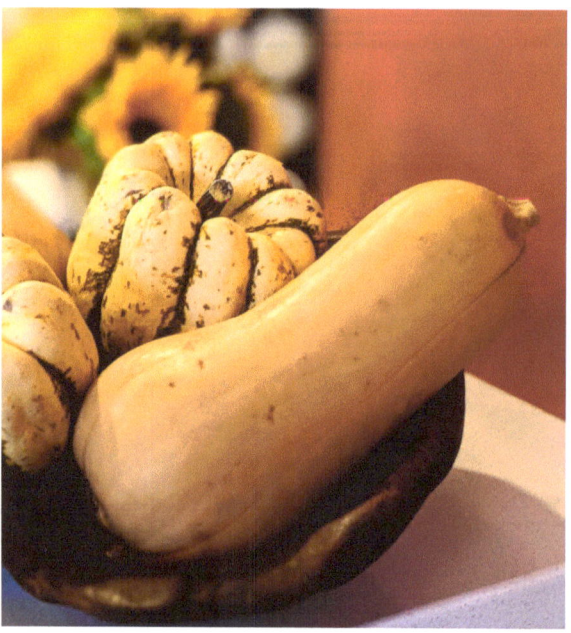

BUTTERNUT SQUASH POTATO TOFU CURRY

We are fortunate here in Fort Collins to have Turmeric, a wonderful Indian grocery and spice shop. This recipe incorporates the bountiful butternut squash and red potatoes which are available in the fall from our local farmers, and is elevated with a new find that takes Indian home cooking to a new level – Kashmiri red chili powder. I have spiced this dish at a medium heat with the red chili powder. You may also choose to substitute a good quality garam masala and curry spice mix for the individual ingredients.

Ingredients
- 1 cup cooked butternut squash, cubed
- 8-10 baby red potatoes, steamed and quartered
- 1 tbsp oil or ghee
- ½ cup finely chopped onions
- 2 garlic cloves, minced
- 1 tsp ground cumin
- 1 tsp ground coriander
- 1 tsp fennel seed, crushed
- ½ tsp fenugreek seed, crushed
- 1 tsp turmeric
- 1 tsp Kashmiri red chili powder
- ½ lb very firm tofu, cubed
- ½ cup coconut milk

Instructions
Heat oil or ghee in a large skillet over medium heat. Sauté onions until soft and golden.
Add garlic and sauté until fragrant – about 30 seconds.
Add the next 6 spices and "bloom" for 30 seconds.
Add the squash, potatoes, tofu and coconut milk.
Simmer until the sauce thickens.
Serve as a filling for dosas, chickpea crêpes, or over rice.

Note: If you do not have Kashmiri red chili powder (which I highly recommend adding to your spice cabinet – it is brilliant in color and taste), the best substitute is combining sweet smoked paprika with a little cayenne for heat. Or use common paprika in addition to a little cayenne.

Elevate This: Top with cilantro or green onions.

Serves 2-3 as a main dish

PASTA WITH PUMPKIN CREAM SAUCE

This is a super easy recipe, assuming you have already cut your pie pumpkin in half or quarters, cleaned out the seeds, and baked until fork tender in the oven at 350°F. I married this sauce with Pastificio Boulder's whole grain zucca pasta that are shaped like pumpkins.

Pastificio Boulder crafts their pastas from whole grain flour which is milled fresh, in-house daily from organic, heritage and ancient grains. What I love about this product is that the ancient grains of Turkey Red, Blue Emmer and White Sonora, are grown by local Boulder farmers. I don't think you can get any fresher than that, unless you live in Italy. The sauce comes together easily, and you can substitute in any other winter squash, such as butternut squash.

Ingredients
- 1 tbsp oil
- 3 garlic cloves, smashed or minced
- ½ cup vegetable, chicken, or vegan chicken broth
- 1 cup pumpkin purée
- 2 tbsp nutritional yeast
- ¼ cup milk (dairy or non-dairy)
- 8 ounces of Pastificio Boulder's pumpkin pasta
- 1 tsp The Spice and Tea Exchange® Fort Collins turmeric pepperberry saffron salt blend
- Additional turmeric if you want a brighter color
- Reserved pasta water

For the Garnish
- Chopped parsley
- Toasted panko bread crumbs

Instructions
Bring a large pot of water to boil. Add salt and boil the pasta to al dente. The pasta will keep cooking a bit once drained and sauced. Rinse, reserve water.

Heat the oil in a large skillet. Add the garlic and warm for 30 seconds. Do not brown.

Slowly add broth and scrape the bottom of the pan. Add the pumpkin purée and skillet mixture to an immersion blender or small blender and briefly purée the mixture. (I wanted a smooth sauce – no chunky garlic pieces.)

Pour the mixture back into the skillet. Cook over medium heat and add the yeast, milk and the turmeric pepperberry saffron salt spice blend. Add additional turmeric if you want a brighter color.

Add some of the reserved pasta water to thin the mixture if necessary.

Add the pasta to the skillet and coat the pasta. Remove the pasta to a serving dish keeping ¼ cup of the sauce in the bottom of the skillet. Add just a touch more pasta water and heat to thicken, then gently pour the sauce on top of the pasta for a better presentation and of course, more sauce.

Garnish with chopped parsley and toasted panko bread crumbs.

Elevate This: This is a basic recipe for you to play with. It is elegant and excellent on its own. Some spices or cuisine blends to consider: cumin, berbere, pan-fried sage bits, or thyme and oregano. You can also try a mixture of crushed fenugreek, fennel, and chile flakes. Golden caramelized shallots and capers will be a nice addition, as well as a gentle drizzle of olive oil.

Serves 2 as a main dish

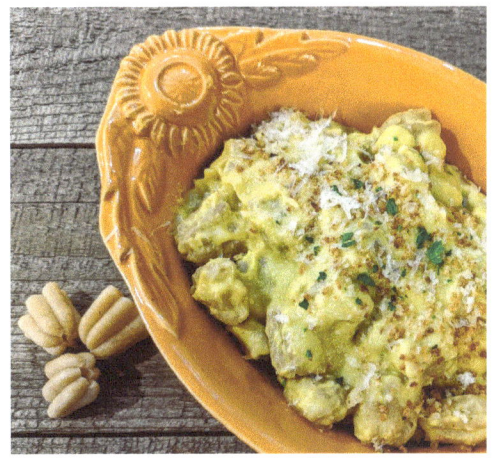

FRENCH APPLE PIE

This is the only apple pie I make, and it elevated when I discovered local Colorado apples, fresh from the orchard. This recipe comes from a magazine back in the 1970s. I was working the night shift in a hospital and started collecting recipes. It took 20 years for me to finally make this recipe, but, since trying it for the first time, I have made it every year.

What makes it special? The custard on the bottom adds a layer of soft decadence, and the apricot preserves glisten through the lattice work. Don't substitute the apricot preserves – the pie needs the tartness to balance the sweetness of the apples and custard.

Ingredients
- 1 package pie crust (or make your own, enough for two crusts)

For the Cream Filling
- ¼ cup sugar
- 2 tbsp flour
- 1 cup milk
- 3 egg yolks
- 1 tbsp butter
- ½ tsp vanilla extract

For the Apple Filling
- 2 lb tart apples (5-6 medium-sized apples; I like a mix of Granny Smith, MacIntosh, Rome and Cameo)
- 1 tbsp lemon juice
- 2 tbsp butter
- 2 tbsp sugar
- Dash of grated nutmeg (about ¼ tsp)
- 1 tsp of cinnamon
- ¾ cup apricot preserves
- 1 egg yolk
- 1 tbsp water

Instructions

For the Cream Filling
In small saucepan, combine sugar and flour. Mix well with a whisk. Stir in milk.
Place over medium heat and bring to a boil stirring constantly. Reduce heat. Simmer until sauce thickens.
In another bowl, beat the three egg yolks.
Temper the eggs by adding ¼ of the hot mixture to the yolks.
Beat for 30 seconds or until incorporated and then pour egg yolk mixture into the milk mixture. Add butter and vanilla.
Cover with plastic wrap and allow the mixture to cool completely.

For the Apple Filling
Core, pare and slice apples into a bowl. Add lemon juice, cinnamon and nutmeg. In a large skillet, heat butter and sugar. Add apple mixture and sauté until tender. Do not overcook! Remove from heat and allow to cool.

Thaw pie crusts on countertop for 15 minutes.
Preheat oven to 425°F.
Place 1 pie crust in a pie pan.
Pour cooled custard filling evenly into pie shell.
Layer the sliced apples on top.
Melt apricot preserves on the stovetop or in the microwave, and spread on top of apples.
With remaining pie crust, slice dough into ½ inch wide strips with a pastry wheel. Arrange strips in a lattice fashion over pie. Crimp edges.
Beat remaining egg yolk and water, and brush onto the latticework.
Bake 30 minutes or until golden brown.
Let cool before cutting.

Serves 8 as a dessert dish

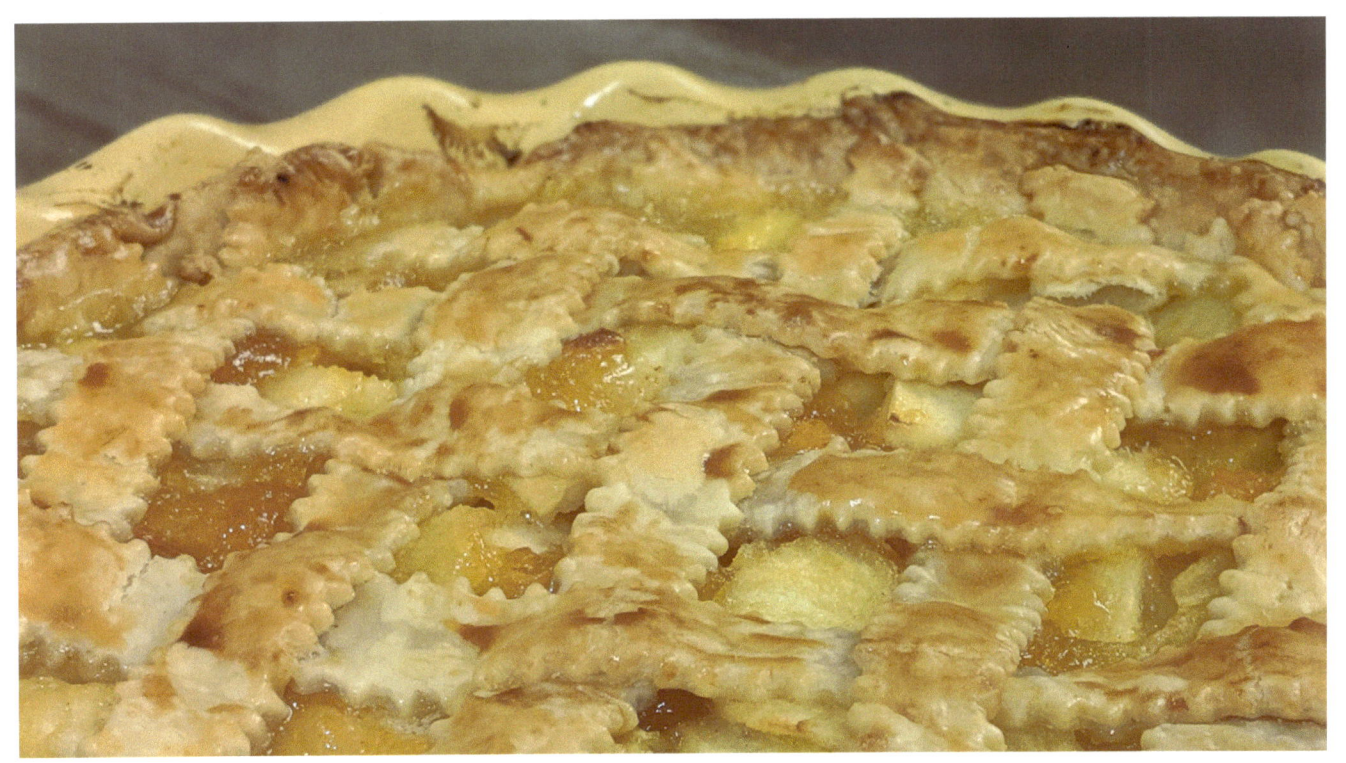

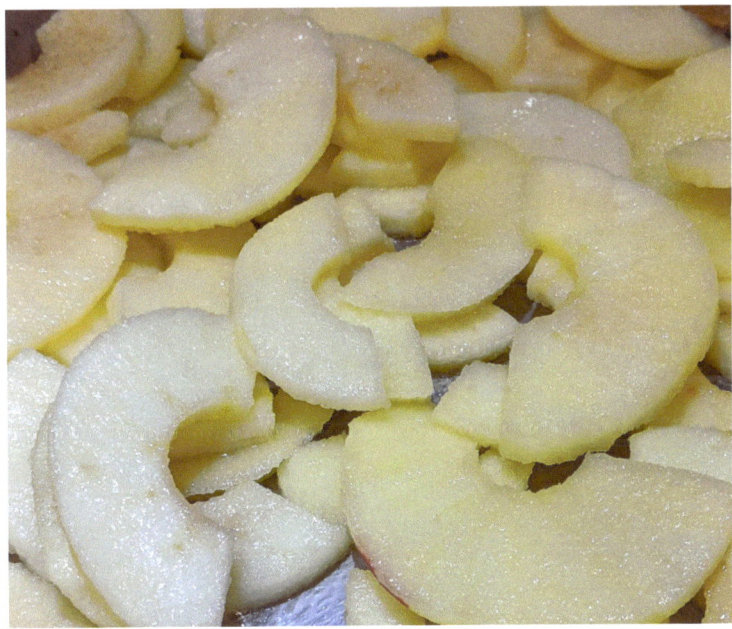

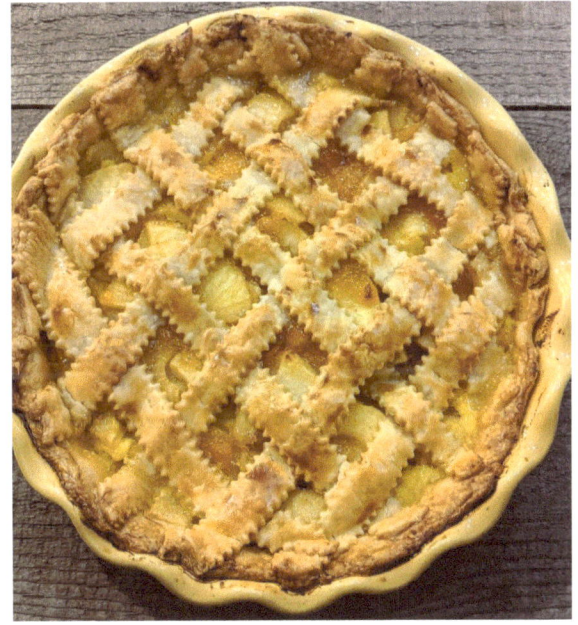

The Beet Goes On

In the early 20th century, Northern Colorado was sugar beet country. It was THE CROP from the 1890s to 1920s, with Colorado having over 20 sugar-refining factories at the peak of sugar beet agriculture. Who knew?

When you bike the Poudre River Trail, you will see a bit of history – a small replica of the real Brooklyn Bridge that transported beet slurry across the river, and the many irrigation ditches that still wind their way across the now grasslands and housing developments, and made this complex land more fertile.

Before mechanization, working the sugar beet fields was incredibly hard work. Beyond the initial field prep, planting, and irrigating, entire families and immigrants of various nationalities would help with the harvest, digging and topping the ideal sugar beet that would weigh about two pounds. Both Fort Collins and Greeley had huge sugar beet industries in the 20th century. It's a bit of a challenge to make a sugar beet recipe, especially when they are not readily available anywhere, so in lieu of sugar beets, I'm giving a culinary nod to the vegetable that sustained many an immigrant family's income and the local economy in the Northern Colorado earlier days.

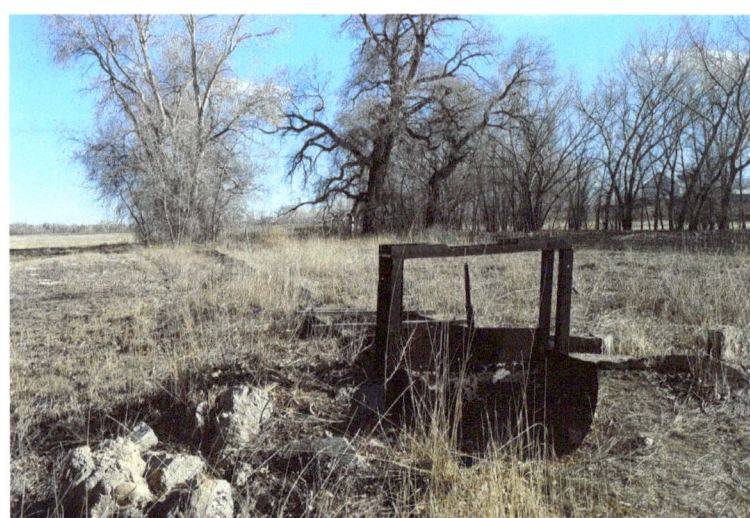
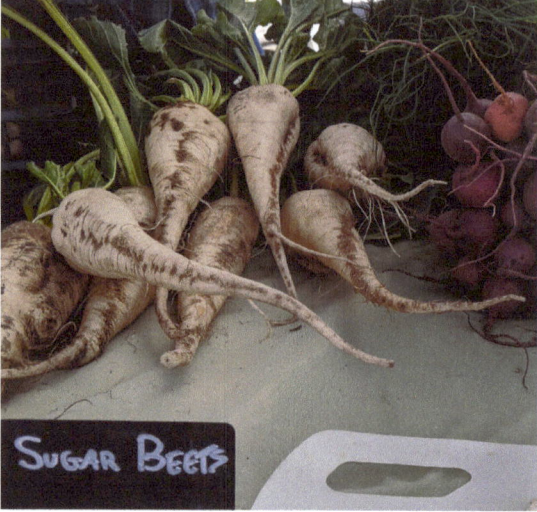
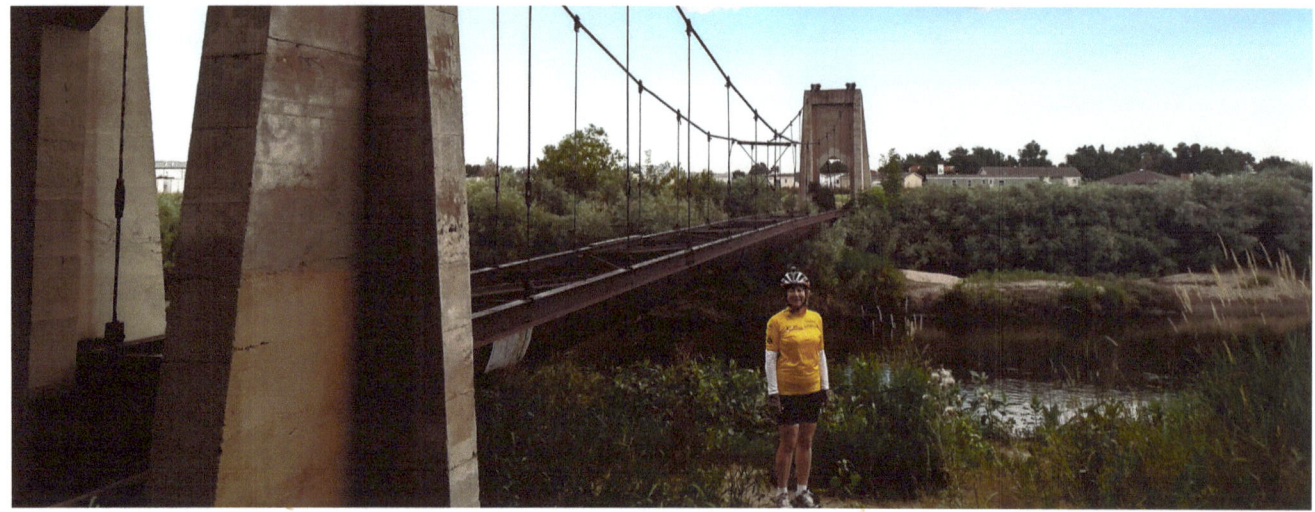

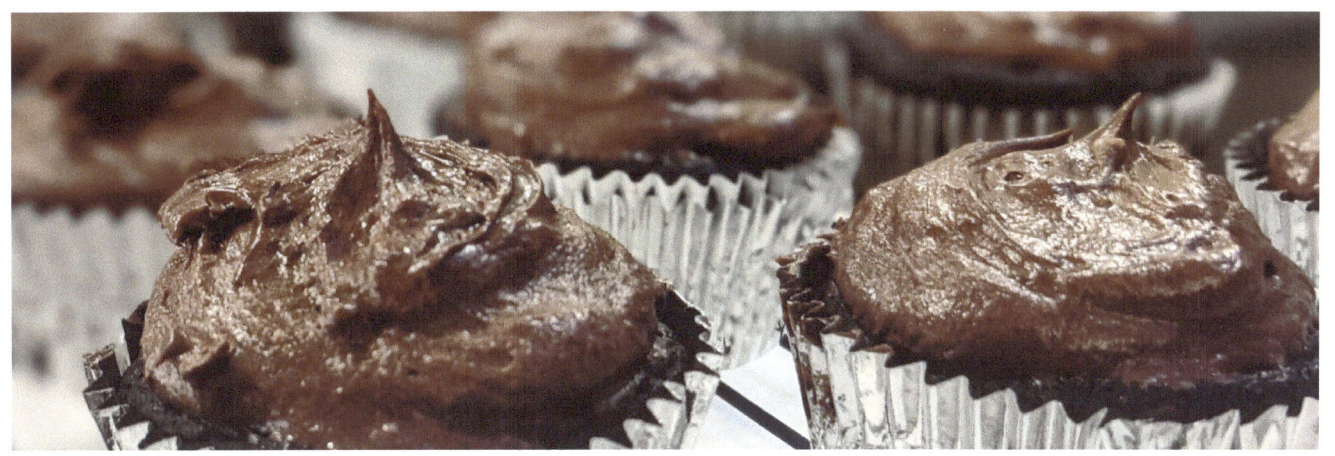

CHOCOLATE BEET CUPCAKES

Who doesn't love chocolate? Beets? Maybe not so much. The batter is entirely made with a food processor. I meant to make a red velvet cake, but I added too much cocoa powder, so I plowed ahead with the batter. The results were moist and amazing. If you get more beets in your CSA than you know what to do with, try this recipe.

Ingredients
For the Cake
- 8 ounces beets; boiled or steamed, cooled, peeled and cut into pieces
- ½ cup eggs (about 2 eggs) or ½ cup liquid egg substitute (ie. JUST Egg)
- 2 tbsp vanilla
- ½ cup milk (dairy or non-dairy)
- ½ cup sugar
- ½ cup flour
- ¼ cup cocoa powder
- 1 tsp baking powder
- ½ tsp salt
- ½ cup mini bittersweet or semi-sweet chips (I used Ghirardelli 60%)
- 1 tbsp vinegar
- 1 tsp baking soda

For the Frosting
- 4 cups powdered sugar
- ½ cup cocoa powder
- ½ cup palm shortening
- ¼ cup milk (dairy or non-dairy)
- 1 tsp vanilla extract

Instructions
For the Cake
Preheat oven to 350°F. Prepare cupcake tins with liners. In a food processor, process the beets until smooth. (They will be beautiful!)
In a small bowl, whisk together the egg or egg substitute, milk, vanilla, and sugar. Process until smooth. In a large bowl, sift the flour, cocoa powder, baking powder, and salt.
Add ⅓ of the liquid mixture to the beets and pulse for 3 or 4 seconds. Alternating dry ingredients and the remaining wet ingredients, pulse the batter just until smooth. Process for 3-4 seconds for each addition, at most. Do not overprocess.
In a small bowl, mix the vinegar and soda. It will foam up. Add the mixture to the food processor and process for 2-3 seconds.
Add the chips and process for 2-3 seconds.
Pour batter into prepared cups and bake for 20-25 minutes, or until a toothpick comes out clean.
Let cool completely before frosting (at least 2 hours).

For the Frosting
Place all ingredients in a mixing bowl and whip until thick and of your desired consistency, about 5-7 minutes. You will have some leftovers, but gosh, it refrigerates well for another cupcake batch.

Makes 12 cupcakes

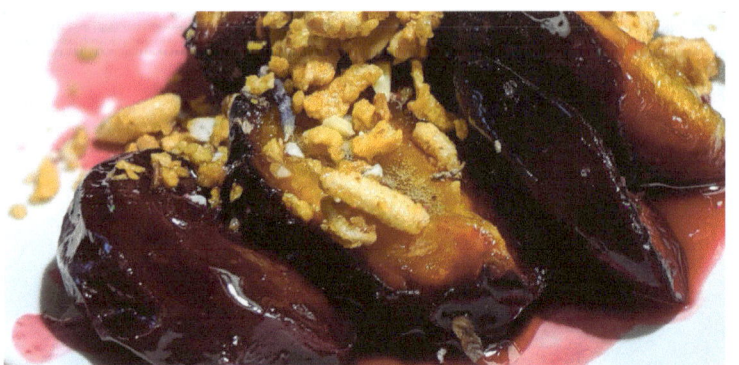
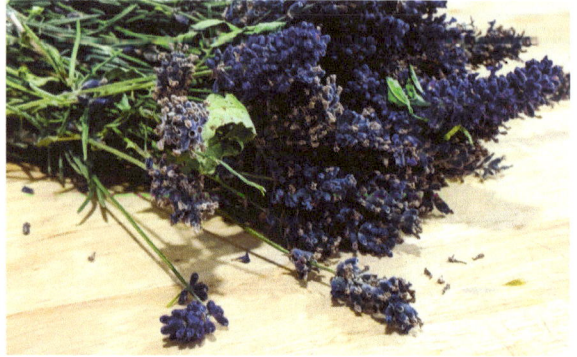
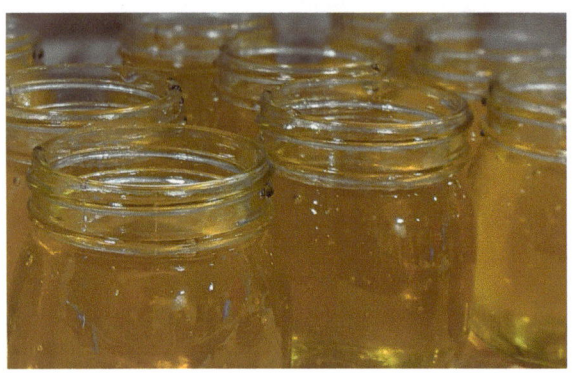
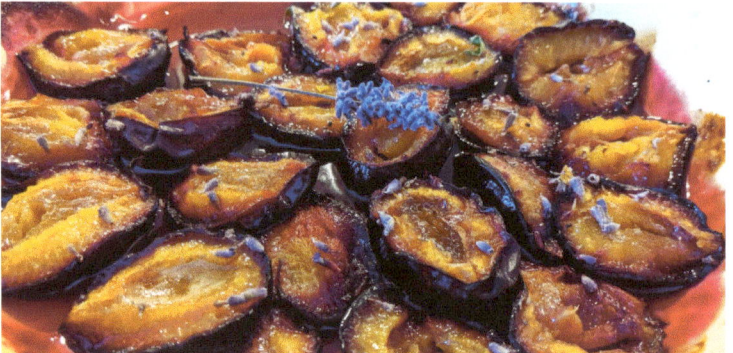

HONEY LAVENDER ROASTED ITALIAN PLUMS

Gorgeous Italian plums grow on the Western Slope and are brought to Northern Colorado farmers markets. They do grow in our area, and passing under a ripe Italian plum tree in late summer or early fall is a wonder to behold – oval orbs of magnificent blue!

Ingredients
- 12-16 Italian plums, halved lengthwise and pitted
- 2-3 tbsp local honey
- 1 tbsp lavender, slightly crushed

Instructions
Preheat oven to 350°F.
Spray a pie plate with cooking spray.
Place the plums in a beautiful pattern in the bottom of the plate.
Drizzle with honey.
Sprinkle with lavender.
Bake for 30-40 minutes, until the plums soften and a lovely, gooey, raspberry-colored syrup develops in the bottom of the pan.

Serve by itself, or over ice cream or a nice shortbread. Leftovers are fabulous when served over a bowl of breakfast oatmeal.

Elevate This: Make add-ons simple so the gentle touch of lavender still shines through. Perhaps some sliced, toasted nut, or a biscotti on the side.

Serves 4-6

CAST IRON SKILLET HONEY ROASTED APPLES

Northern Colorado and the Western Slope offer more than 200 varieties of apples to eat refreshingly raw, roasted, baked, or pressed into cider. This recipe is super easy and combines the sweet and tart of local apples with the sticky earthiness of local honey. I chose a mix of Northern Colorado apples for this honey-roasted apple recipe - it just makes the dish more interesting. A gentle topping of toasted almonds is all you need to present this dish to your friends or family, or to enjoy on your own. Leftover honey-roasted apples are also yummy in your breakfast oatmeal or chai pudding. You might want to make extra! I prefer using a cast iron skillet for these types of dishes, but it will work with any skillet that is oven-safe.

Ingredients
- 3 slightly tart or mixed-use apples; peeled, cored and diced into ½-inch pieces. (I used a mix of Cameo, Winesap, and Jonathan. Avoid Red Delicious as they will get mushy.)
- 2 tbsp butter (dairy or non-dairy)
- ⅓ cup local honey

For the Garnish
- 2 tbsp toasted almond slices, hazelnuts or pecans would do nicely as well

Instructions
Preheat oven to 375°F.

Heat the butter (dairy or non-dairy) in the cast-iron skillet over medium heat until bubbly. If you are using real butter, a nice touch is to let it heat until browned. Add the apple pieces, stirring occasionally until nice and golden, with slightly caramelized edges. The pieces should still be firm.

Once the apples are golden, add the honey. Stir and cook for 5 minutes or until sticky and more golden. They should still be firm.

Place the skillet in the oven and bake for another 15-20 minutes until the apples are done to your preference. I prefer a bit of a firmer apple, but you may prefer a softer result.

Serve in a bowl or pudding cup.

Top with toasted almonds or your topping of choice.

Elevate This: Use a dash of smoked salt or pepper, cardamon sugar, or salted caramel sugar sprinkled gently on top.

Serves 3-4

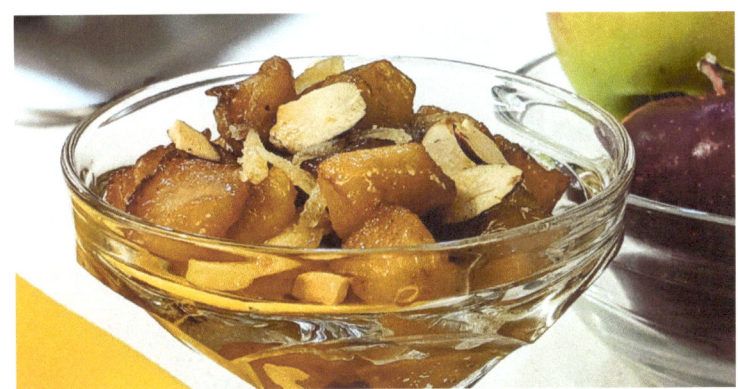
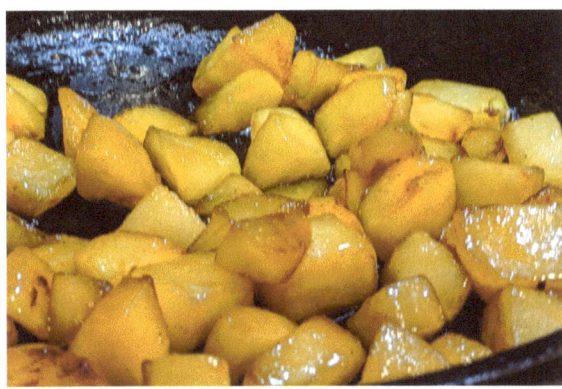

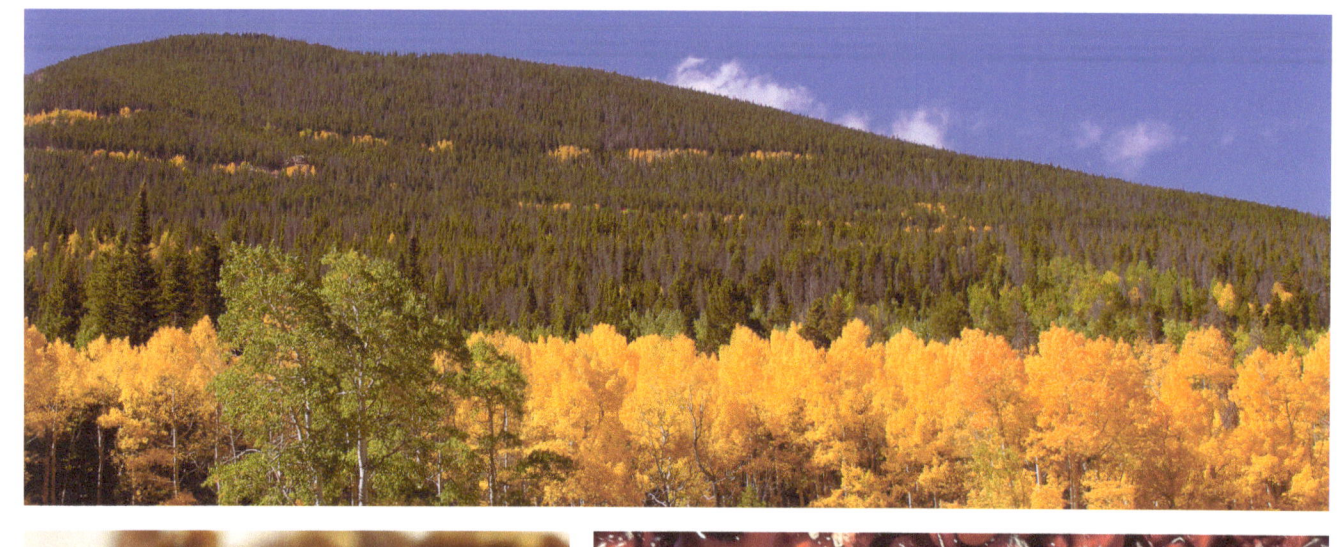
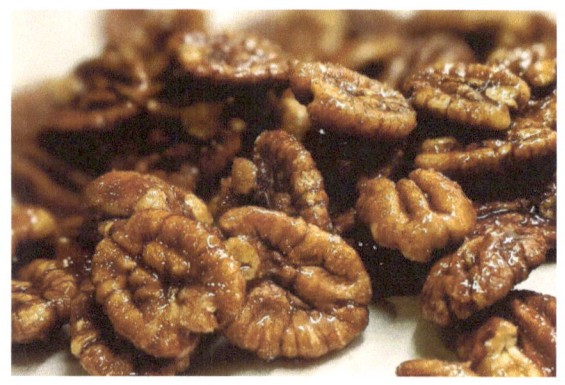
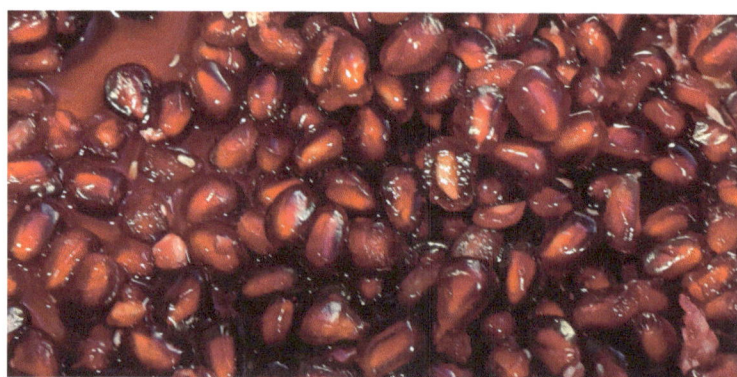
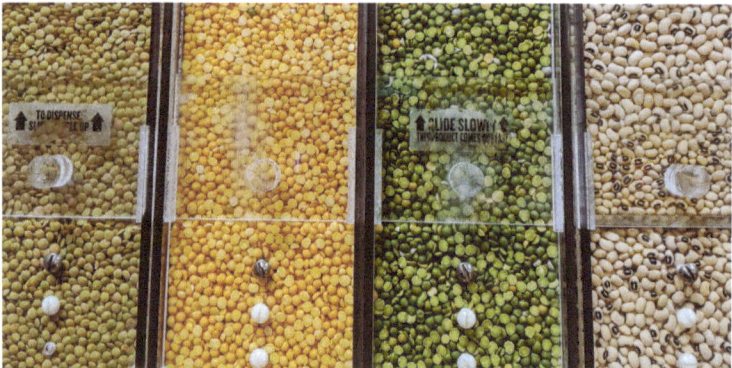
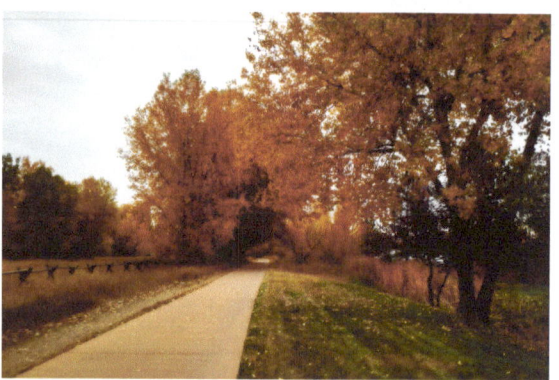
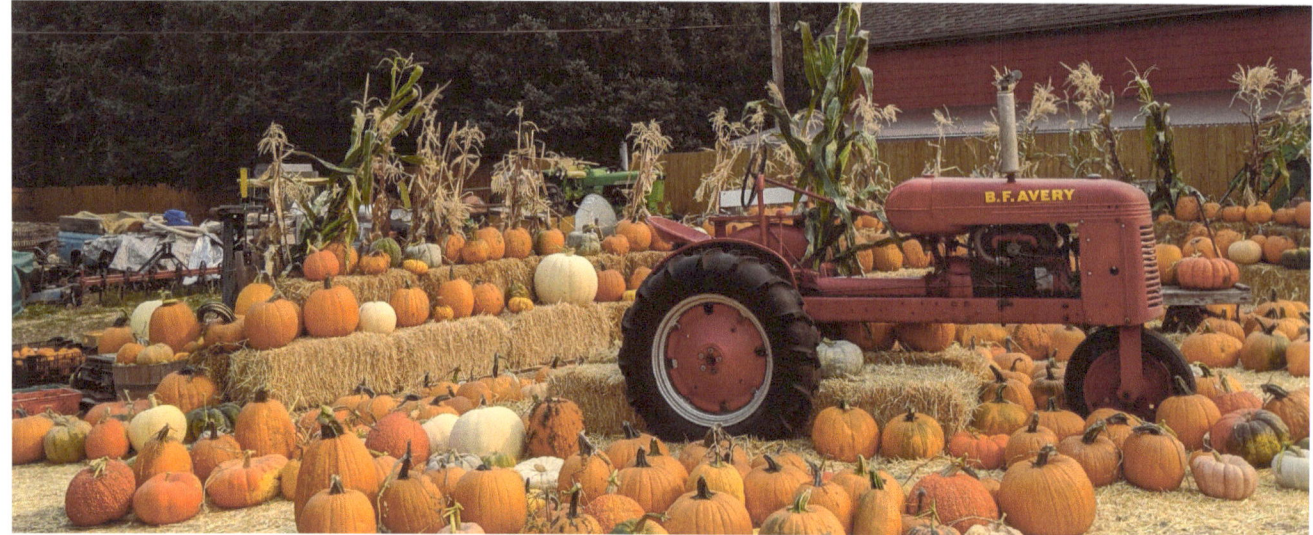

WINTER

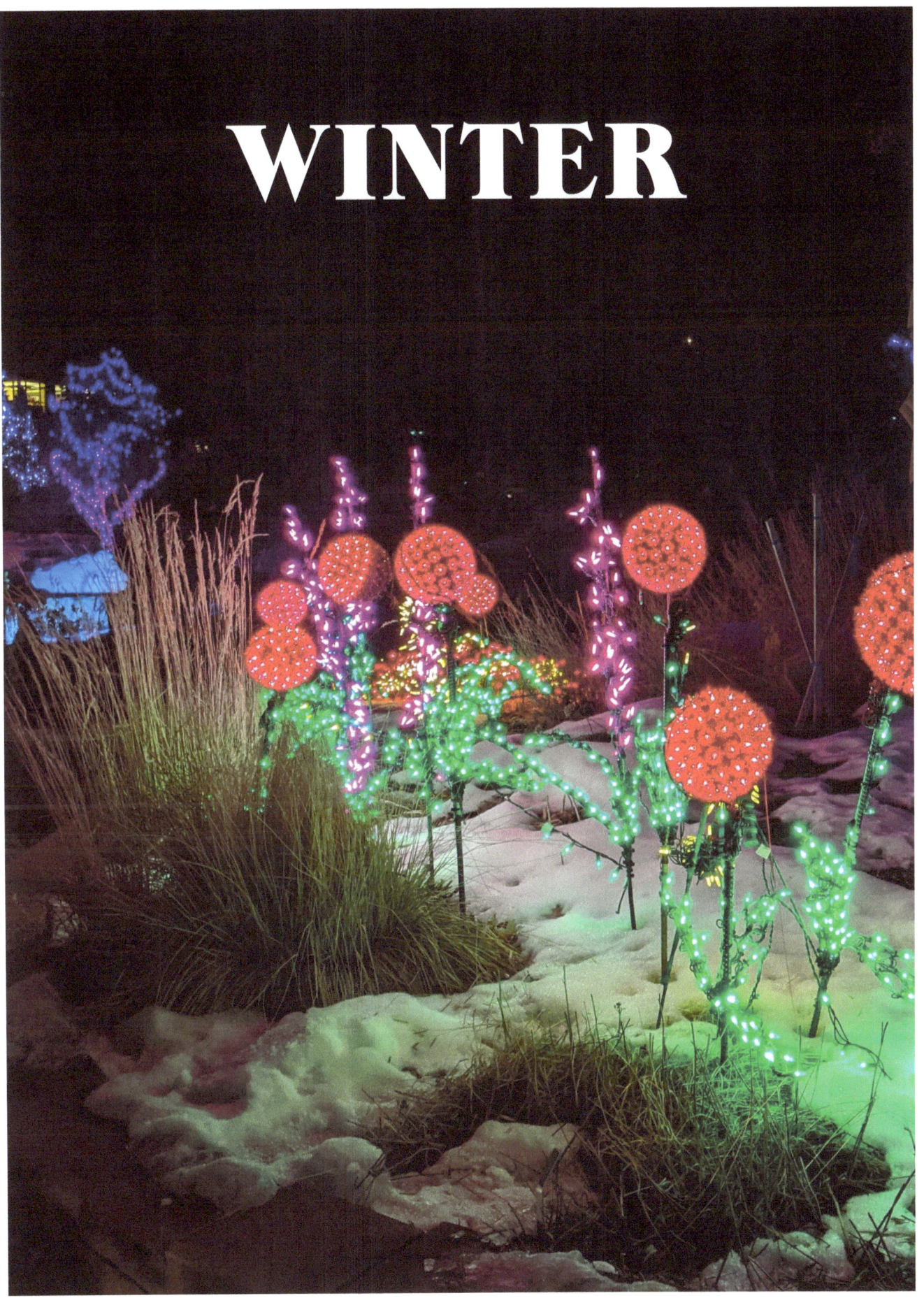

The farmers were snuggled all warm in their beds, with visions of summer dancing in their heads.

A farmer's work is never done. In the words of a local grower, "Sure, I take a European vacation from January to August, and come home in time for harvest." Not quite. But the winter months in Colorado are the time to take pause, plan, clean equipment, prepare to start seeds, or plan soil amendment once the ground softens from the Spring warmth. Other smaller gardeners start planning for pollinator flowers or perhaps an Audubon Rockies Habitat Hero garden.

With December comes adjustment and the farmers markets transition – the weekly events move indoors. Hardier root and vine vegetables that withstand cold storage are still available. Dried, packaged, canned, and prepared goods are plentiful. It's time to discover local crafters pasta, kombucha, and roasted coffee. Spice mixes, olives from Greece, olive oils from Tuscany, leafy greens, and fall and winter produce. There are condiments, dairy, cheese, and responsibly raised beef, lamb, chicken and eggs. Did I mention mushrooms and microgreens?

Fort Collins downtown brightens up with holiday lights and the Gardens on Spring Creek begin their holiday Garden of Lights extravaganza. The 18 acres of multiple gardens are transformed into a winter wonderland for visitors to enjoy in December through the end of the year.

The bees are cozied up in their hives. The holidays are around the corner. The new year is coming. It's winter sport time or hibernation for others, and we want to eat healthy. How shall we celebrate?

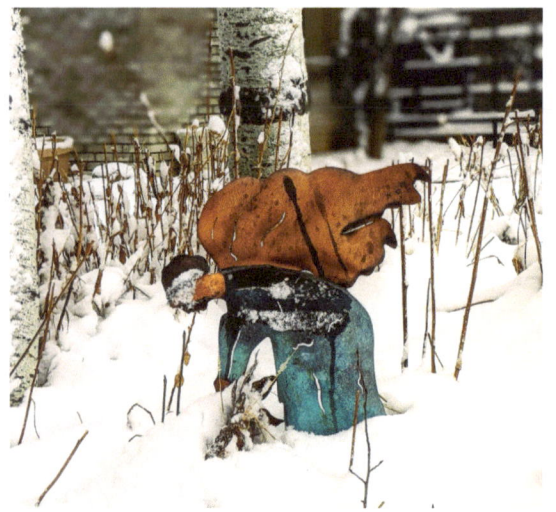
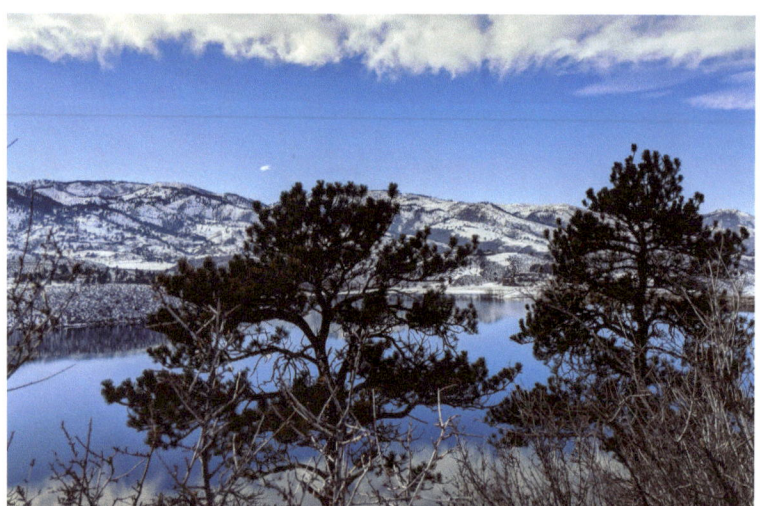
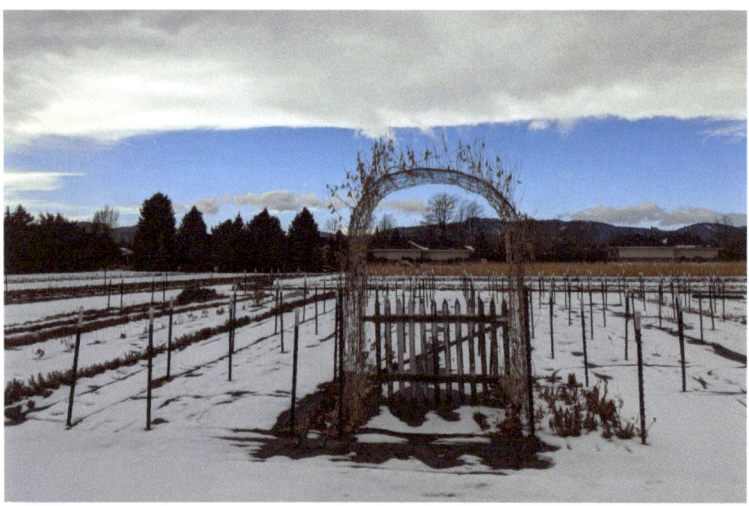
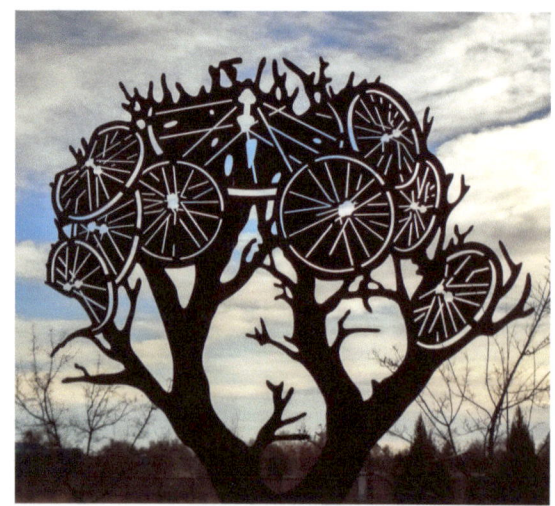

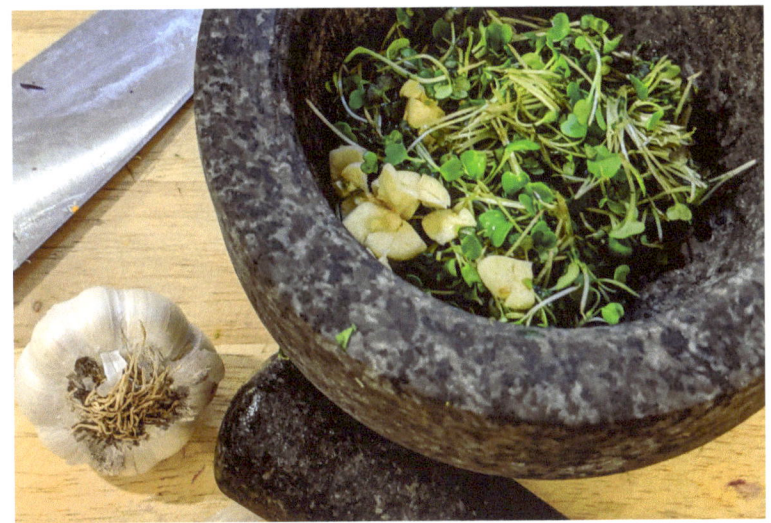
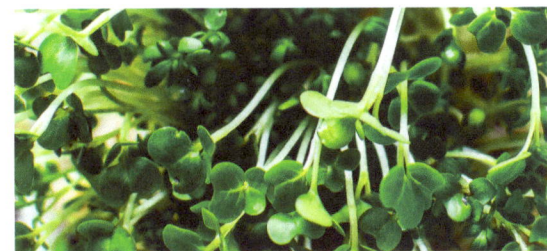
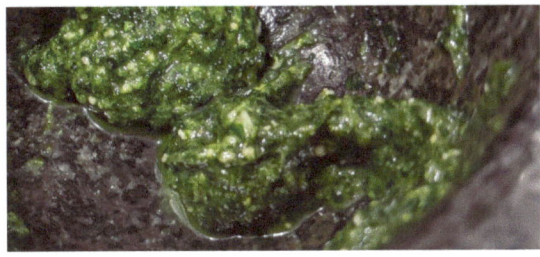

MICROGREEN GREMOLATA, PISTOU, AND PESTO

After much research and determining which terminology is correct for these three garnishes or sauces, I'm giving you all three. Add lemon – it's a gremolata. Add some pine nuts and maybe some cheese, you have pesto. The sky is the limit once you have the technique.

Why so many recipes with microgreens in this cookbook? Because they are micro-powerful in nutrients and add some splashes of horseradish-y spiciness depending on the microgreen used. If you want the taste of the microgreens, but are a bit tired of whole stems in your salad or sandwich, you can use these easy elevations for any dish. Plus, in the winter, you get a refreshing taste of summer!

Ingredients
For the Basic Mash
- 1 cup microgreens
- 3 garlic cloves, peeled and coarsely chopped

Instructions
For the Microgreen Gremolata
Finely chop the Basic Mash ingredients. Mix with the juice of ½ a lemon or 2 tsp lemon juice. in a bowl. Stir well. Salt to taste.

For the Microgreen Pistou
Mash the Basic Mash ingredients into a fine mash in a mortar and pestle. Stir in 1 tbsp extra virgin olive oil. Salt to taste.

For the Microgreen Pesto
Mash the Basic Mash ingredients in a mortar and pestle. Add 2 tsp toasted pine nuts and mash until creamy. If desired, stir in 1 tbsp grated parmesan (dairy or non-dairy) and 1 tbsp olive oil.

Makes 2-3 tbsp, enough for a quick dip or garnish.

TOUM

This delectable Lebanese dip or garnish is a mindbender. It is basically mayo without the egg – a chemical reaction of garlic, lemon juice and oil. Shak Shouka, a vendor at our farmers markets, offers functional Middle Eastern food. The owner, Fauzi Silbaq, and family, are at the market selling their fabulous food craft, rain or shine. My recipe is not Fauzi's secret recipe, but if you are in Northern Colorado, it is worth a trip to the Larimer County and Fort Collins summer and winter markets to taste Shak Shouka treats for yourself. His products are also available at the local Mountain Avenue Market. Fauzi is ever-expanding his offerings beyond babaganoush, toum, and harissa – they are creative, inspiring, and will get you eating more veg.

As stated on Shak Shouka's Facebook page, Middle Eastern food has been influenced by and evolved from Aramaic, Assyrian, Phoenician, Asian, and North African, as well as Arabic cuisine. I know it is hard to believe, but it is herbs and spices that elevate food—particularly vegetables and grains—not the fat content.

This recipe works only in a small 2-4 cup food processor – it will not work in a blender. It is possible to use an immersion blender, but you will need to add ¼ tsp xanthum gum at the end to create the desired texture.

Ingredients
- 1 full head or bulb of garlic, peeled and roughly chopped
- Juice of 1 lemon
- ½ tsp salt
- 2 tsp water
- 1 cup canola oil, or a mix of canola or avocado oil
(Do not use straight olive oil – it will not emulsify.)

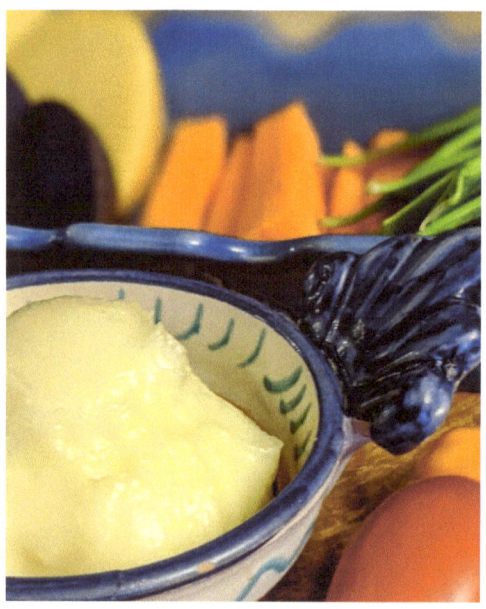

Instructions
This is the most important step: In a 2-4 cup food processor, purée the garlic, lemon, salt and water for about 5 minutes. You will need to stop to scrape down the sides of the bowl frequently. Process until a paste consistency – no chunks or pieces. You can't process too much, but you can process too little.

Add the oil 1 tbsp at a time. Process very well for the first 4 additions – for at least 2-3 minutes between each addition.

The mixture will begin to emulsify after the third or fourth addition of 1 tbsp oil each. Continue to add the oil in larger quantities, emulsifying well after each addition until the mixture thickens. Start watching texture after ½ cup total oil is added. Depending on the size of the head of garlic, the mixture may thicken after ¾ cup of oil. At this point it should have the consistency of a very thick mayonnaise.

If for some reason the puréeing and emulsifying failed, and your mixture is still separated, sprinkle ¼ tsp xanthum gum to pull it together. It will have a slightly different texture, but it will save the dish.

Note: Toum can be a topping for grilled vegetables, meat, toast, mixed with avocado, used as a sandwich spread or used as a veg dip. It elevates anything, including almost any recipe in this cookbook.

Makes ¾-1 cup

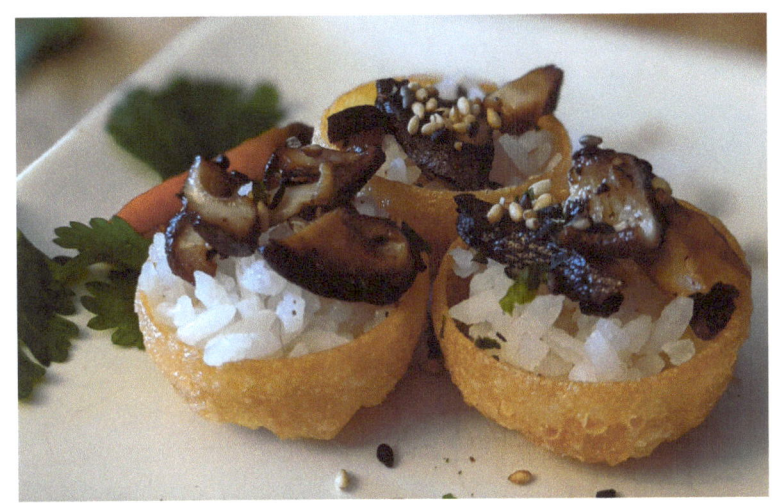
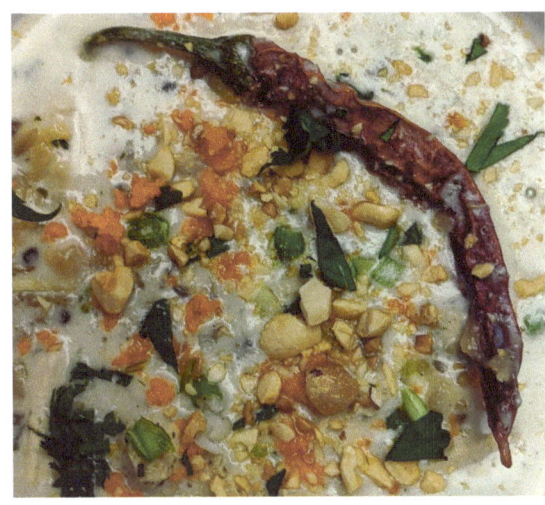

ROASTED SHIITAKES TWO WAYS

ROASTED SHIITAKE RICE CUPS

Ingredients
- 8 ounces shiitake mushrooms, stems removed and sliced
- 1 tbsp smoked soy sauce
- 1 tbsp oil
- 1 tsp smoked black pepper
- ½ cup cooked white rice
- Silijams croustades or phyllo cups

For the Garnish
- Chopped cilantro and furikake

Instructions
Preheat oven to 425°F (I used a toaster oven).
Prepare sheet pan with foil and non-stick spray.
Combine the soy sauce, oil and pepper in a bowl and mix well. Add the mushrooms and stir to coat well.
Spread on the baking sheet and roast for 15 minutes, stirring to coat every 5 minutes.
Using a 1 tbsp food scoop, fill Siljans croustades or phyllo cups with cooked white rice.
Place chopped or sliced roasted mushrooms on top.
Garnish with chopped cilantro and furikake.

Serves 2 as a small plate

ROASTED SHIITAKE COCONUT THAI SOUP

Ingredients
- ½ can of full-fat coconut milk
- ½ cup milk (dairy or non-dairy)
- 2 tbsp The Spice and Tea Exchange® Coconut Thai Spice Blend
- ½ cup vegetable broth
- 1 tsp white miso
- ½ cup cooked white rice
- ½ cup roasted shiitakes (as prepared in above recipe)

For the Garnish
- Chopped peanuts, cashews, lime, cilantro, grated carrot, and furikake

Instructions
Place first 5 ingredients in a saucepan.
Heat this soup base over medium heat until the spices blend and the mixture thickens.
Split the cooked white rice and roasted shiitakes into two serving bowls, then pour the soup base over the bowls of rice and shiitakes.
Garnish with chopped peanuts, cashews, lime, cilantro, grated carrot, and furikake.

Serves 2 as a soup dish

Greens, Grains, and Veg Goodness

This is not so much a recipe as it is an idea for crafting a beautiful dish. Salads can be works of art from the color wheel of nutrition, thus, no measurements. Think color variety, texture, grain, veg, fruit, seeds, nuts, spice and more. Salads do not need to be tossed. Non-tossed salads or bowls allow a bit of pause in your life to examine the beauty of a veg – its texture, its characteristics, and how it will fit the taste and design of the dish. Refer to the *Elevations* section of this book (p. 168) for more cuisine-based ideas, easy mixes and garnishes to have on-hand.

To eat mostly plants, it is helpful to parboil or batch-cook veggies and grains. My favorites to keep in the fridge are beets, potatoes, carrots, Brussels sprouts, sugar peas, broccoli, and the Giardiniera (p. 63). Toum (p. 130) and hummus are always in the fridge as well. Sprouts and peas have a decent shelf life. In our household, potatoes and beets are steamed, and I parboil broccoli to extend its life as much as possible.

For this bowl, I had the following on hand:
- Local kale; stem removed, chopped and massaged
- Beets, steamed for 20 minutes in an Instant Pot
- Purple potatoes, steamed for 12 minutes in an Instant Pot
- Leftover black rice and a bit of quinoa
- Mixed-color grape tomatoes, halved
- ¼ cup or so chickpeas from another project
- 1 carrot; cut in small batons for color, or grated
- Dried cranberries
- Italian nutritional yeast mix (Nutritional yeast, Tuscan spice mix, and pine nuts – mixed together)

Elevate This: Dress with the Grated Garlic Dressing (p. 50). Think colors – yellow or purple carrots, orange yams or sweet potato chunks, a leafy purple and green lettuce. If you have leftovers or want a more substantial dish, wrap your bowl ingredients in a whole grain flatbread. Spread Toum or aioli, harissa and/or Microgreen Pistou (p. 129). It will be beautiful and healthy.

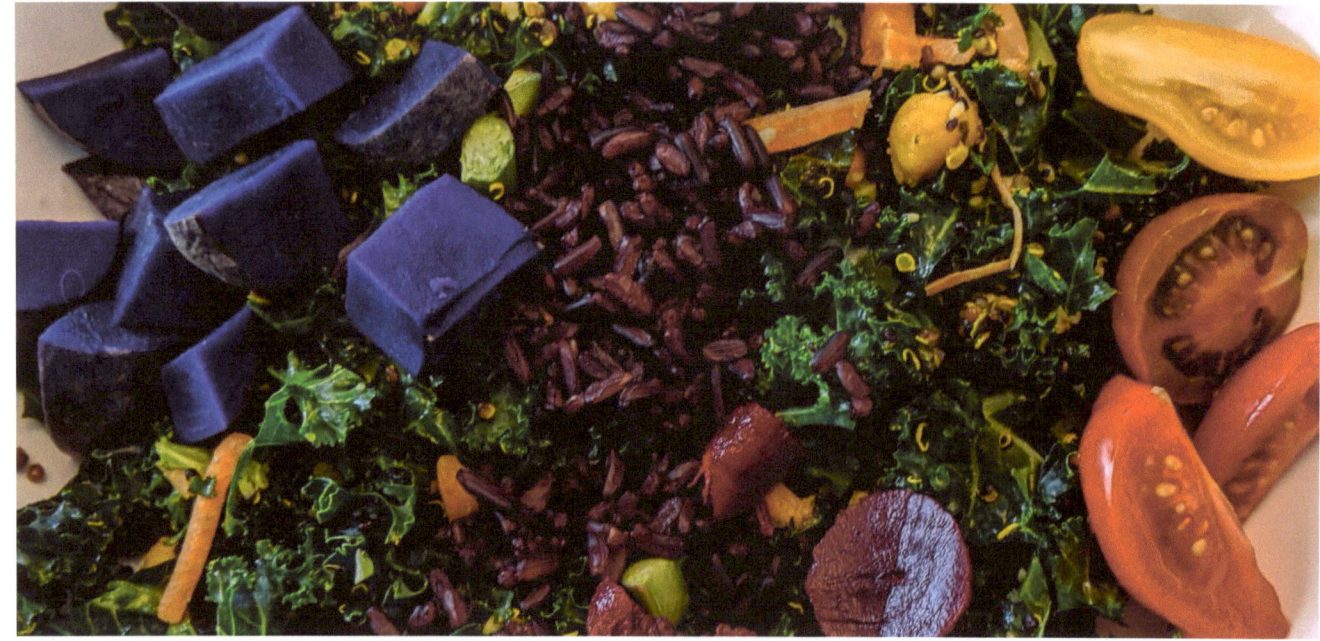

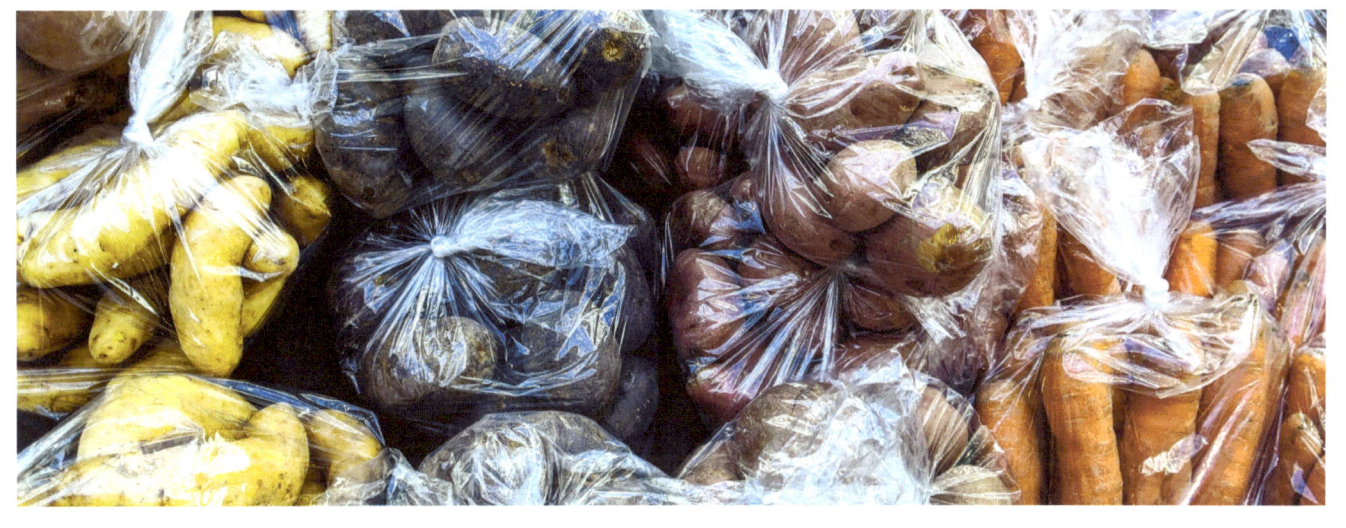
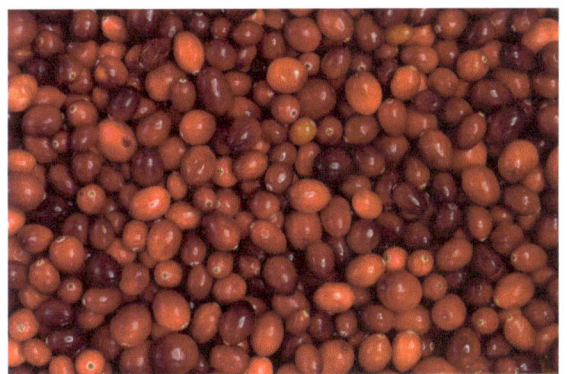
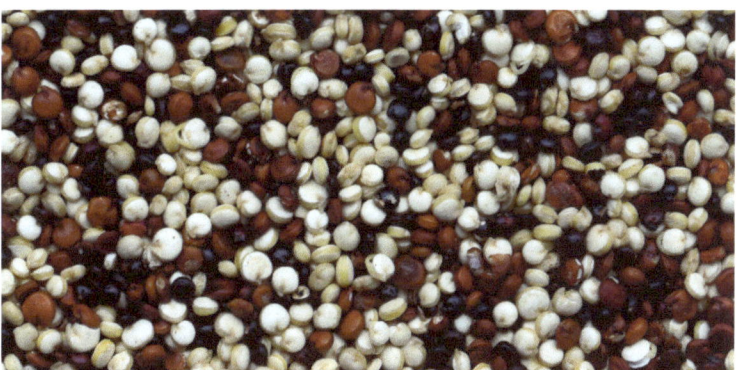
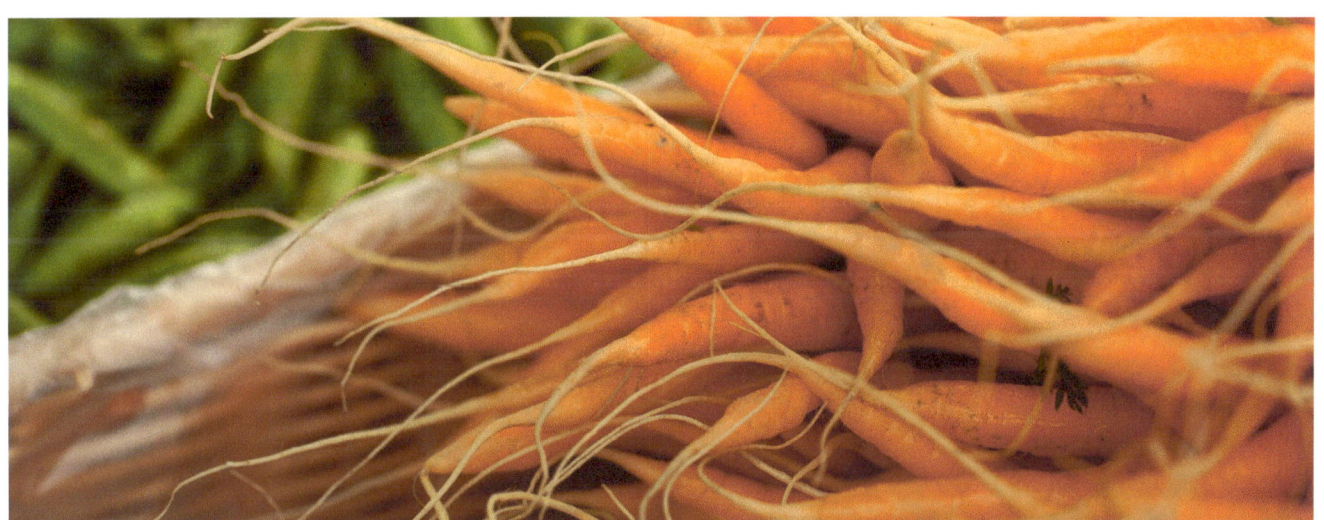
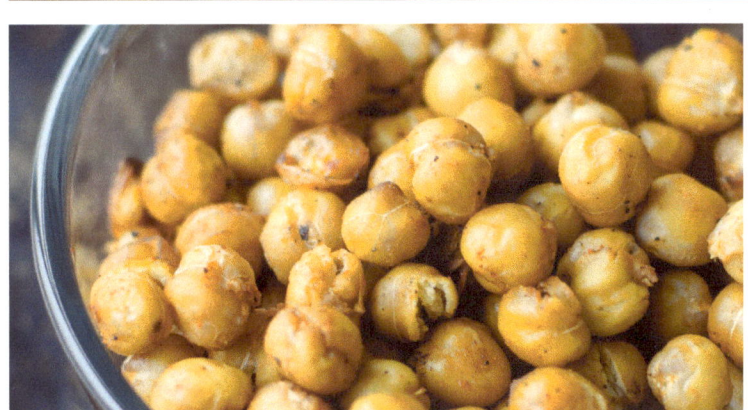
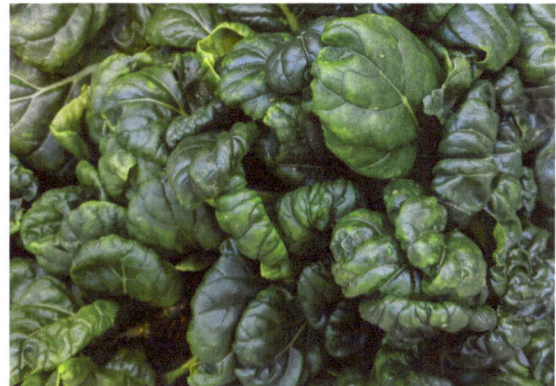

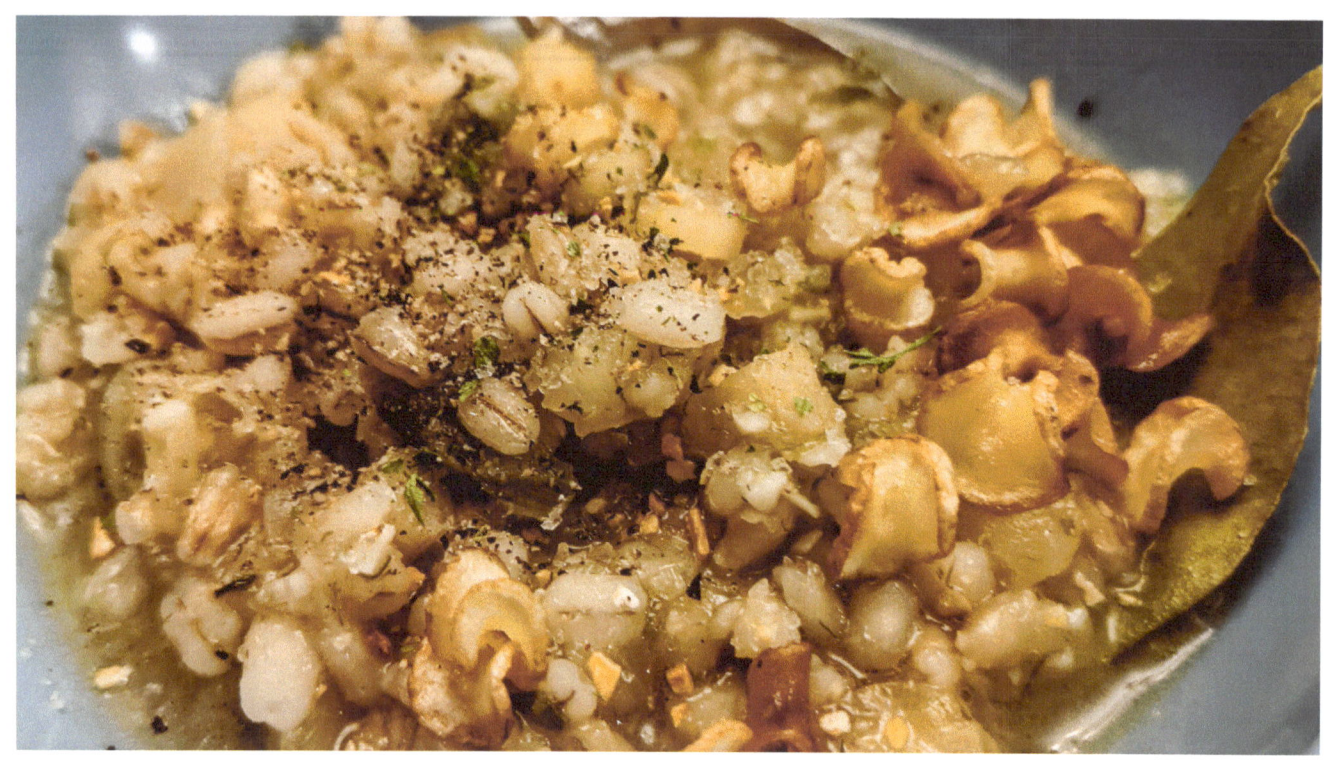

VEGETABLE BARLEY SOUP

This recipe is a nod to the barley agriculture that was, and still is to some degree, prevalent in this area in the first half of the 20th century. Early on, most of the barley grown was for the large breweries in the area, but many of these lands have been subject to urban growth. Businesses such as Root Shoot Malting of Olander Farms in Loveland still manage barley production from seed to final kilning. Using newer techniques, regenerative farming, and partnership leasing with Larimer County, they are able to still farm the lush lands of the Front Range and bring grain goodness to the local brewing and distilling industry.

Root vegetables are the epitome of fall and winter. Parsnips, carrots, beets, potatoes – they all conjure up visions of Laura Ingalls and her family taking hardier, sturdier vegetables to the root cellar for the winter. Nowadays, pretty much any root vegetable is available year-round. But I love salivating over the buckets of winter vegetables our area farmers produce during the season and offer during the long days of winter.

I think parsnips are under-appreciated. They have a lovely sweetness to them when roasted, or in this case, when added to a warm, cozy, "creamy" soup.

There are a lot alliums in this recipe, but don't leave out the leeks. Every allium has its treasure flavor and leeks have their own. I generally keep sliced leeks in the freezer. Rarely do I need crunchy leeks, so when I need to add their wonderfully garlicky, slightly oniony, leek flavor to a soup, frozen ones are perfect.

The beautiful velvety texture comes from puréeing the first five ingredients – do not forget the puréeing technique. The magic ingredient is the nutmeg at the end.

Ingredients
- 1 tbsp oil
- ½ large onion, minced
- ¼ cup chopped celery
- 1 leek, white and tender green parts only, sliced
- 2 garlic cloves, minced
- 2 cups vegetable broth (divided in half)
- 1 cup cooked pearled barley
- 2 bay leaves
- 1 thyme sprig or ¼ tsp dried thyme
- 1 parsnip, peeled and cut into ½-inch pieces
- 1 medium Yukon potato, peeled and cut into ½-inch pieces
- ¼ tsp grated nutmeg
- Salt and pepper to taste

For the Garnish
- Chopped parsley

Instructions
Heat oil in a saucepan over medium heat.
Add the onion, celery and leek and sauté until soft and golden, about 5-10 minutes.
Add the garlic and sauté for 30 seconds.
Add 1 cup of broth, the bay leaves and thyme, and simmer for 10 minutes.
Remove the bay leaves and thyme sprig. Place mixture in a blender, or use a hand immersion blender in the saucepan, and blend the mixture until smooth.
Add the mixture back to the saucepan. Add the remaining 1 cup of broth, the parsnip, and potatoes.
Return the bay leaves and thyme sprig.
Simmer the soup until the vegetables are soft.
Remove the bay leaves.
Add the cooked barley and heat for 5-10 minutes.
Add the nutmeg and salt and pepper to taste.
Garnish with chopped parsley.

Elevate This: Grated carrot will provide color and sweetness. Add croutons, a gentle sprinkling of parmesan (dairy or non-dairy), or a handful of spinach.

Serves 2 as a soup dish

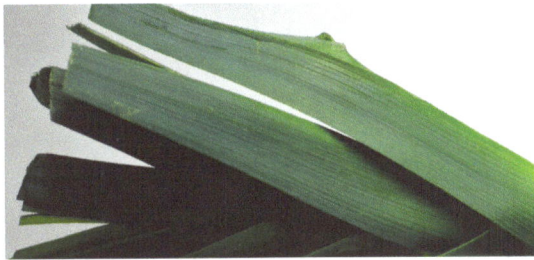
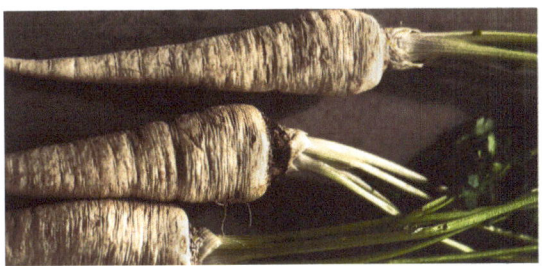
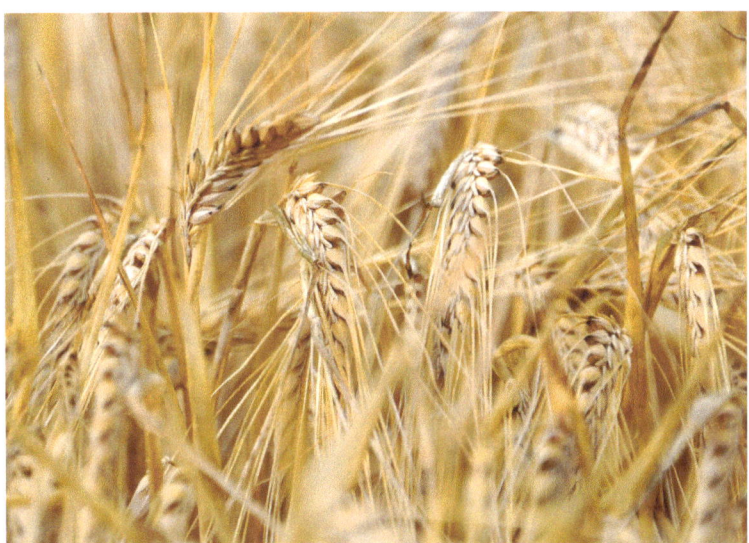

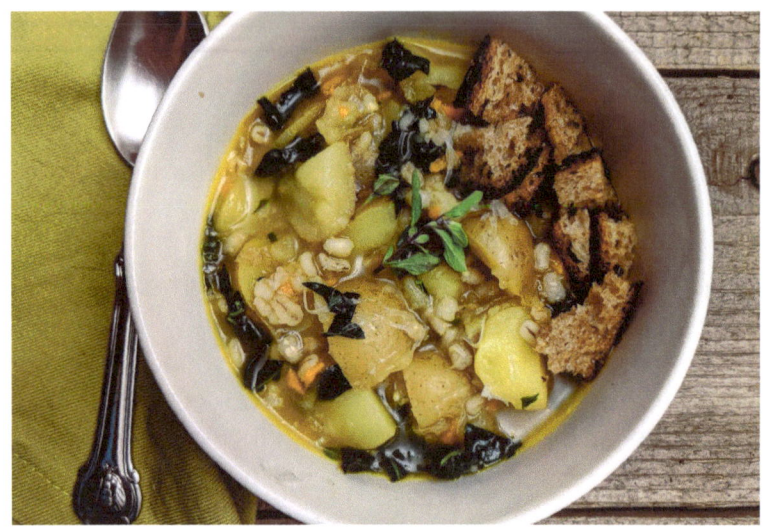
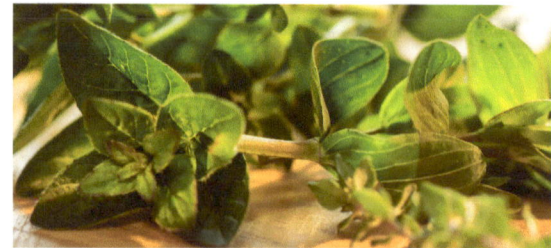
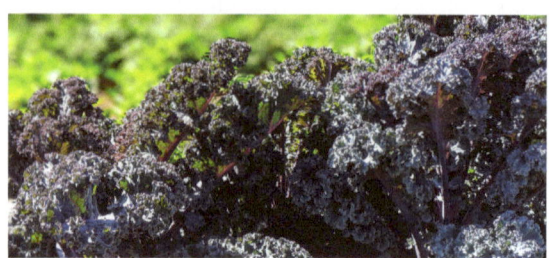

KALE, BEAN, POTATO, AND MARJORAM SOUP

Here in Colorado, it's amazing what the small farmers are able to overcome to grow beautiful vegetables. The soil is marginal in some areas, especially backyard and community gardens. It may require amendment through soil regeneration or biodynamic farming, shifting to raised beds for backyard gardeners, and using hoop gardening or green houses for the cooler months. We are at altitude, and contrary to the number of trees, lakes and green grasslands in view, we are classified as an arid climate getting roughly 14 inches of precipitation per year. Houston, the city that I moved from, is known to get that much precipitation in one day.

I bought some kale and potatoes at the Larimer County Farmers Market. The kale was so beautiful, and the potatoes reminded me of digging up potatoes in my grandmother's garden in Texas. After scoping out what I had in the fridge, I discovered leftover cannellini beans and marjoram. I love marjoram and its sweet yet earthy flavor. When I rub the leaves between my fingers and smell it, it reminds me of my mother. It is the gentler member of the mint and oregano family but really has neither flavor. It's popular in middle European cooking – think Czech Republic, Slovakia, Eastern Russia. If you use fresh marjoram, add it at the end. If you use dried, add it before the simmering process to allow time for the leaves to rehydrate a bit.

Ingredients
- 1 tsp oil
- ½ onion, minced
- 2 cloves garlic, minced
- 2 cups chopped and massaged kale (Massaging helps break down the cell structure so you won't have tough greens in your soup. This is particularly helpful if you are in a hurry and don't have time for your soup to simmer. The extra few minutes of massaging really does help speed up your soup.)
- 1 cup cannellini beans (canned are fine); rinse and drain, reserve the liquid
- 6-8 baby Dutch or baby red potatoes, steamed and quartered
- 2 cups vegetable broth
- 1 tbsp chopped fresh marjoram, or 1 tsp dried marjoram
- 1 tbsp porcini powder

For the Garnish
- Grated carrot

Instructions
Heat the oil in a saucepan over medium heat.
Add the onion and sauté until golden.
Add the garlic and sauté 30 seconds. Do not let burn.
Add the vegetable broth and bring to a boil.
Add the kale, beans, potatoes, porcini powder and dried marjoram (or, if using fresh marjoram, see instructions below). Lower heat and simmer for 15-20 minutes until kale is tender.
Check your broth – if you prefer a thicker soup, add ¼-½ cup of the reserved bean liquid and simmer the soup another 10 minutes or so.
If using fresh instead of dried marjoram, add the fresh marjoram now.
Garnish with the grated carrot.

Elevate This: Serve over farro or brown rice for a fuller dish. Top with parmesan (dairy or non-dairy). Add a crunchy topping using nutritional yeast, seeds, and nuts. Substitute oregano, thyme—or both—or a sprig of rosemary, although the experience of marjoram is out of this world and the intention of this recipe.

Serves 2 as a soup dish

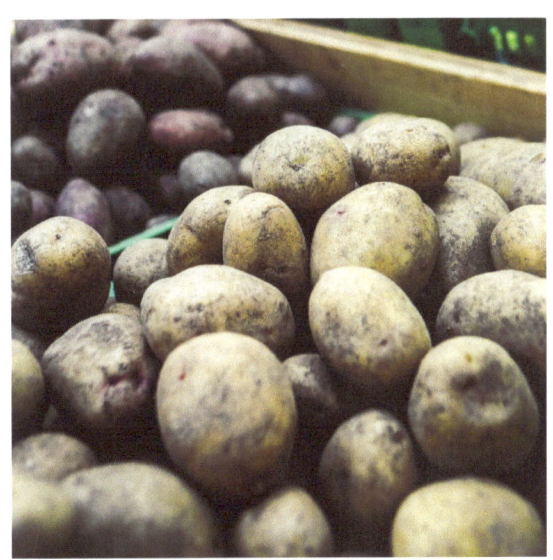

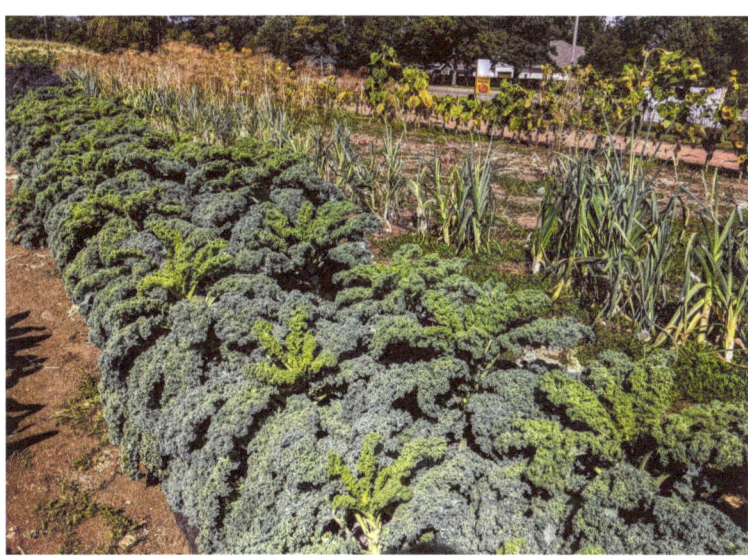

PORCINI WHITE BEAN ROSEMARY SOUP

When I think of an Italian winter soup, my mind goes to this soup. I have made this soup for years, and it continues to evolve. This dish calls for two kinds of mushrooms – porcini, which are usually found dried, and shiitakes. Multiple mushroom growers offer these options through our local farmers markets. Hope Farms focuses on wild-foraged morels, chanterelles, and dried Oregon porcini (boletes), as well as fresh varieties. This is a simple soup that packs a lot of flavor. The fresh rosemary adds special warmth to an already comforting soup.

Ingredients

- 1 cup boiled water
- 1 ounce dried porcini mushrooms
- 1 cup vegetable or chicken broth
- 1 tbsp olive oil
- ½ small onion, minced
- 2 garlic cloves, minced
- 4 ounces fresh shiitake mushrooms, stems removed and sliced
- ½ cup chopped fresh tomato (or canned tomatoes will work)
- One 4-inch sprig fresh rosemary
- 1 can cannellini (or similar) white beans, rinsed and drained
- Salt and pepper to taste

Instructions

Place the dried mushrooms in the hot water and steep for 10 minutes.
Drain the mushrooms through a sieve and reserve the liquid.
Slice the porcini mushrooms.
Add the mushroom liquid to the vegetable broth.
In a saucepan over medium heat, heat the olive oil.
Add the onion and garlic and sauté until golden.
Add the shiitake mushrooms and sauté until soft.
Add the tomatoes and porcini mushrooms and sauté for 2-3 minutes.
Add the broth, rosemary and beans. Cover and cook over low heat for 10-15 minutes to allow the rosemary to permeate the soup. Salt and pepper to taste.
Garnish with more rosemary and serve in soup bowls.

Elevate This: Serve this over a grain such as barley or farro. Sprinkle with Crispy Capers (p. 168) or lentils.

Serves 2 as a soup dish

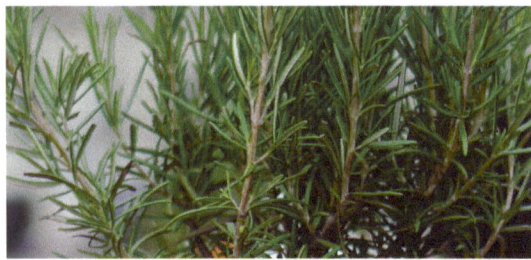

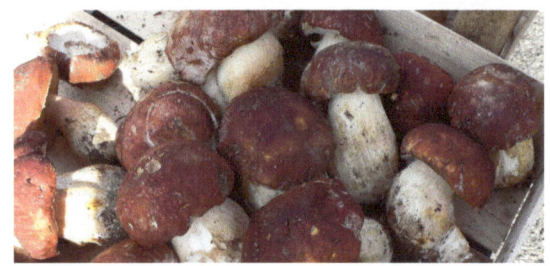

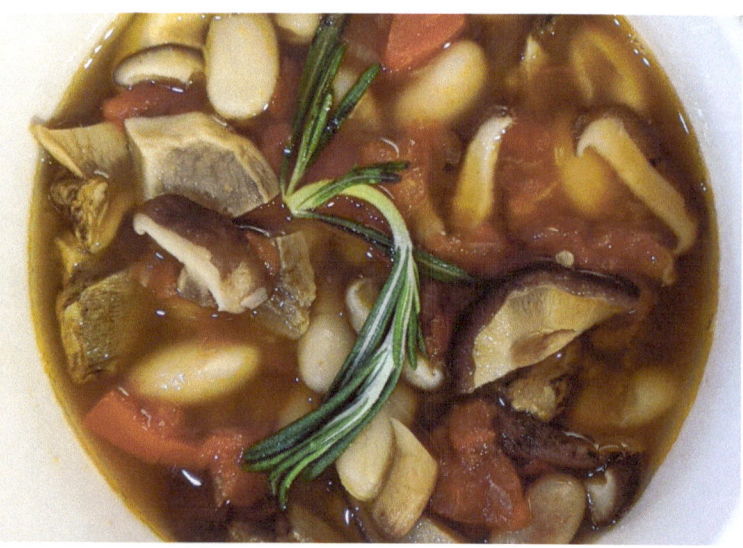

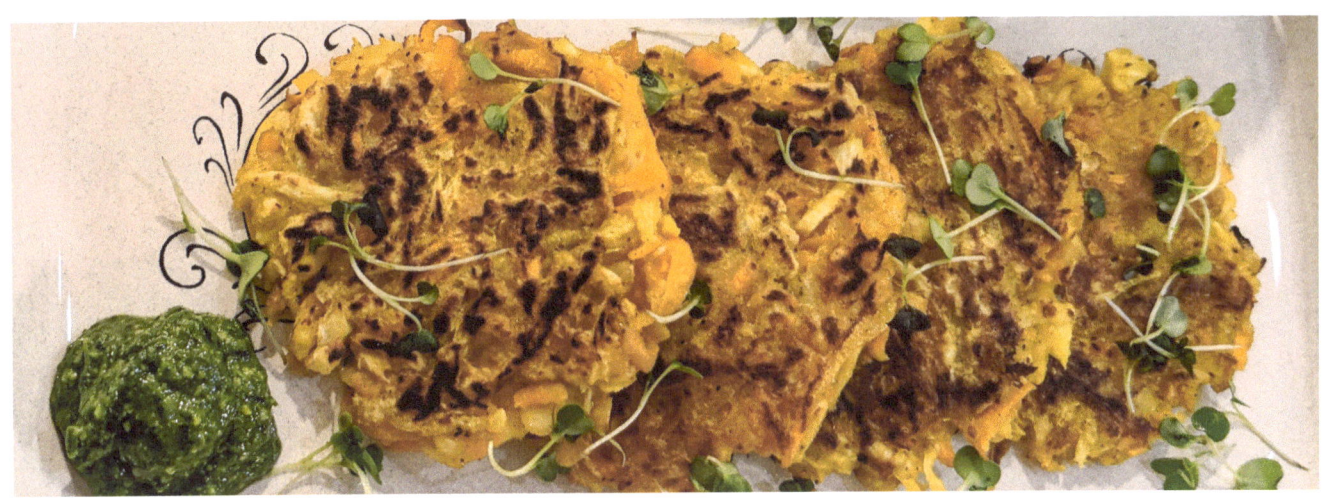

PARSNIP CARROT LATKES

Latkes are of Russian, German, Austrian, and Polish origins. Our hash brown patties in the freezer section are a nod to this lowly peasant food that can be elevated with different vegetables, spices and toppings. These are super easy to make. Enjoy this version with the sometimes passed-over parsnip.

Ingredients
- 1 carrot, peeled and grated
- 1 parsnip, peeled and grated
- 1 tbsp minced onion or shallot
- ¼ tsp salt
- 1 tbsp flour or cornstarch
- 1 egg or 1 tbsp egg replacement (ie. JUST Egg)
- ½ tsp baking powder
- 1 tsp asafetida
- 1 tsp turmeric
- ½ tsp black pepper
- Oil for pan frying

Instructions
Preheat oven to 300°F (for warming).
Place the grated carrot, parsnip, onion and salt in a paper towel and squeeze out any moisture.
Let stand for 15 minutes. Pat dry.
In a bowl, add the drained vegetables to the next 6 ingredients and mix thoroughly. The mixture should hold together but not be mushy. Add a little more flour if mixture is too wet.
Add 1-2 tbsp of oil to a skillet and heat over medium. Make round balls using 2 tbsp of the mixture, then flatten into 3-inch latkes and place onto heated skillet. Cook only 3-4 latkes at a time (do not crowd), flattening with a spatula. Cook until crispy on one side. Flip, flatten again, and cook until golden and crispy. Place cooked latkes on a sheet pan and keep warm in oven until all latkes are cooked.

Elevate This: This is a basic recipe to learn the latke technique. Instead of asafetida and turmeric, play with different spice mixtures to create a different cuisine experience. Russet or Yukon Gold potatoes are traditional, but sweet potatoes, purple potatoes, and colorful yams work well. Squeeze out as much moisture from the veg as possible for a crispier result.

Makes 8 3-inch latkes

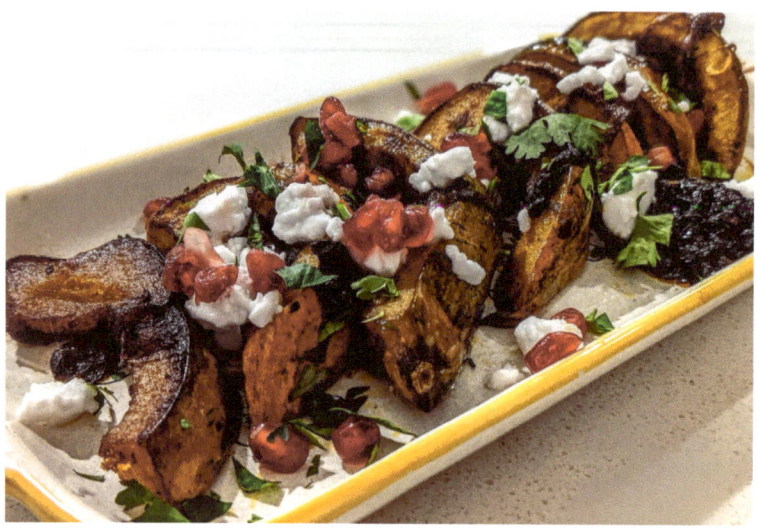
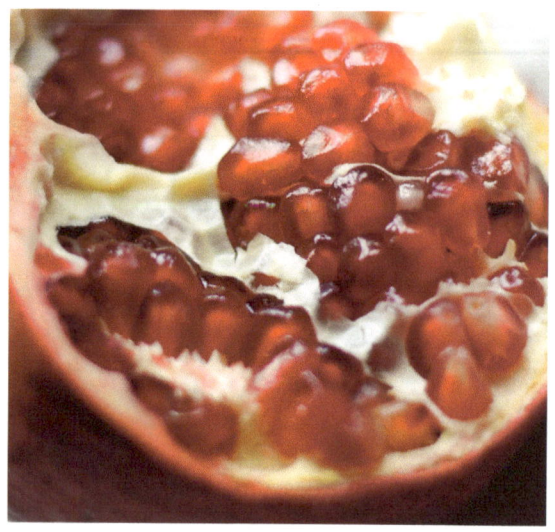

SMOKY ACORN SQUASH WITH POMEGRANATE AND FETA

Many of us may have memories of growing up with the usual brown sugar and cinnamon acorn squash. I was not a particular fan of this type of squash. An acorn squash from my CSA had been staring at me for a week, so I gave it a try with a Middle Eastern touch. Roasted in a smoked paprika chile pomegranate molasses wash, topped with feta (dairy or non-dairy), poms, and caramelized onions is a well-rounded tasty blend of sweet, spicy, salty, and a bit of tartness. Pomegranate molasses is a reduction of pomegranate juice. Do not substitute regular molasses. A reasonable substitute is an infused dark balsamic vinegar, such as Black Mission Fig Dark or Cinnamon Pear Dark – although not quite the same, it will still be delicious.

Ingredients

- 1 acorn squash, sliced into wedges and seeds removed
- ½ red onion, thinly sliced
- 2 tbsp olive oil
- 1 tbsp smoked paprika
- 2 tbsp pomegranate molasses (do not substitute regular molasses)
- ¼ tsp dried chile flakes
- ½ tsp salt

For the Garnish
- Feta (dairy or non-dairy), crumbled
- Chopped cilantro
- Pomegranate arils (seeds)

Instructions

Preheat the oven to 350°F.
Prepare a sheet pan with foil and non-stick spray.
In a large bowl, mix together the oil, paprika, pomegranate molasses, chile flakes and salt.
Add the squash and onion, and coat well. You may use a silicone brush or spoon to help coat the squash.
Place the squash and onion mixture on the sheet pan and bake for 25-30 minutes until the squash is tender.
Place the squash in a serving dish and top with the bits of remaining caramelized onion from the pan.
Sprinkle squash with crumbled feta (dairy or non-dairy), chopped cilantro, and pomegranate seeds.

Elevate This: Sprinkle roasted and chopped pistachio nuts. Lightly drizzle with a medium or bold extra virgin olive oil.

Serves 2-3 as a side dish

KURBIS STUMFUS

(Pumpkin and Potato Mash) *This dish popped up during my research of Germans from Russia. "Kurbis" is an old German word for pumpkin. Google cannot find the translation for the word "stumfus," but the Germans from Russia blog indicated that stumfus is "potatoes". Regardless, I think Kurbis Stumfus sounds much more interesting than pumpkin and potatoes, don't you? Some serve this dish as a mash. Others add a bit of flour and cottage cheese and reimagine the mash into dumplings. I went with mash. I love combining two vegetables and improving the taste of one of the veg substantially. I know, it's too simple to put in a cookbook, but that is the point – start simple, then elevate. The original recipe calls for lard, but we won't go there.*

Ingredients
- 1 cup pumpkin or winter squash, puréed (see p. 101)
- 2 Yukon Gold potatoes
- Salt and pepper to taste
- 2-3 tbsp butter (dairy or non-dairy), melted
- ½ onion, minced (optional)

Instructions
Steam or boil the potatoes until a fork easily pierces the flesh. Cool and peel.
Place the pumpkin, potatoes, and optional onions in a food processor and gently pulse the vegetables until lumpy. Do not overprocess.
Add the melted butter (dairy or non-dairy) to the mixture. Pulse gently again until smooth.
Salt and pepper to taste.

Elevate This: Garnish with crispy shallots or Crispy Capers (p. 168). Sprinkle with smoked paprika, crispy lentils, or toasted panko bread crumbs. A drizzle of garlic olive oil will be a nice touch.

Serves 2 as a side dish

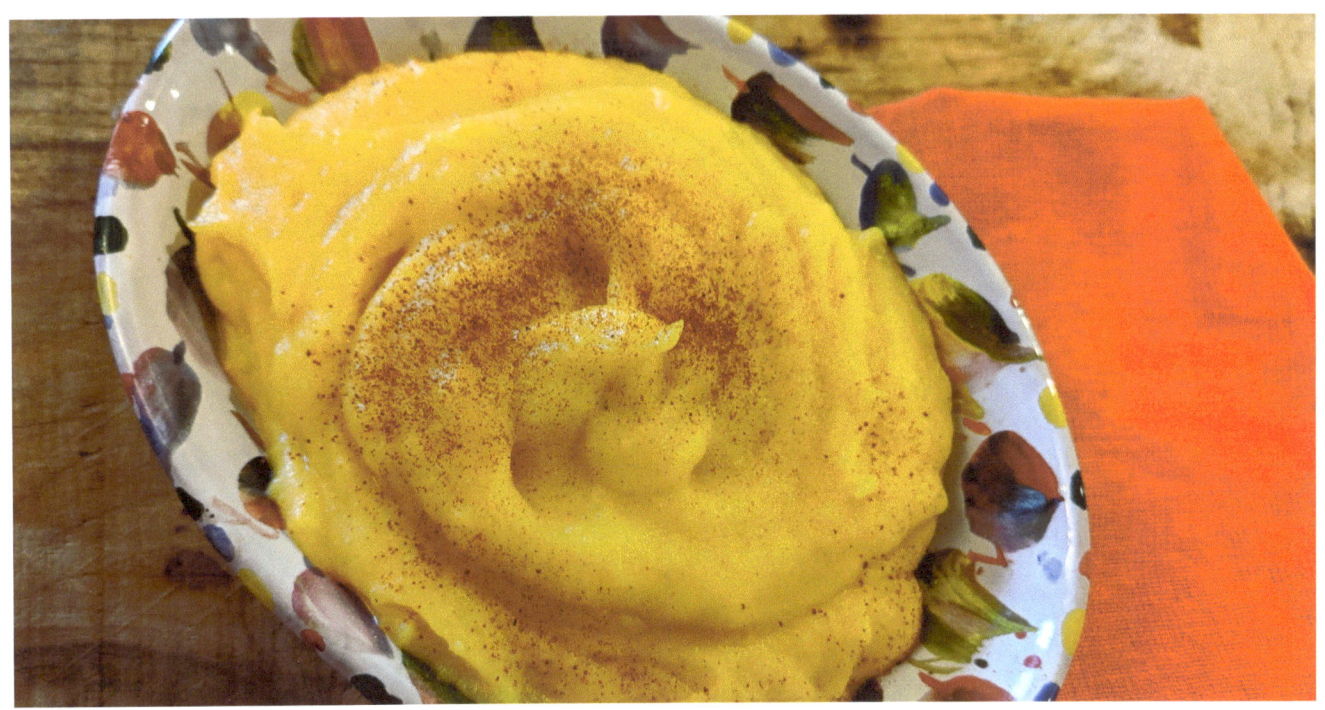

FRENCH STYLE LETTUCE AND PEAS

You are simply not going to believe that braised lettuce is good. Not just good, but even great. Lettuce has a very short season here, unless of course you are growing tender greens via hydroponics, green house, or hoop beds in Winter. This recipe comes together easily on the stove top and may be a new technique to add to your repertoire. These vegs look exceptionally beautiful in this artfulbowl, handmade by Danyelle Butler of ArtHausCeramics.

Ingredients

- 1 head butterhead-style lettuce (such as Mervailles des Quatres Saisons, Passion Brune, or similar)
- ½ cup shelled peas (frozen or fresh)
- 1 tsp olive oil
- ½ cup vegetable broth
- 1 tbsp flour
- 2 tsp butter (dairy or non-dairy)
- Salt and pepper to taste

Instructions

Make a *beurre manié* by combining the flour and butter (dairy or non-dairy) with your fingers into a thick paste.

Heat the oil over medium heat in a skillet. Add the lettuce and sauté for 2-3 minutes.

Add the peas and ½ the vegetable broth. Cover with a lid and let steam for 2-3 minutes.

Remove the lid and add the remaining broth and *beurre manié*.

Mixture will thicken, become nice and glossy, and will coat the lettuce and peas. Do not overcook. Braise just until nicely wilted.

Salt and pepper to taste.

Elevate This: Garnish with white or black sesame seeds, sliced and toasted almonds, or toasted panko bread crumbs. Add some pea shoots or curls.

Serves 2 as a side dish

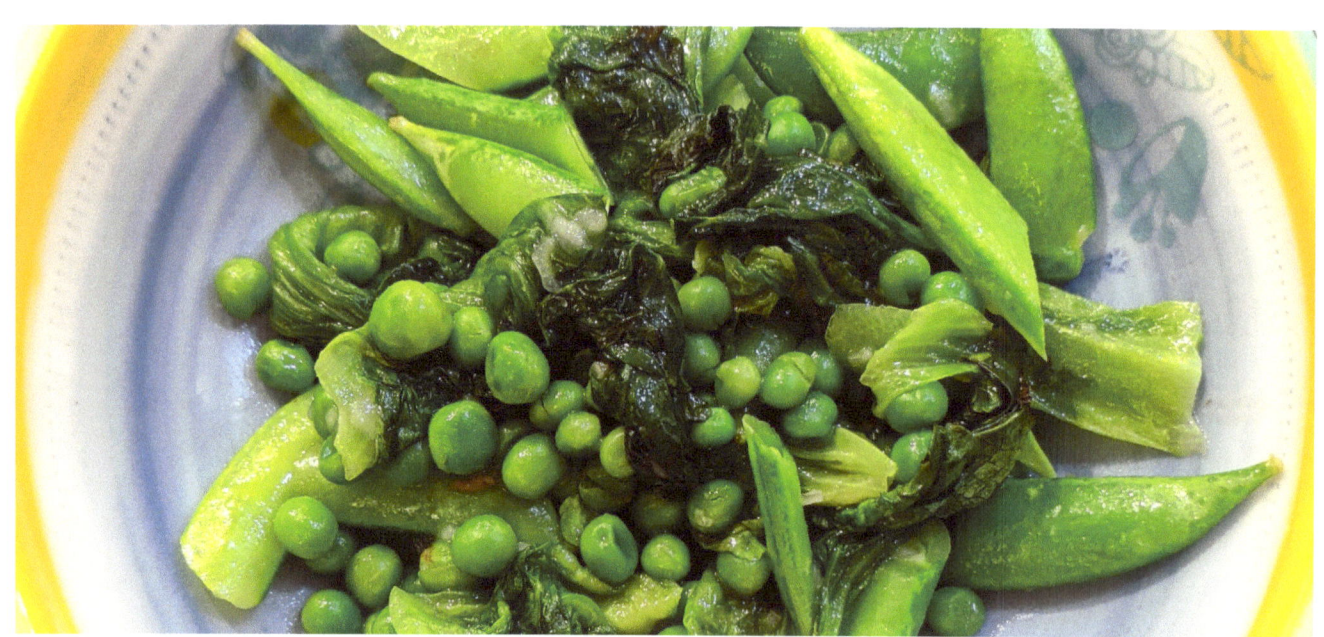

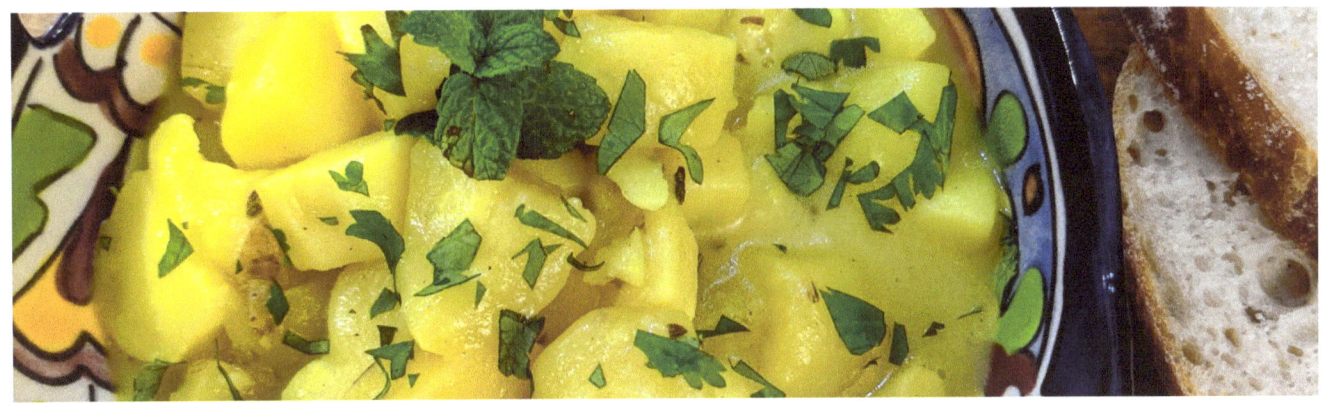

INDIAN SAFFRON POTATOES IN COCONUT MILK

Since our trip to Ireland, my husband and I have eaten a LOT of potatoes. Potatoes have been given bad press in the past, but they provided primary sustenance to the Irish throughout the 19th century, and to the Prussian Army in the 18th century. They are loaded with vitamins and minerals; and if steamed, offer a nice quick snack with a bit of sea salt. Multiple CSAs and growers offer different varieties of local potatoes including purple and steak fingerlings. My favorites are purple, but I don't think that would have been a good color match for this dish. To speed up this dish, purchase ready-made garlic paste and ginger paste from Olive Tree Market or your favorite local Mediterranean market.

There are at least five recipes with saffron in this cookbook – as you can see, I love saffron. Although expensive, it doesn't take a lot to flavor a dish. Whenever I have leftover saffron water, I freeze or reuse it in another dish.

Ingredients
- 1 lb baby Dutch potatoes, steamed for 12 min. in Instant Pot
- 1 garlic clove, minced
- 1-inch piece of fresh ginger, minced or grated
- 1 tbsp oil
- 1 tsp fennel seed, crushed
- ½ tsp ground turmeric
- Freshly grated nutmeg
- 5-6 saffron threads (or ½ cup of saffron water you may have saved from the saffron pasta, p. 74)
- ½ can full-fat coconut milk
- ½ cup milk (dairy or non-dairy)

For the Garnish
- Chopped mint or cilantro

Instructions
If using saffron threads, gently crush the saffron with your fingers and immerse in ½ cup hot water.
Heat the oil in a skillet over low heat. Add the garlic, ginger, fennel seed, and spices. Stir until fragrant.
Add the potatoes, increase the heat to medium, and stir for 2-3 minutes.
Add the coconut milk, milk (dairy or non-dairy), and the saffron water. Simmer for about 15 minutes.
Garnish with fresh mint or cilantro and serve.

Elevate This: Serve alongside other favorite vegetables, chickpeas, or on top of rice for a complementary grain medley. Other white vegetables will come together with the potatoes, such as kohlrabi or parsnips, or white yams. Purple or dark orange veg will change the color, so a note of caution on mixing veg in this dish. Just enjoy its golden beauty.

Serves 2 as a side dish

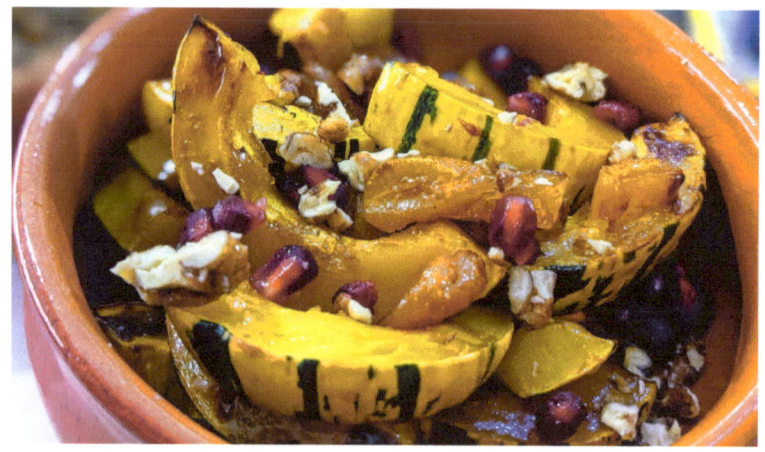
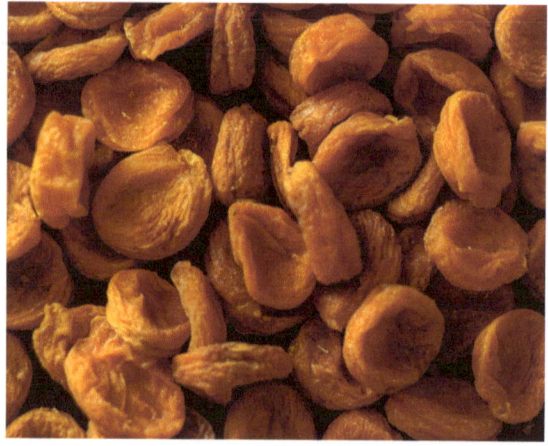
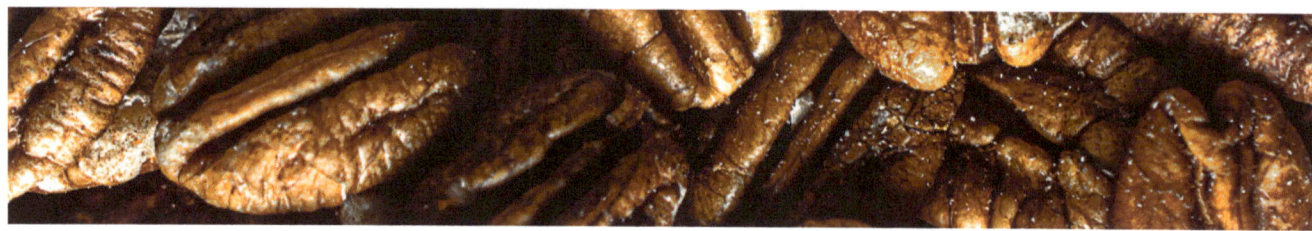

DELICATA SQUASH WITH APRICOTS, POMS, AND PECANS

There are a myriad of squash varieties available – striped, green, yellow, orange, squatty shaped, round, and oblong. My goal this year was to try as many types as possible, in different methods and cuisines. The delicata squash skin is soft enough to eat, so don't take the time to peel – especially since they are a bit small and you may lose some of the soft, golden flesh. I love this technique as the squash is steamed in the oven and then allowed to caramelize for the last 15 minutes. You may find it useful with other vegetable dishes.

Ingredients
- 1 tbsp oil
- ¼ cup water
- 1 delicata squash; sliced into rings, seeds removed, then cut in half moons
- 5-6 dried apricots, slivered
- 2 tbsp honey

For the Garnish
- ¼ cup candied or honey pecans
- ¼ cup pomegranate seeds

Instructions
Preheat oven to 375°F. Prepare a sheet pan with aluminum foil and non-stick spray.
Add the water and oil to the pan.
Arrange the squash on the tray and sprinkle the apricots around the squash.
Drizzle the honey over the squash and apricots.
Cover tightly with foil.
Bake for 15 minutes or until the squash can be pierced easily with a knife or fork.
Uncover the pan, and bake another 15 minutes until the water evaporates and a glaze forms on the squash. Garnish with pecans and pom seeds and serve.

Elevate This: Top with chopped herbs, a bit of feta, a seasoned spice, salt or pepper.

Serves 2-3 as a side dish

SAGE ROASTED SHIITAKES

Roasted shiitakes are a great substitute for meat. Mushrooms have umami, that lovely meaty "je ne sais quoi" – that "thing" that makes you think you are eating something with four legs. The addition of sage elevates these mushrooms. When eating, be sure to get a bite of crunchy sage with your hearty shiitake.

Ingredients
- 8 ounces shiitake mushrooms, sliced if large
- 8 large sage leaves; roughly chop 4 leaves, keep 4 leaves whole
- 1 tbsp oil
- Salt and pepper to taste

Instructions
Preheat oven to 375°F. Line a baking sheet with aluminum foil and spray with cooking spray. Combine all ingredients in a bowl and stir well. Spread on the prepared baking sheet.
Roast for 20-30 minutes until mushrooms have shrunken a bit, but are still soft and have absorbed the liquid. Roast to your preferred consistency and taste. Salt and pepper to taste.
Serve these as a side with rice or over creamy mashed potatoes, or as an elevation to other recipes such as a soup or stir fry.

Elevate This: Alternatively, add 1 tsp soy sauce, 1 tsp mirin, 1 tsp liquid smoke, 1 tsp black pepper, 3-4 shakes of Maggi sauce, and 1 tsp Marmite for a smoked rendition of this dish. Roughly chopped rosemary is also a nice addition.

Serves 2 as a side dish

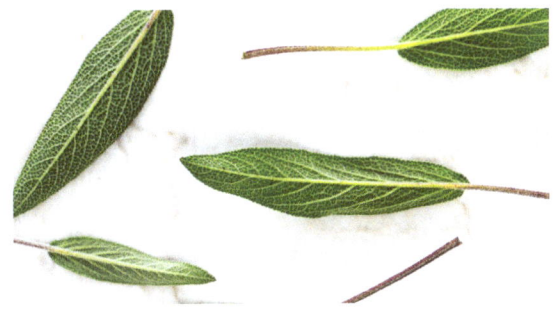
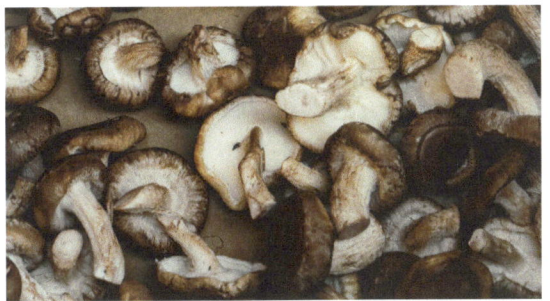
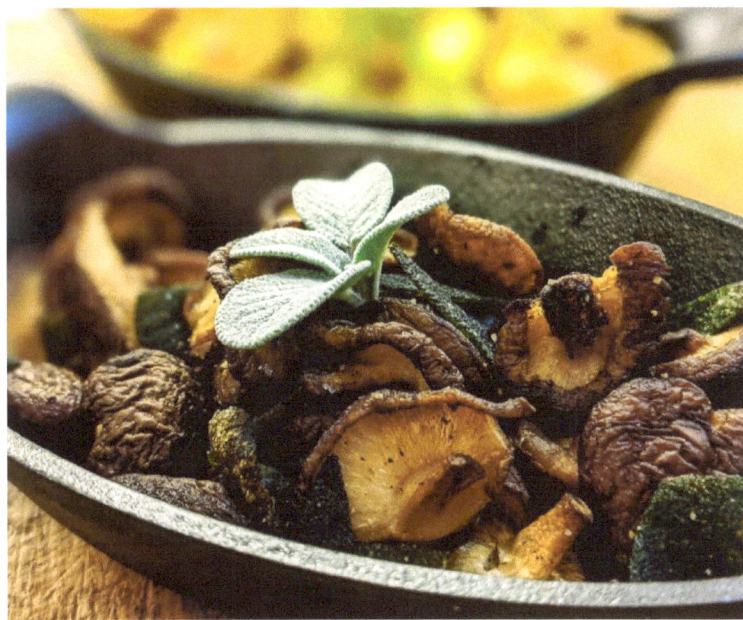

ROASTED BRUSSELS SPROUTS WITH AMARETTO CHERRIES

Brussels sprouts are good just about any way but puréed. For a Thanksgiving dinner, I brought a bag of Brussels sprouts to my in-laws' and decided to wait and see what they had in the pantry. Some of the "fun" in cooking is garnering things from someone else's pantry and testing my knowledge of what might be good together. Sliced, roasted Brussels sprouts were definitely the foundation, but what else did Marg have that would make them stand out? There was a shelf of liquor, a half box of raisins, and a can of fried onions. Sweet, savory, salty, nutty, fruity, veg. Add pepper for some spice. The recipe below is the improved version of the original Raisin Amaretto Roasted Brussels Sprouts using locally grown Brussels sprouts. Can you see the pattern for pulling together a plant-dish? Remember fruit, veg, seed, nut, herb, spice, and grain.

Ingredients
- 1 lb or 12 Brussels sprouts, cleaned and thinly sliced (you can buy bags of shaved sprouts)
- ½ cup dried cherries (or raisins, cranberries, etc.)
- ¼ cup amaretto (Cointreau works well too)
- 1 tbsp olive or avocado oil
- ½ shallot, finely sliced
- 1 tsp oil
- Salt and pepper to taste

For the Garnish
- ¼ cup candied or honey pecans

Instructions
Preheat the oven to 375°F.
Cover a sheet pan with aluminum foil and spray with cooking spray.
Combine the cherries and amaretto in a bowl. Heat them for 60 seconds in the microwave, then allow to cool and rehydrate for about 10 minutes.
Place the sprouts in a bowl. Sprinkle with the olive or avocado oil. Stir. Salt and pepper to taste.
Drain the cherries and reserve liquid. Add the soaked cherries to the sprouts and stir.
Pour the Brussels sprouts onto the prepared baking sheet and bake for 10-15 minutes, stirring every 5 minutes. The edges should be brown but not burnt. (I used a convection oven and the sprouts were done in 10 minutes.)
Remove sprouts from the oven and stir in 1 tbsp of the reserved amaretto.
Place the shallots in a small bowl. Add 1 tsp oil and a dash of salt, and mix well. Microwave for 1-minute intervals until soft and caramelized.
Place the Brussels sprouts in a serving dish and sprinkle them with the caramelized shallots.
Garnish with candied or honey pecans.

Elevate This: Sprinkle a bit of dairy or non-dairy feta, blue cheese, or queso fresco. Think about different textures, complementary tastes and colors. Use crispy beets or jalapeño strips, chopped and roasted pistachios, or pine nuts.

Serves 3-4 as a side dish

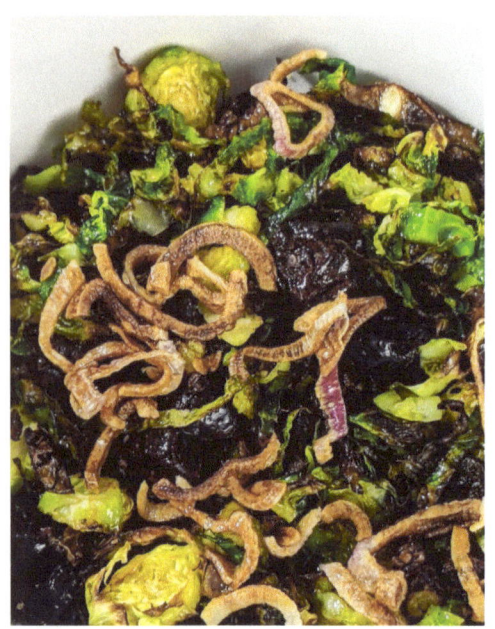

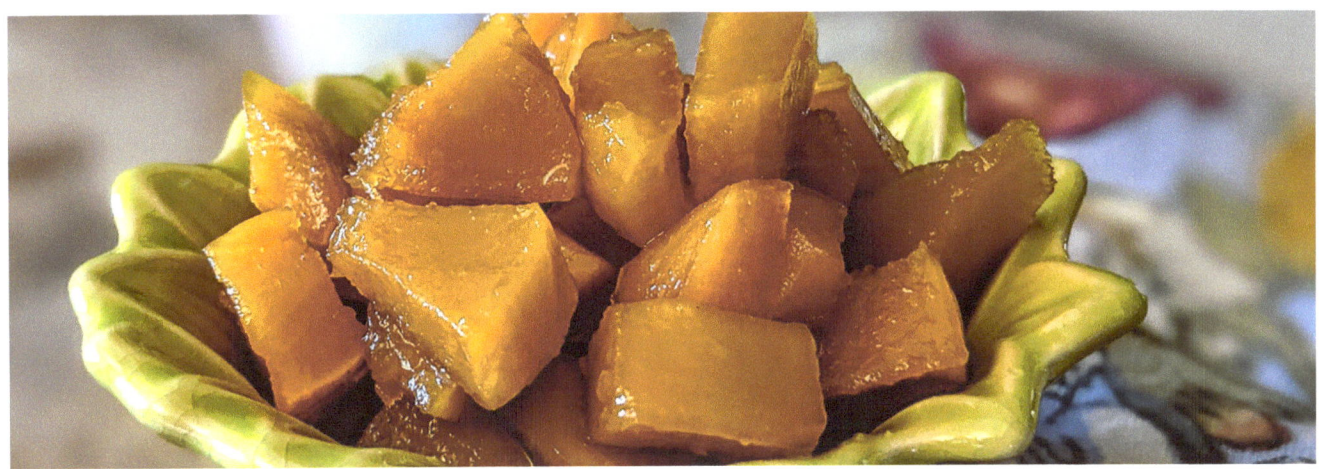

GOLDEN PUMPKIN CHIPS

Northern Colorado was home to many small farmers, and their legacies—in many cases—were having a housing development in their name. I live in Nelson Farm, which was once a dairy farm. Rigden Farms is nearby. The original farmers, Cora and Ed Johnson, owned several hundred acres of land, which is now midtown Fort Collins, and has transitioned to housing developments including Parkwood East, English Ranch, Rigden Farms, and the Jessup Farm Artisan Village. In the day, the Johnsons farmed sugar beets and soybeans, corn for feed, and barley for Coors. In addition, they raised sheep and cattle. One of their final legacies to the area is the wonderful Edora Park – artfully named for Ed and Cora.

Rigden Farms has one of the original farmhouses utilized as a community building. It also has one of the most magnificently managed community gardens in the area. Walking or cycling by, one can take pause and enjoy pumpkins and melons peeping out under leaves, vines laden with tomatoes and a multitude of flowers and herbs.

During my research of Rigden Farm, I discovered this recipe in a 1948 Timnath Columbine Club vintage cookbook the Johnsons' grandson gave me to peruse. Among all customary post-war recipes of cakes, pies, meatloaf, and dinner in a dish, this recipe from Mrs. Paul Peasley caught my eye. Per the website, The Columbine Club is Timnath's historical society. Organized by Helen White Rigden and Alta Lewis Bush, this women's club first met in the Timnath home of Mrs. Tom Black in September 1907. The club was originally a study group that met to discuss timely topics such as gardening, homemaking, children, fine arts, patriotism, and education. Meetings were held the first and third Thursdays of the month, and dues were fifty cents. In 1908, the Club became affiliated with the Colorado Federation of Women's Clubs and the General Federation of Women's Clubs. The club flower was the Columbine, and the colors were lavender and yellow. Edna Wilkins Elliott suggested the club motto: "The measure of our growth is not what we gain, but what we give." Fun Fact: Per Mrs. Peasley – use fresh not crystallized ginger. In 1948, you may have had to find the fresh ginger root at the drug store.

Ingredients
- 2 cups fresh pumpkin, peeled and diced
- 2 cups granulated sugar
- Juice and grated rind of ½ lemon
- 1-inch piece of fresh ginger root, peeled and grated or finely chopped

Instructions
Place all the ingredients in a bowl and mix well.
Cover and place in refrigerator overnight.
Cook in a saucepan or skillet until the pumpkin has a clear and transparent gold color.
Pairs well with meat or served with vanilla ice cream, although I found it delightful on a spoon!

Serves 2 as a side dish

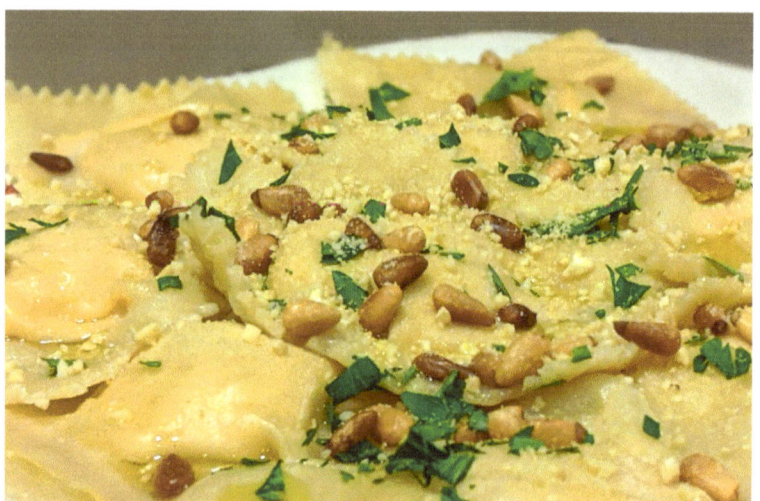
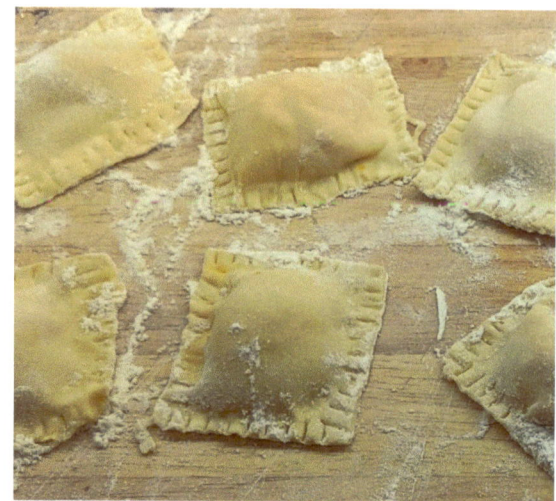
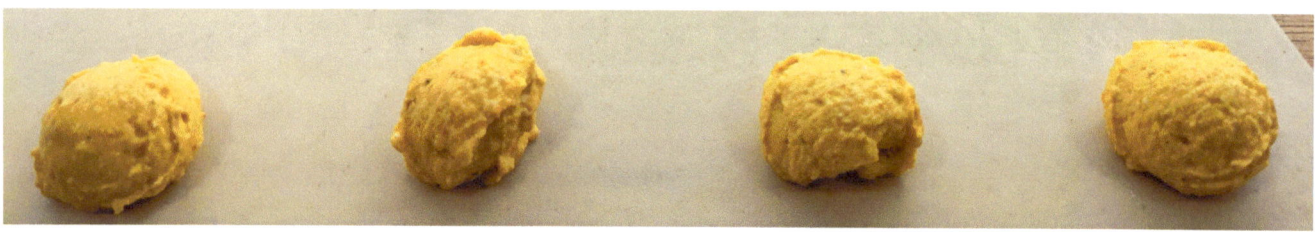

PUMPKIN RAVIOLI

Making fresh ravioli can be a labor of love, but it is worth every bit of effort. Playing with the dough and working with your hands to bring it together is part of the art. This is a tender ravioli made with pumpkin purée, but this recipe will also work well with butternut squash. These are rustic ravioli – they don't have to be perfect, except in taste!

Ingredients

For the Pasta Dough
- 1 ½ cups flour
- 2 whole eggs or 4 tbsp liquid egg replacement (ie. JUST Egg)
- 1 tbsp oil
- Water

For the Filling
- 1 cup pumpkin purée
- ½ cup ricotta cheese (dairy or non-dairy)
- 1 tsp ultimate umami spice mixture from The Spice and Tea Exchange®, or similar

For the Garnish
- Olive oil
- Grated parmesan (dairy or non-dairy)
- Toasted pine nuts
- Chopped parsley

Instructions

For the Pasta Dough
Add the first 3 pasta ingredients in a food processor, and pulse until combined.
Add enough water to bring the dough together.
Use either the food processor or hand knead the dough on a board until the dough is light to the touch (not sticky), and springs back just a bit when you dent with your finger.
Flatten the dough into a disk, place on a plate, cover, and let sit for 30 minutes to an hour.
Combine all the filling ingredients in a bowl. Mix well.

Assemble
Cut the dough in half and keep the remaining half covered on the plate.
Roll out the dough into a ⅛-inch thick rectangle, or less. Cut the dough into 4-inch-wide lengths.
Using a small scoop or spoon, place a 1-inch round of filling 2 inches apart on the rolled-out dough.
With a pastry brush, wet the edges of the dough and in between the filling balls.
Fold the dough over and press the dough well, between each ball of filling. Pat the filling down just a bit, then cut the dough into ravioli squares.
At this point, you may leave as is, crimp with a fork, or cut the edges with a rolling pastry design cutter. Place the shaped ravioli on a sheet pan and refrigerate until ready to cook.

Let's Cook
Bring a large pot of water to boil. Add salt.
Boil 3-4 ravioli at a time so they have room to move around and not stick to each other.
When they float to the top, they are ready. Scoop out and drain well.

Plate the ravioli and garnish with a drizzle of olive oil, grated parmesan (dairy or non-dairy), toasted pine nuts, and chopped parsley. Less is more.

Elevate This: This ravioli is very mild in taste, but very full-bodied. The extra flavor should come from the garnishes, so consider a flavorful oil varietal with a bold or spicy taste.

Makes 12-15 ravioli. Serves 6 as a small plate, or 3-4 as a main dish.

ESPINACAS CON GARBANZOS

(Chickpeas with Spinach) *This tapas dish is a great small plate for dinner. Kale can also be used as a leafy green replacement for the spinach. Practice and play with different types of smoked paprika, or combine them for your own unique take on this dish.*

Ingredients
- 1 tbsp olive oil
- 3 garlic cloves, minced
- 1-2 tsp hot smoked paprika
- ¼ tsp chile flakes
- ¼ tsp cinnamon
- 1 tsp cumin
- ½ tsp dried oregano
- Dash of freshly grated nutmeg
- Dash of cinnamon
- Pinch of sugar
- ½ cup plain tomato sauce or crushed tomatoes
- 4-5 saffron strands, melted in ⅛ cup hot water
- 1 can garbanzo (chickpeas), drained and rinsed
- 1-2 handfuls baby spinach, or stemmed and roughly chopped large spinach or kale
- Salt and pepper to taste

Instructions
In a large skillet, heat the oil over medium heat.
Add the garlic and warm for 30 seconds.
Add the rest of the spices to the pan and allow the spices to bloom.
Add the tomatoes and sugar to the pan, and cook the mixture until it thickens.
Add the garbanzo beans, spinach or kale, saffron water and salt.
Cover and simmer over medium low heat for 20-30 minutes.
If necessary, add small amounts of water if the mixture becomes dry or too thick to cook the leafy greens.
Salt and pepper to taste.

Elevate This: If you have leftovers, they marry well in a whole grain wrap with leftover potatoes, winter squash, more fresh spinach or kale, Microgreen Pistou (p. 129), and a drizzle of harissa. A perfect lunch or dinner for a busy day.

Serves 2 as a small plate

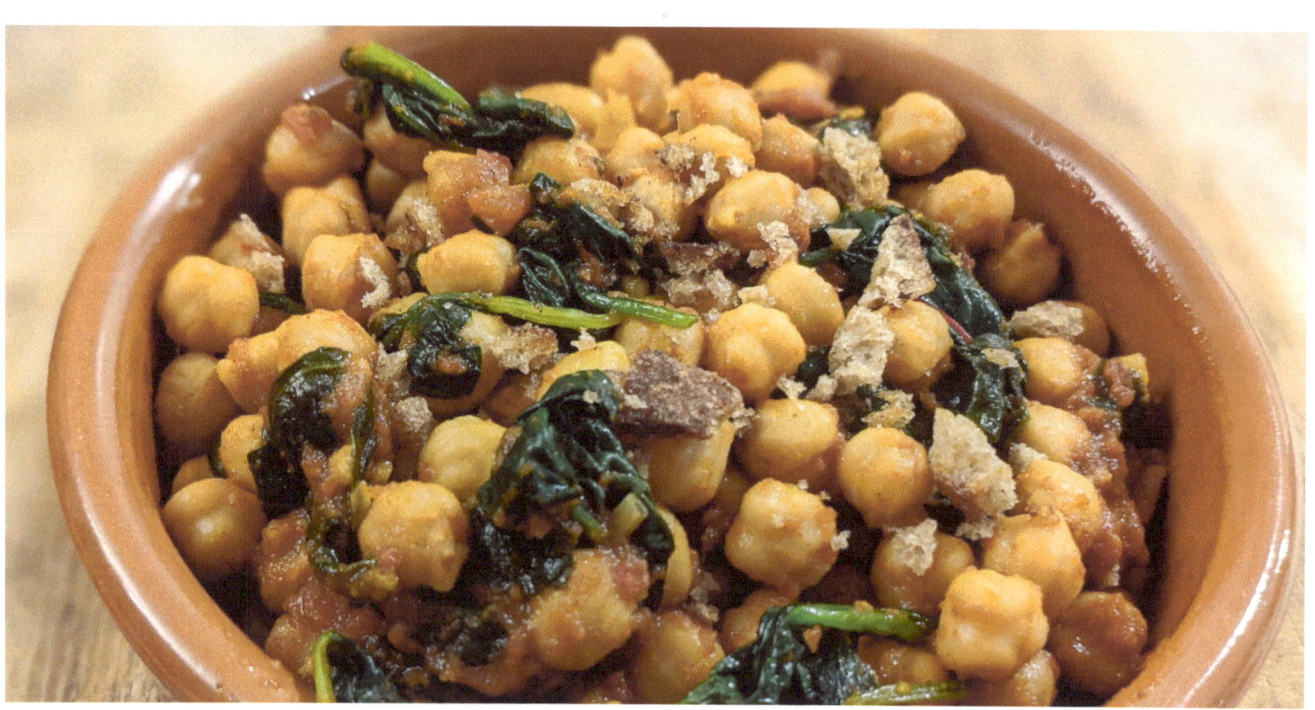

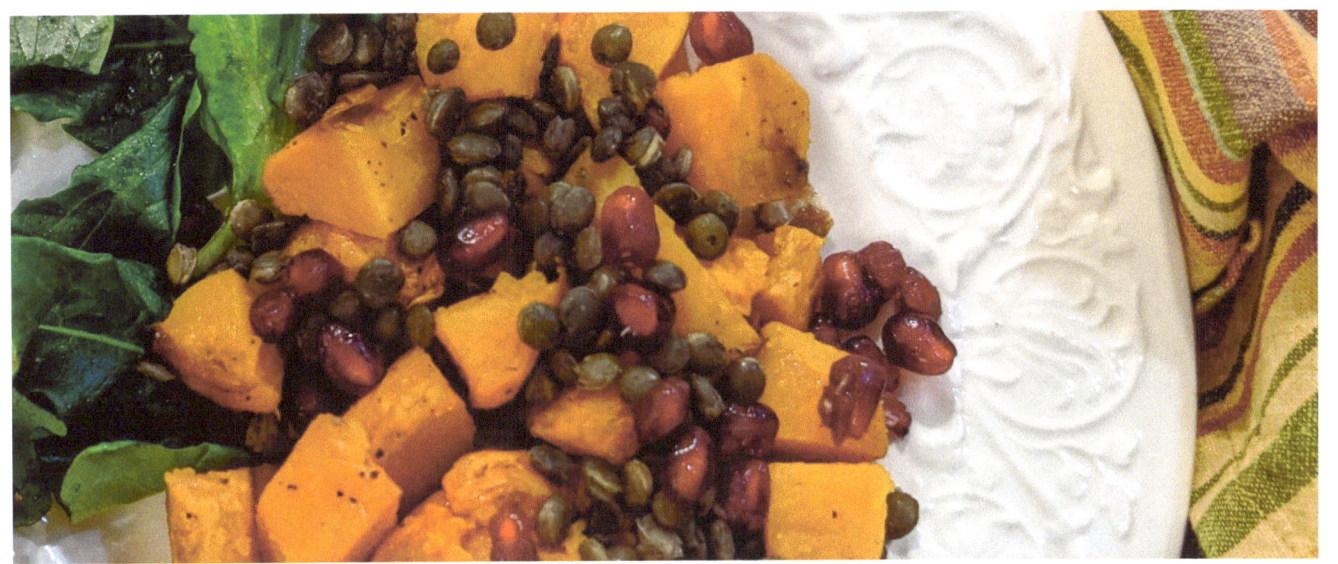

BUTTERNUT SQUASH, TOASTED LENTILS, AND POMS

This dish can be a salad or small plate, or part of a larger main dish. It's also colorful enough for a holiday small plate, especially at Thanksgiving when a pop of orange on the dining table ushers in the harvest look. To save time, refer to the briefing in this cookbook on how to prep and store squash (p. 100). Pumpkin or sweet potatoes are great substitutes for butternut squash.

Ingredients
- 2 cups butternut squash, cut into ½-inch or 1-inch cubes
- 1 tbsp oil
- 1-2 tsp interesting spice mixture (Mediterranean blend, Tuscan, Italian, berbere, etc.)
- 1 tsp brown sugar
- Salt and pepper
- ½ cup French lentils, cooked and drained
- 1 tbsp nutritional yeast (optional but gives depth)
- Dash of garlic powder
- Dash of onion powder
- A few lettuce leaves

For the Garnish
- 2-3 tbsp pomegranate arils (seeds)
- Extra virgin olive oil

Instructions
Preheat oven to 400°F. Prepare 2 sheet pans with aluminum foil, parchment paper, or a silicone mat. Place the first 5 ingredients in a bowl and mix well. Spread on the first prepared baking pan and roast for 20-30 minutes or until the squash is fork tender and caramelized. Stir every 10-15 minutes.

In a bowl, mix the lentils, yeast, garlic and onion powders, and salt and pepper. Spread on the second sheet pan and roast with the pumpkin for 10-15 minutes until crunchy, but not burned.

On a salad plate, lay a couple of colorful lettuce leaves on the plate. Spread 1 cup of the roasted butternut squash on the lettuce. Place the toasted lentils on the squash. Garnish with the pomegranate arils and drizzle lightly with a bold extra virgin olive oil.

Elevate This: Review the *Cuisine-Related Pairings* chart (p. 167). Pair fresh or dried herbs, and a nut, seed, or spice with your selection. Use the Grated Garlic Dressing (p. 50) to add some zest to the lettuce.

Serves 2 as a main plate

Beans - They're What's For Dinner

Colorado has an amazing bean history. On the Southwest side of Colorado, known as the Four Corners, the Dove Creek area is the self-proclaimed Pinto Bean Capital of the World. The bean fields—with enriched (albeit dry) soil—made of a red, sandy loam blown in from Utah's Monument Valley, were prime bean growing for the La Platas, Sleeping Ute, and the Abajo Indian tribes. The entire region once housed the Anasazi, the original masters of dryland agriculture, for whom beans were a staple crop.

The majority of beans produced in Colorado are pintos (80-85%), with light red kidney, Great Northern, black and navy beans providing the remaining acreage. Currently, Weld County in Northern Eastern Colorado produces the largest amount of dry beans – primarily speckled or pinto beans. Boulder County farmers, such as Aspen Moon Farm, are growing unique culinary varieties as well.

For primarily plant-based lifestyles, beans are one of the best ways to get fiber and protein. A half cup of beans will give you approximately 15 grams of protein and 5 grams of fiber.

What You Need to Know About Beans

Soaking: Pick over the beans for rocks and debris and soak overnight in salt water. (I have studied this and can confirm salt does not harden them). Alternatively, place dried beans in a bowl, cover completely with boiling water (at least two inches) and let sit for several hours until cool. Rinse.

Cooking: Put soaked beans in your Instant Pot or pressure cooker and cover with water so there is at least one inch above the bean line. Then, depending on the bean, use the "Bean" option and cook for 15 minutes. I use the low pressure setting. Err on the side of undercooked. You can always add more time, but you can't put the skin back on a bean once it is blown off. If they are still a little al dente (hard to the teeth), I cover and cook on the sauté mode on low for another 15-20 minutes. Truthfully, I did not like my Instant Pot at first – but now I use it to speed up the process of cooking beans. Pressure cooked beans (which is what an Instant Pot primarily is), does make better beans than canned beans.
Note: Read the instructions for your cooking device.

Storing: If you prefer not to drain the liquid, divide up the cooked beans into containers and freeze. I prefer to drain, spread the beans gently on a sheet pan lined with a thin silicone mat, and freeze them on the sheet pan. When frozen, fold the liner up like a funnel and pour the beans into freezer bags.

How to Create a Bean Dish

Color: Beans have color. Think of that before you put them in a dish. If you want the final product brown or gray, use pintos, black, or black-eyed peas. If you are using potatoes or want a lighter color finished product, use cannellini, Northern, cream peas, or similar. For a touch of contrast, choose black beans; or for a real pop of color, use edamame.

Texture: Beans have varying textures. White beans such as cannellini and Great Northern are softer and lend themselves to smoother things like a sauce or mash. White bean varieties seem to cook a bit faster than red or black beans. Experiment and play with the texture for different dishes. Think whole beans, slightly mashed, or full-on puréed. Whole, soup, or a dip.

Elevate This: Add sautéed onions and garlic as a base to your bean dish. It always helps. Be sure to add umami when you aren't using pork, chicken, or beef. See the lists on p. 153 for spices, seasonings, and foods to successfully pair with beans. **Helpful Tip:** To speed up onion prep, slice or chop your onions, then put in a microwavable bowl with a small amount of oil and salt. Cover with a paper towel and microwave for 2 minutes. This will save you several minutes of sautéing if you are on a time budget.

Bean Flavor Boosters
- Porcini mushroom powder or similar
- Marmite
- Soy Sauce
- Maggi Seasoning
- Kitchen Bouquet
- Any kind of canned or boxed broth (I like Better Than Bouillon concentrate in a jar.)

Supportive Bases and Toppings
- Nutritional yeast
- Nuts, seeds, and herbs
- Dried fruit
- Farro, millet, barley, bulgur, or polenta
- Vegetable purées to serve as a base or bowl for the beans
- Brown rice
- Any whole grain mixture found in the freezer section, like quinoa, rice, millet, etc. – there are so many options now!

For more helpful tips to make beans more nutritious and interesting, review the *Cuisine Table* in the *Elevations* section of this cookbook (p. 168).

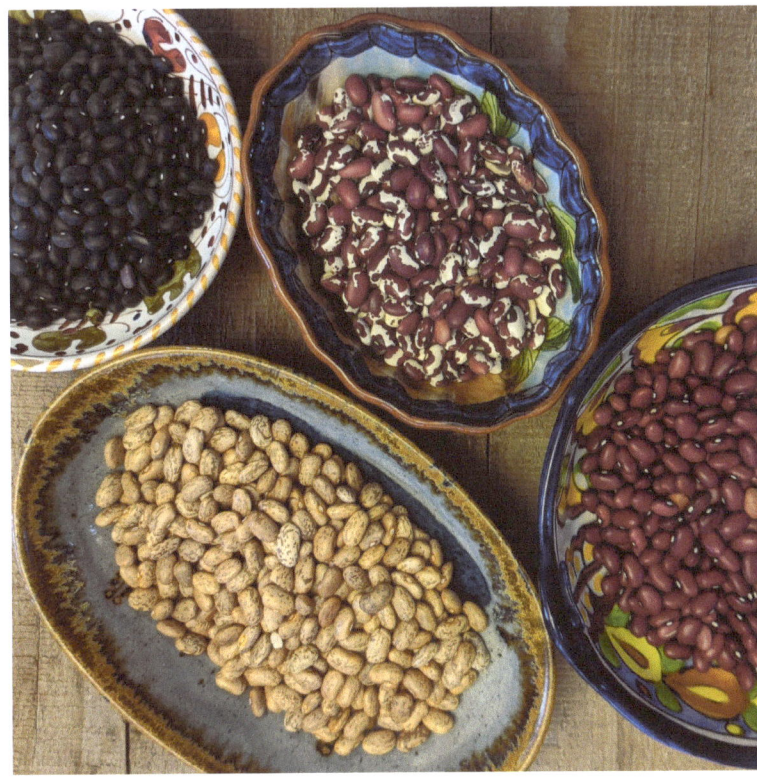
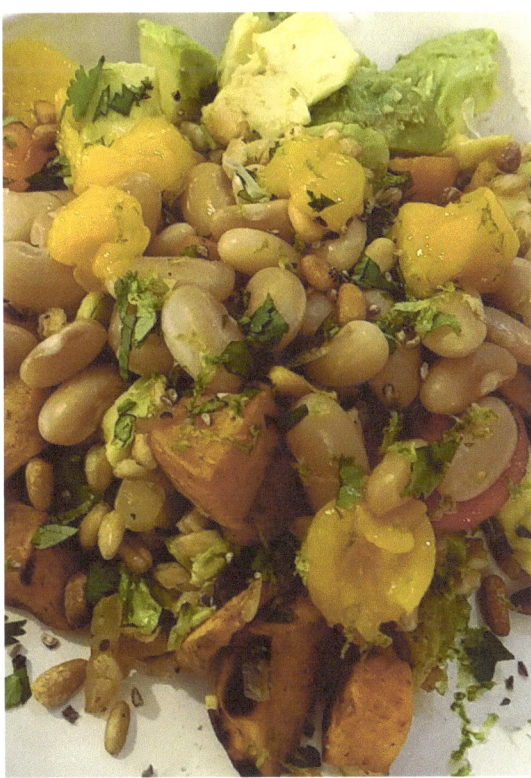

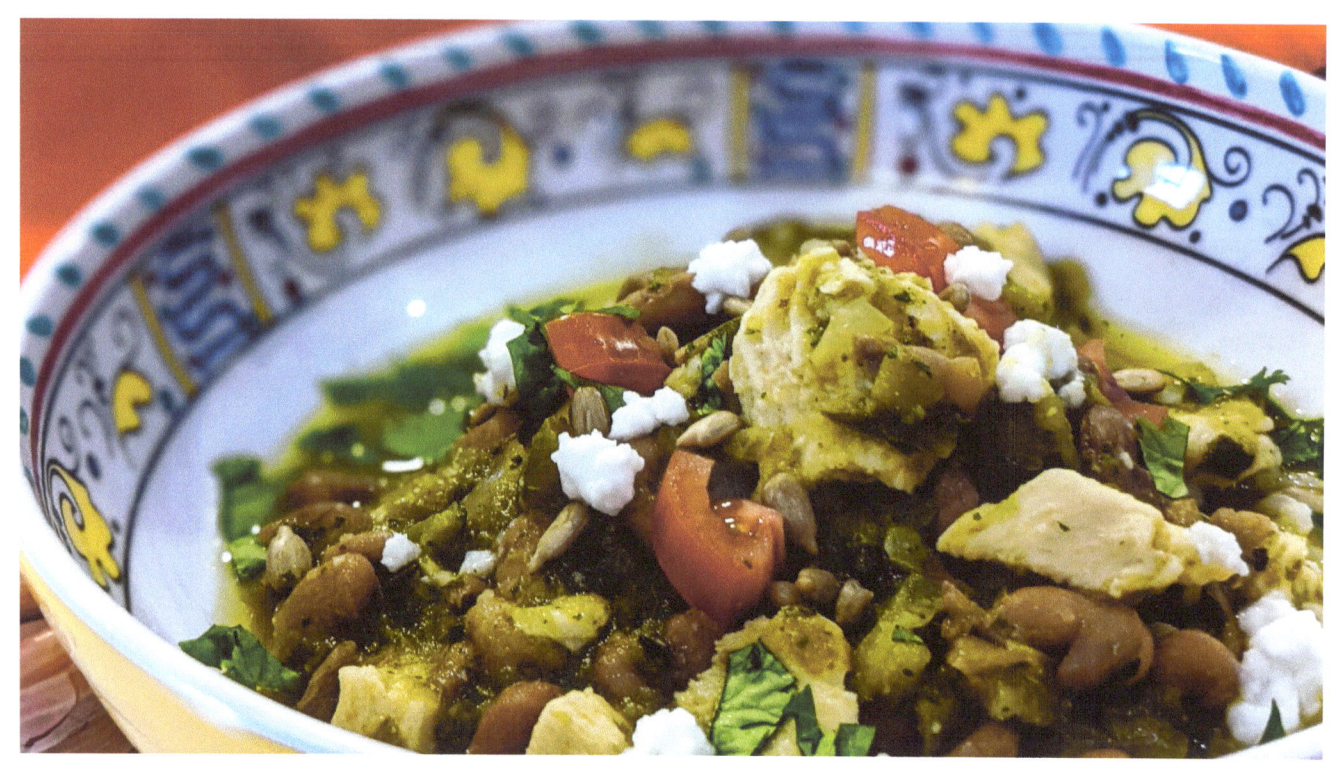

COLORADO SMOKED GREEN CHILI

What is real Colorado chili? Is it green or red? Some even come in a shade of pink. I'm solving the rivalry by giving you recipes for both. New Mexico has the Hatch chile. We have the Pueblo chile, not to be confused with another green chile from Pueblo, New Mexico. Grown in Pueblo, Colorado, this chile has roots that go back to the Oaxaca region of Mexico. The Pueblo chile as we know it is actually a strain of Mosco chile bred to have a thicker wall for roasting. It is a larger size and has a meatier texture, more capsaicin than an Anaheim or Hatch chile. If you don't have access to the Pueblo chile, Hatch chiles will work.

This is a fully plant-based dish. I was playing around with smoking chiles instead of roasting them. The smoked chiles were much easier to peel than the roasted ones, and it elevated the dish with more depth. I was also experimenting with some of the new plant-based protein substitutes, hence the look of meat in the dish. Feel free to sub out chicken or pork cubes.

You can explore many different types of chiles at the Pueblo Chile Festival, which occurs every September in Pueblo, Colorado.

Ingredients

- 5 fresh Pueblo chiles, roasted, peeled and seeded; or 2 small cans of Hatch green chiles
- ½ medium onion, finely chopped
- 5 garlic cloves, minced
- 1 tbsp oil
- 1 tbsp ground cumin
- 1 tbsp ground coriander
- 1 tbsp Mexican oregano (do not substitute Italian oregano)
- 1 tsp salt
- 1 tsp black pepper
- If not using smoked chiles, add 1 tsp of liquid smoke or mesquite smoke powder
- 2 cups vegetable broth
- 1 handful of fresh cilantro leaves
- 2 cups of cooked Colorado pinto beans or Anasazi beans; or 1 can pinto beans, drained and rinsed

For the Garnish
- Chopped cilantro
- Queso fresco (dairy or non-dairy)
- Sunflower seeds
- Grape tomatoes, quartered

Instructions

If using fresh-roasted chiles, chop the chiles into ¼-inch pieces.

In a medium pot, heat the oil over medium heat. Add the onions and sauté until golden and soft. Add the garlic and heat until aromatic.

Move the onions to the side of the pot, and add the spices and herbs to bloom for 60 seconds (This is a technique called blooming).

Add the chiles and mix thoroughly.

Add 1 tsp salt and 1 tsp pepper. Add liquid smoke or mesquite smoke powder if not using smoked chiles.

Add the broth and cook over medium low heat for 15 minutes.

Using an immersion blender or similar device, blend 1 ladle full of the soup base with the cilantro leaves until smooth. (This is a technique for creating a creamy soup without the cream.)

Add the blended mixture back to the pot.

Add the cooked or canned beans, and cook for another 10 minutes.

Serve in bowls over brown rice. Garnish with cilantro, queso fresco (dairy or non-dairy), sunflower seeds, and grape tomatoes.

Elevate This: Serve with a meat or meat substitute of choice (as pictured). Top with nutritional yeast, crunchy tortilla strips, or pepitas for a more traditional approach. Pink baby radishes will add a nice bite.

Serves 4 as a main dish

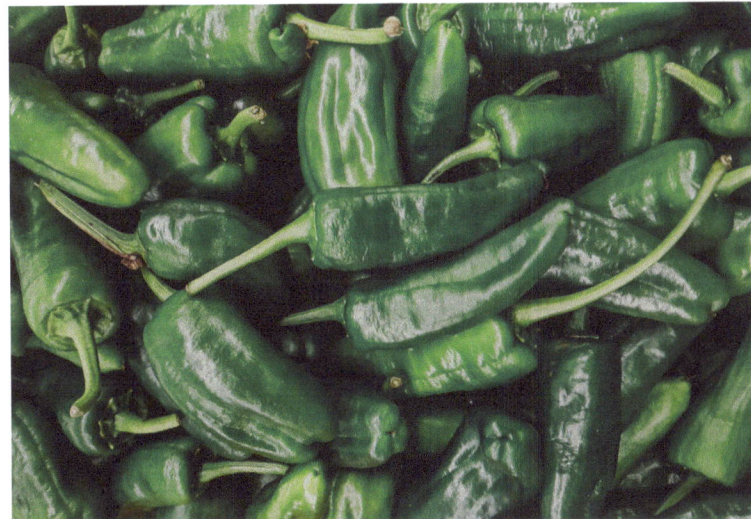
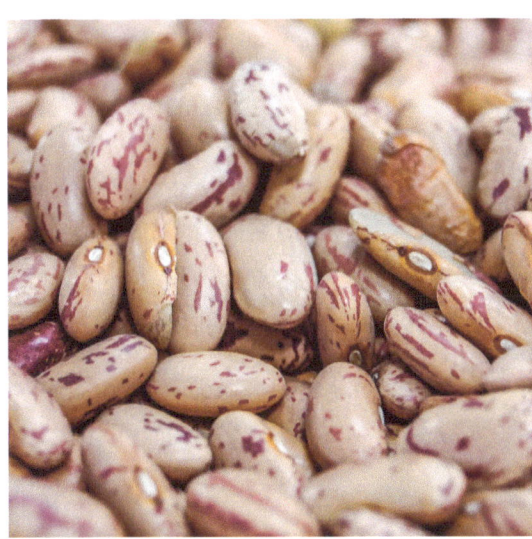

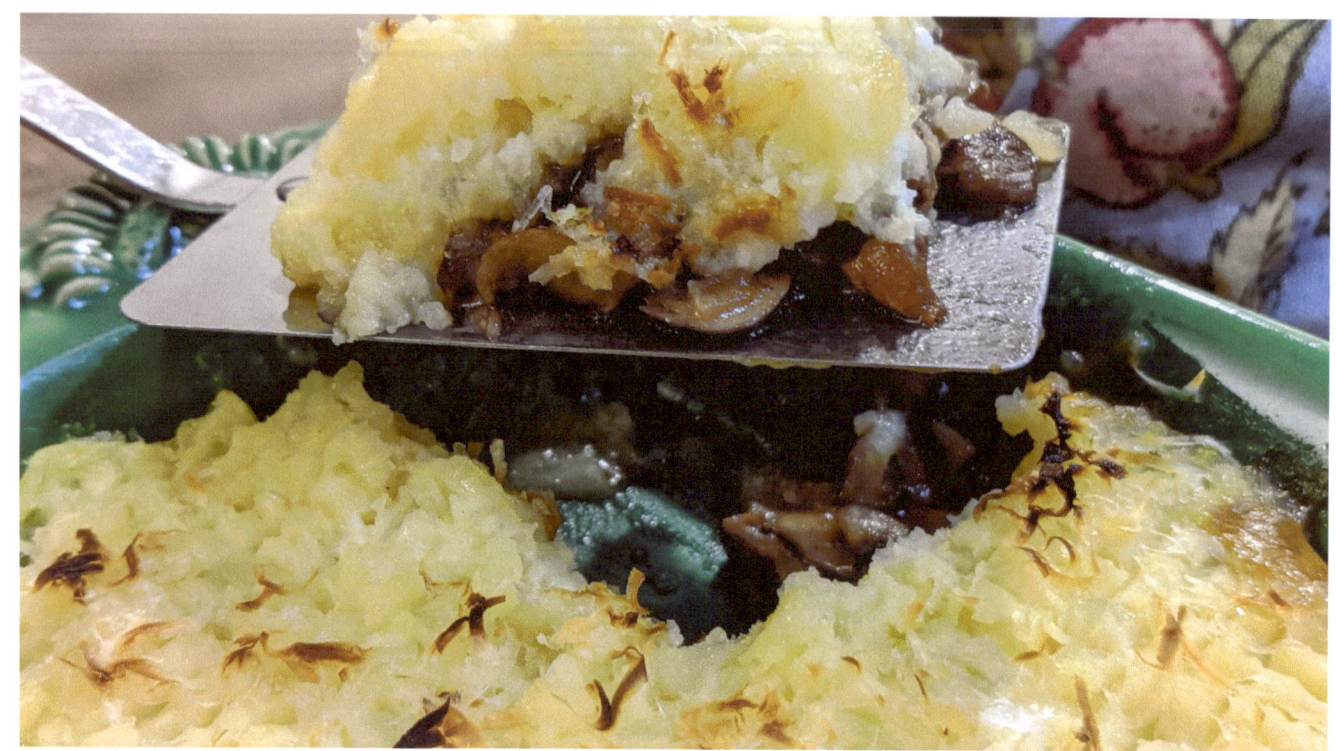

MUSHROOM PARMENTIER

Antoine-Augustin Parmentier was a French scientist and agronomist who promoted potatoes as a food source for humans in France and throughout Europe. He also pioneered the extraction of sugar from sugar beets – a very important factoid given the local sugar beet industry history. I could add much more, but I want you to try this recipe. Mushroom Parmentier sounds much better than Shrooms and Taters, don't you think? I served this at our French Food Belgian Beer party and it was gone before I could taste it. And, no one even knew I had made it plant-based.

Ingredients

For the Mushrooms
- 1 tbsp butter (dairy or non-dairy)
- 2 tbsp oil
- ½ onion, minced
- 2 garlic cloves, minced
- 1 lb mixed mushrooms (I used chanterelles, cremini, and shiitake)
- ½ cup red wine
- ¼ cup vegetable or chicken stock
- 1 sprig fresh thyme (or ⅛ tsp dried thyme)
- 1 tbsp butter (dairy or non-dairy) and 1 tbsp flour, mixed together in a small bowl
- Salt and pepper to taste

For the Potatoes
- 3 medium Yukon gold potatoes
- ¼ cup milk (dairy or non-dairy)
- 2 tbsp butter (dairy or non-dairy)
- 2 ounces Comté cheese (dairy or non-dairy), cubed; or 2 ounces Gruyere (dairy or non-dairy), cubed
- ¼ cup grated Parmesan (dairy or non-dairy)
- Salt and pepper to taste

Instructions

For the Mushrooms
Preheat oven to 425°F.
Heat the butter (dairy or non-dairy) and oil in a skillet.
Add the onion and cook slowly to caramelize.
Add the garlic and heat for 30 seconds.
Add the mushrooms and sauté for 5 minutes until soft.
Add the wine, stock, and thyme, and slowly cook until the mixture is reduced and the mushrooms are glossy.
Knead together the flour and butter mixture with your fingers, then add to the skillet. Continue to cook until the mixture thickens. Salt and pepper to taste.
Spread the mixture into the bottom of a small casserole dish.

For the Potatoes
Steam or boil the potatoes until fork tender. Allow to cool enough to handle and peel.
In a large bowl, mash the potatoes, butter (dairy or non-dairy), and milk (dairy or non-dairy) until blended well. Salt and pepper to taste.
Dollop the potatoes on top of the mushrooms and spread until mushrooms are covered.
Sprinkle the cheese (dairy or non-dairy) on top.
Bake until the dish is bubbling hot and the cheese is browned, for about 18-20 minutes. If using vegan Parmesan cheese, cover with aluminum foil for the first 15 minutes, then uncover and bake the last 5-7 minutes.

Elevate This: Make this dish with half potatoes, and half sweet potatoes or pumpkin, for an elegant holiday side dish or main course. Mix and match mushrooms. Cinnamon cap mushrooms would be a pretty and artful addition.

Serves 2 as a main dish

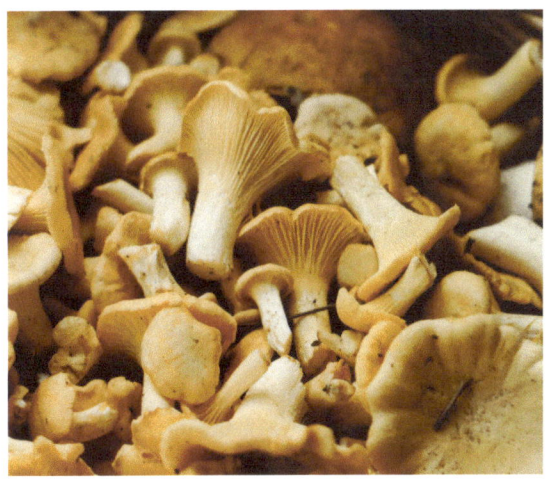
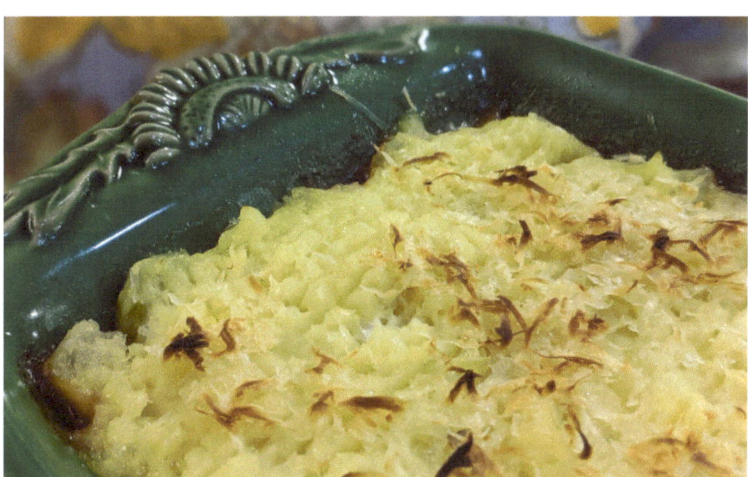

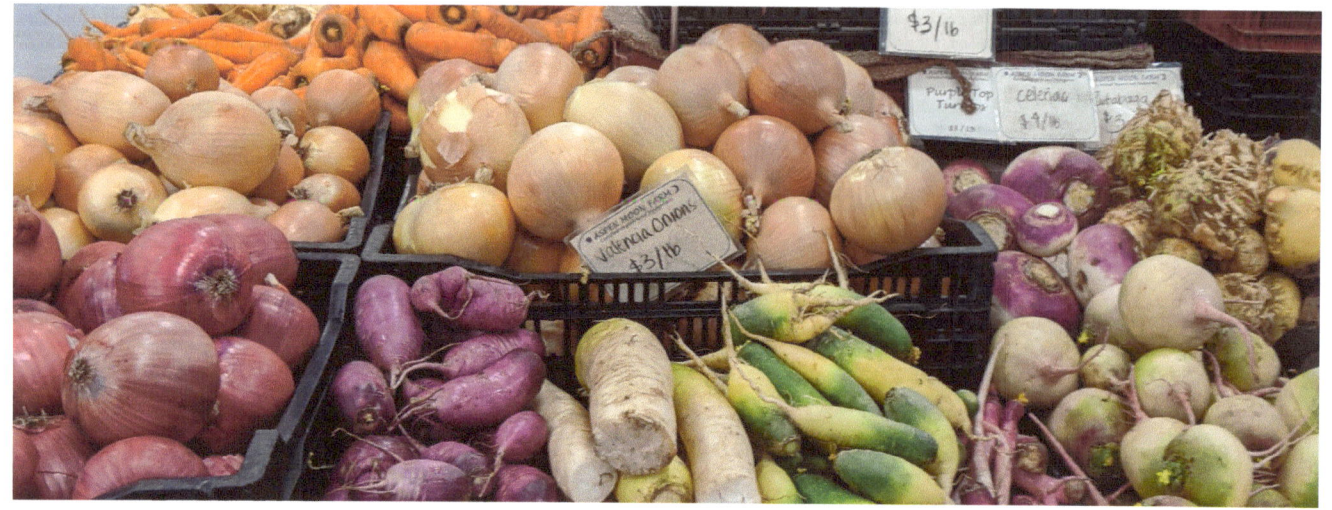
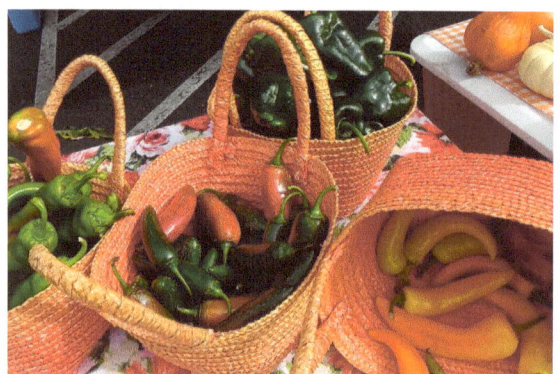
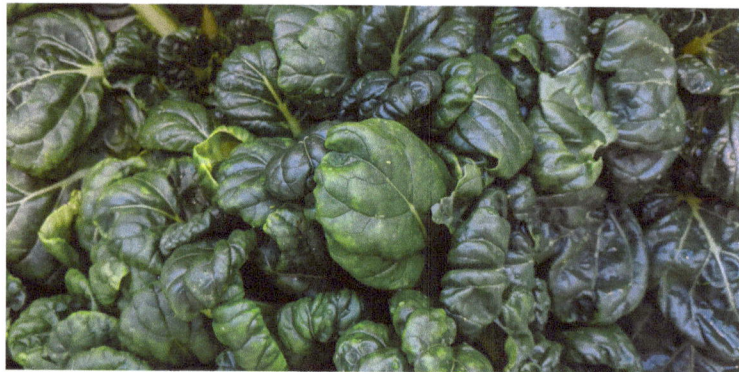
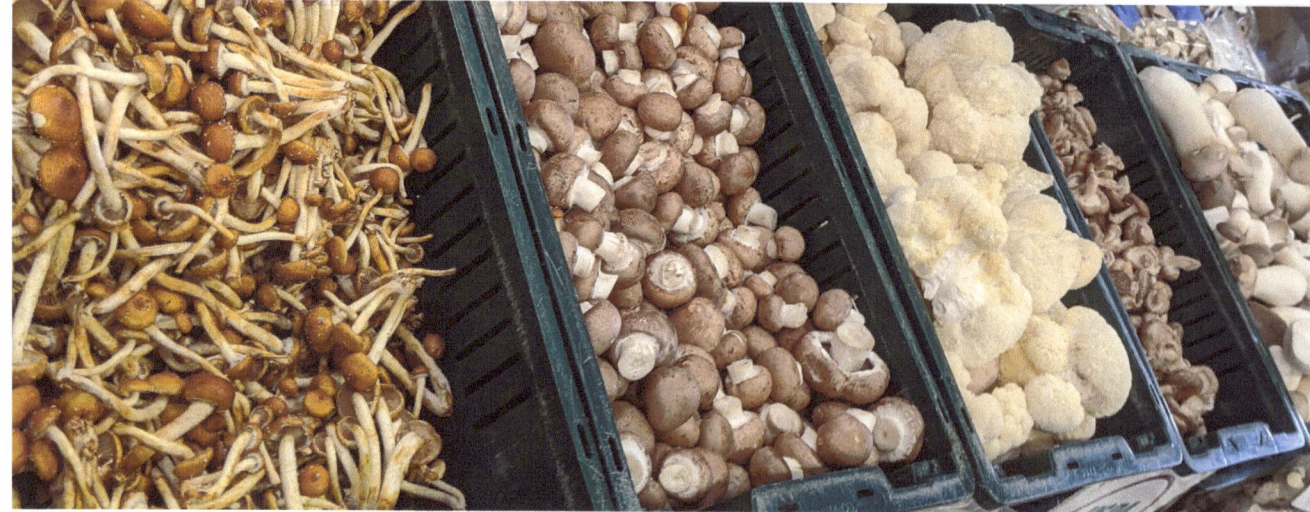
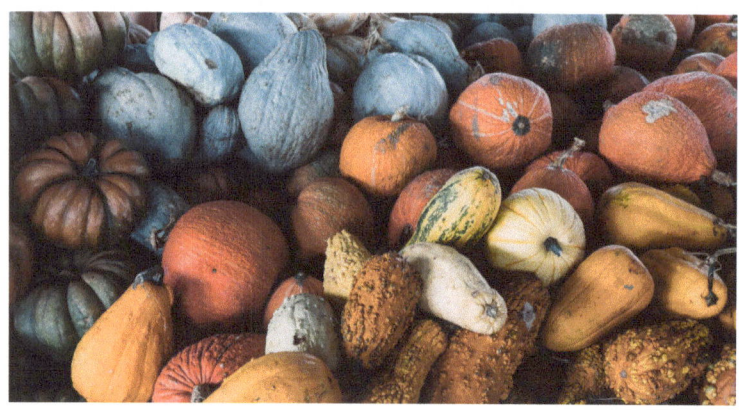
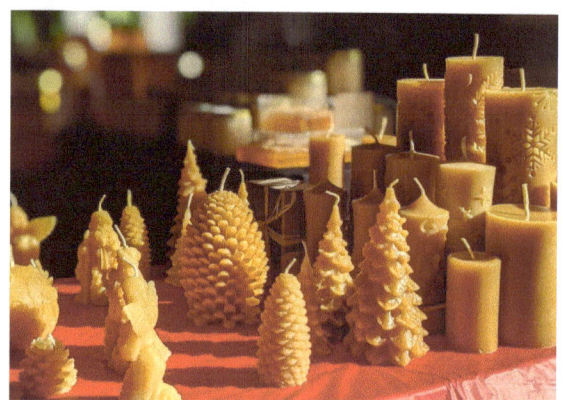

FOUL MUDAMMAS

I love our local Mediterranean market, Olive Tree Market, in Fort Collins. The fresh-frozen, double-peeled fresh beans that they carry are the best, but, when the supply chain hiccups, or it is off season, there are dried or canned options. Upon further exploration of their store, I discovered multiple cans of fava beans, unique to specific nationalities. I had no idea. The market owner encouraged me to make this Egyptian dish and pair it with the Iraqi flatbread they receive from a Denver baker. I hope you enjoy. The sauce is a keeper too!

Ingredients
- 1 can of plain fava beans (pintos will work in a pinch)
- ½ tsp salt
- 1-2 tsp cumin to taste
- 1 jalapeño pepper, seeded and chopped
- 3 garlic cloves, peeled and chopped
- Splash of lemon juice

For the Garnish
- Extra virgin olive oil
- Chopped parsley
- Grape tomatoes, quartered
- Sliced jalapeños

Instructions
Drain the beans and reserve the liquid.
In a saucepan, warm the beans and ½ the liquid.
Add the salt and cumin, and mash the beans to your desired consistency.
In a mortar and pestle, mash the jalapeño pepper and garlic to be as smooth as possible. Add the lemon juice and mix with a spatula.
Transfer the beans to a serving dish or a small, heated cast iron skillet to keep warm. Drizzle the beans with the jalapeño and garlic mixture.
Garnish with olive oil, parsley, tomatoes and jalapeños. Serve with a beautiful flatbread or pita.

Elevate This: Serve with a small plate of Kalamata or Koroneiki olives, Giardiniera (p. 63), and whole almonds. Add dates or figs for a touch of sweetness.

Serves 2-3 as a main dish

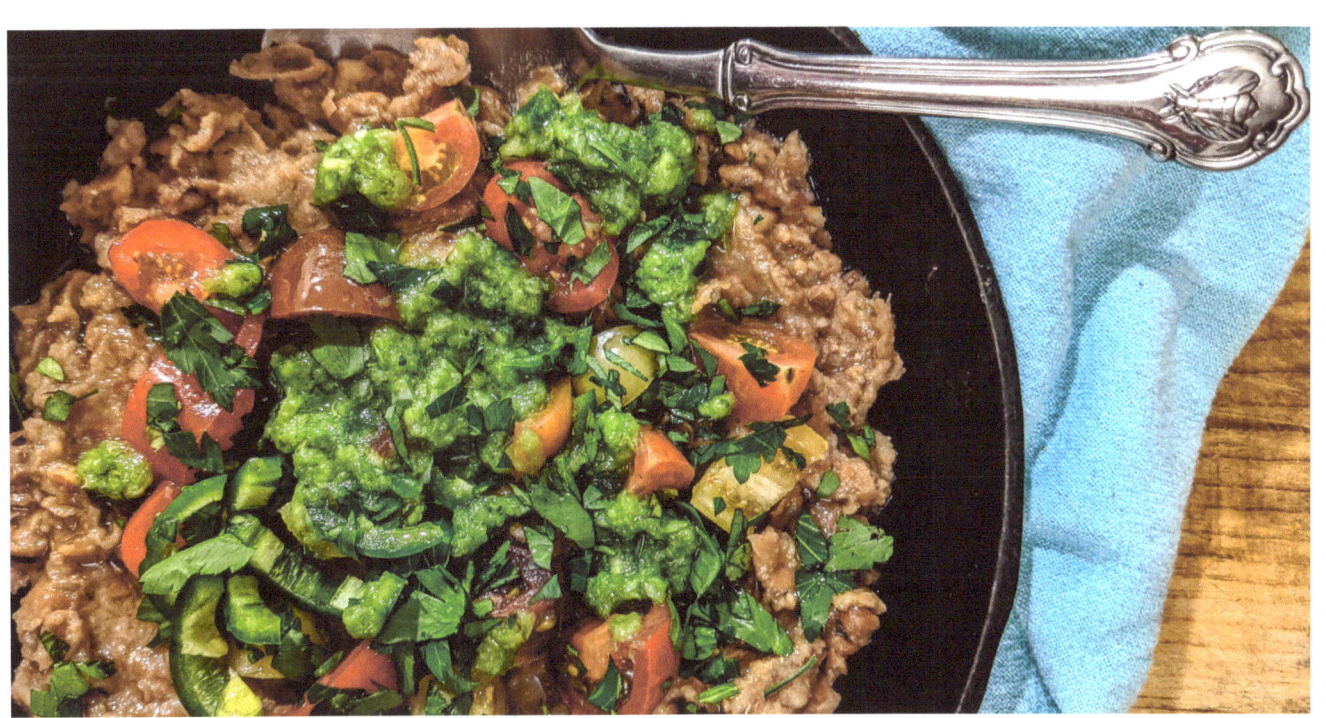

Health for the Holidays

The holidays are a time for joyful celebration, gatherings, and of course, treats. They are a time to rejoice and enjoy an occasional bite of an artisan cheese, a well-prepared, sustainably raised tasting of meat, a touch of smoked trout, or a lovely egg custard. As a family member of mine says, "It's all about the sides!" Well, what do the sides look like? From a starter soup and artful, easy salad, to marriages of root vegetables, fruits and nuts – you will now have some stand-out dishes to bring to a holiday table.

I have enjoyed creating small takeaway bites for my guests – that way I can manage amounts, servings, and layering of flavors by taking traditional dishes and paring them down to one or two-bite sizes. I enjoy having a friend come over to help with the assembly and visit before the holiday hubbub begins.

Helpful Tips to Create the Perfect Bite-Sized Side

For the Base: I love the Siljans Croustades available on Amazon and sometimes locally at World Market. They are quite sturdy and the perfect size for a bite. I also use phyllo cups and French mini toasts.

For the Filling: Repurpose recipes to be used as filling! To fill bite-sized pastry cups, I highly recommend using a very small serving scoop (1 tbsp capacity or less). Two spoons will work, but a scoop makes filling the cups so much easier – which is a game changer in the holiday kitchen.

A: Since you now know how to make Pumpkin Flatbreads (p. 107), these can be made into street taco size flatbreads to support a Costa Rican beef or pork shoyu filling.

B: To make an Ikarian-style bite, add some oregano or Greek spice mixture to ½ cup black-eyed peas and 8-10 steamed baby Dutch potatoes. Mash slightly. Using a 1 tbsp scoop, scoop into pastry cups. Garnish with chopped nuts, parsley, and slices of a good quality black olive.

C: Indian potatoes – mash the Indian Saffron Potatoes in Coconut Milk (p. 143) or Butternut Squash Potato Tofu Curry (p. 118), add some chickpeas, and scoop into pastry cups. Drizzle on the Cilantro Green Dip (p. 21) and Tamarind Sauce (see *Elevations* section, p. 168) for added flavor. Garnish with cilantro leaf.

D: Go Asian. Fill the cups with a bit of cooked rice, Roasted Shiitake Mushrooms (p. 131), sprinkle with some furikake and garnish with a microgreen sprig.

E: Now that you have learned how to roast red peppers, you can make this beautiful and simple red pepper dip. Oven roast a red bell pepper (p. 62) and blend the pepper in a blender with ¼ cup walnuts, ¼ cup cashew cream or milk, 2 tbsp olive oil, and ½ tsp red pepper flakes. Salt and pepper to taste. Blend until smooth. Garnish with pomegranate seeds and serve with flat crackers.

F: I realize it is super easy to just purchase a vegetable tray from the store, but isn't this more colorful? This is a small plate version, but of course you can expand it to be a large tray. Think color, sweet, tart, texture, and of course Toum (p. 130) on the side!

G: Local baby bok choy and avocado mashed with a touch of Toum and sea salt, topped with tomatoes spiced up with The Spice and Tea Exchange® adobo spice mix. Round out the tray with gorgeous, steamed-to-perfection purple potatoes, plantain chips, Boulder Blue Corn Tortilla Chips, a bowl of Toum, and lima bean dip.

H: Lima Bean Dip – My friend who can't stand lima beans still enjoys this dip. Hopefully you will too. Drain 1 can of lima beans, reserve liquid. In a food processor, blend the beans with 2 tbsp olive oil, 1 tsp lemon juice, ¼ tsp dried thyme, and ½ tsp sea salt. Purée until smooth. This is lima beans – ELEVATED.

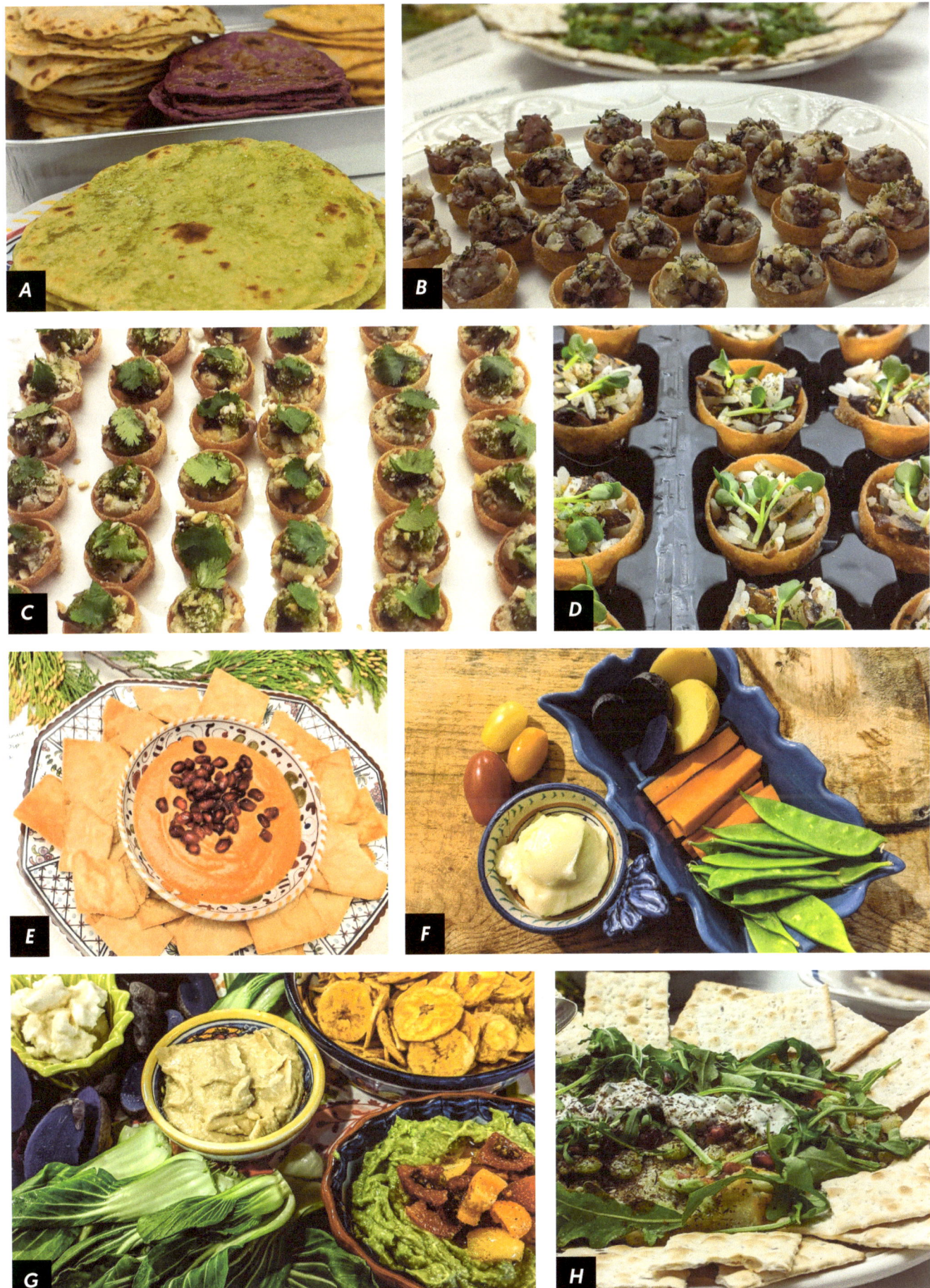

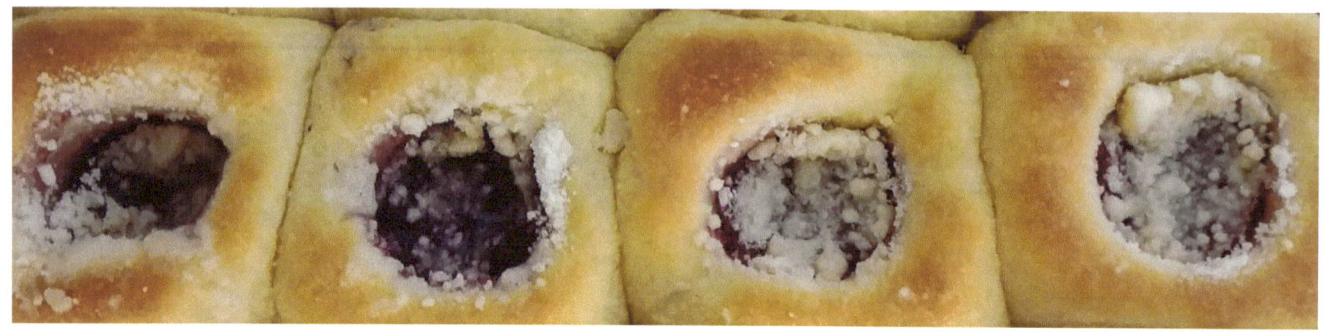

KOLACHES

Since we have been doing so great at eating 95% veg most of the time, let's have a little treat – kolaches! Growing up, kolaches were reserved for holidays, birthdays and other get togethers – mostly because they are time-consuming to make, and you generally don't bake just one dozen at a time. If it takes four hours to bake something, you might as well bake three dozen.

Let's be honest, some treats just don't translate perfectly to primarily plant-based cooking, and we do live in the land of diary and fresh, sustainably raised eggs. Whether it is an apple fritter, (for my husband), or a kolache (for me), there is probably one dish that you keep in your repertoire for some reason – memories of your grandmother, a special vacation, who knows what gets plugged in our brain in regards to comfort food. I have encouraged you to get plugged into primarily veg with most of the recipes in this cookbook, but for this recipe I want you to at least understand how much work goes into making a soft kolache that melts in your mouth.

Kolaches are a part of my Czech heritage. If you live in Colorado, you may have purchased kolaches from The Kolache Bee – that was me. This is 99% of grandmother's recipe. I have pared down the recipe to make a dozen. Unless you need three full dozen (which is temptation at its greatest), one dozen will do you nicely.

I will say, since I stopped baking kolaches and started eating 95% (or more) plants, I have lost 15 lbs and feel better than ever. If you are full-on vegan, just skip this recipe. In the future I will test some plant-based kolache recipes to make sure they are as good as this recipe.

Ingredients
- 1 cup milk
- ¾ tsp Red Star Platinum Yeast (seriously, the only yeast to make these with)
- 1 tsp sugar
- 1 ¾ cup flour
- 1 egg + 1 egg yolk
- 3 tbsp white sugar
- 1 ounce lard (makes them fluffy)
- 2 ½ tbsp butter, softened
- 1 tsp salt
- Enough flour to keep the dough manageable, but not tough
- Butter for basting

Overview
There are four risings for a chemistry reason. This is the only recipe I have researched that calls for this first yeast rise. Don't skip it – if you skip it, your kolaches will be okay, but they will not be fluffy. Do not over work the dough. Use your hands. You will be picking up dough throughout the process. so err on a slightly wet dough. Like sourdough, as the flour absorbs the liquid over the three rises, it will smooth out.

Instructions

Heat the milk to 110°F. Add the yeast, 1 tsp sugar and flour, and mix well.

First Rise

Cover the mixture and let rise until bubbly and doubled, about 30 minutes to 1 hour. At this point it should be a bubbly, thin-ish mixture.

Now you can start making your filling – flip the page to find recipes for a few filling options.

In a separate bowl, beat the egg and egg yolk, 3 tbsp sugar, lard, butter and salt. You can use a hand mixer for this.

With a wooden dough spoon, fold the egg mixture into the milk and flour mixture. Keep mixing until the flour becomes incorporated.

Add additional flour, 1 tbsp at a time, until the dough becomes thicker, but not stiff. Beat until the dough pulls away from the sides.

You can use a small electric mixer just to help pull the dough together, but do not use the kneading option on an electric appliance – you may create too much gluten and the dough will get stiff.

Pour the dough out onto a floured board and gently knead the dough only 2-3 minutes, just to the point that it starts holding shape. It should still be soft.

Grease a large bowl and weigh the bowl.

Second Rise

Place dough in the bowl and let the dough rise in a warm place until double in bulk. Be patient. Depending your area, it could be 30 minutes or it could be an hour.

Weigh the bowl and dough. Subtract the weight of the bowl from the total – that is your dough weight.

Pour out the dough onto a floured board and cut into 12 pieces, weighing each piece to 1/12th of your final dough weight. Mine traditionally are around 1.5 ounces.

Roll each piece into a ball –I roll and then pull the dough underneath and tuck it into the bottom of the dough ball. You want each ball of dough to be smooth. No cracks, or the dough will rise with imperfections for the next step.

Place the dough balls in a greased roughly 9x11 inch baking pan, spacing them out evenly. The disposable aluminum pans work great.

Third Rise

Baste the dough balls with melted butter and let rise into double in bulk.

Fill the Kolache

Use a shot glass – dip the bottom of the shot glass into flour, and insert the glass into a dough ball to make an indention large enough to hold 1 tbsp filling. Do not puncture the bottom of the dough.

Use the floured shot glass to gently spread the dough balls out so they touch each other and the side of the pan. If you are at altitude, gently prick the bottom of each kolache. Do not go all the way through to the bottom of pan, or your filling will drip through to the bottom of the pan.

Fill each kolache with 1 tbsp filling. Do not overfill. Drizzle pocepka on top (flip the page for recipe).

Fourth Rise

Set the kolaches aside and let rise for 30 minutes to 1 hour, until they are nice and fluffy looking.

Let's Bake

Preheat the oven 400°F.

Bake the kolaches for 15-20 minutes, rotating at 10 minutes and watching closely. Depending on your oven and altitude, your kolaches may brown more than you want.

When done, remove from the oven and immediately baste with butter.

I know it's difficult, but let cool 30 minutes before eating – the filling needs to set.

Prost!

Makes 12 kolaches

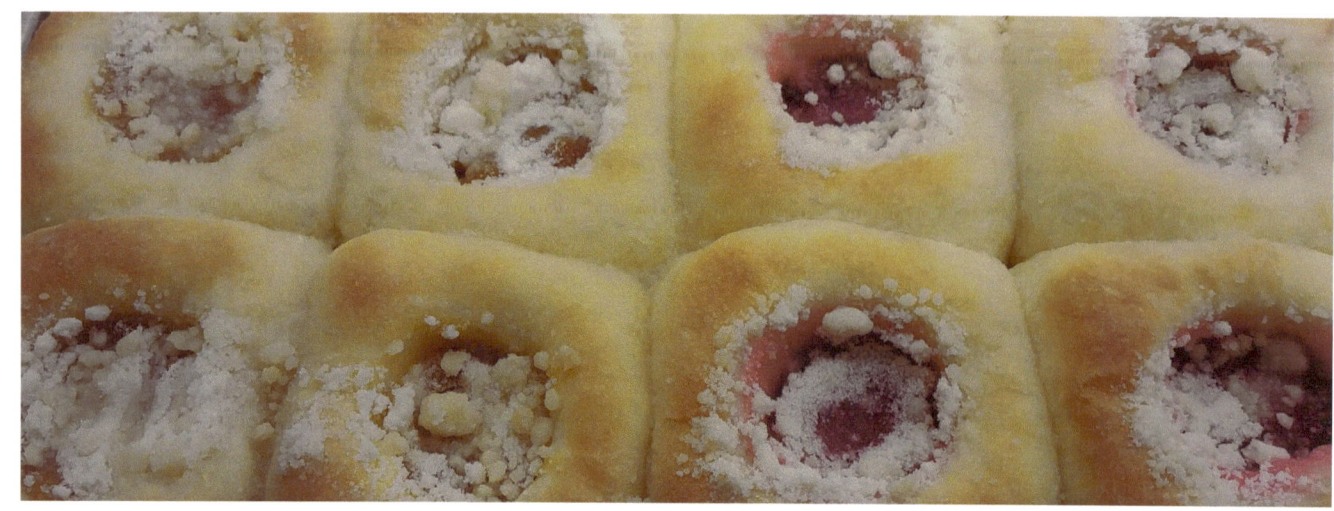

KOLACHE FILLINGS TWO WAYS AND POCEPKA TOPPING

Do not use regular fruit jam or jelly as a filling for your kolaches. It may not work, and the filling may blow up out of the kolaches. Either make your own, or use Solo brand fillings for your kolaches. I included two of my favorites from what I called The Colorado Sampler Dozen – Vanilla Peach Bourbon and Sour Cherry.

VANILLA PEACH BOURBON KOLACHE FILLING

Ingredients
- 1 cup slightly mashed fresh or frozen Palisade peaches
- 1 ½ cups sugar
- 1 tsp Sure-jell
- 1 tsp plain gelatin dissolved in ¼ cup water
- 2 tsp vanilla
- 1 tbsp bourbon

Instructions
In a large pot on the stove, or in an Instant Pot, mix peaches and Sure-jell together. Let sit for 5-10 minutes. Bring the mixture to a boil. Reduce heat to medium heat. Cook for 5-10 minutes to reduce liquid by half. Add the sugar and continue to cook over medium heat until the mixture reaches 200°F, or when you can run a spoon on the bottom of the pot and leave a channel. You will also see the bubbles become larger and the sound and movement of the bubbles will become slower and more resonant.

Remove pot from heat and stir in the gelatin. Mix well. Add the vanilla and bourbon. Be careful – the hot mixture may spatter. Mix well.

Place the pot back on the heat and rapidly bowl for 2-3 minutes to reduce the mixture.

You should be able to put 1 tsp or so in a small bowl and it will firm up to a gelatin consistency in 2-3 minutes. Remove from heat and cool completely before filling kolaches. Leftovers can go in the fridge or freezer.

Fills 12-18 kolaches

SOUR CHERRY KOLACHE FILLING

Ingredients
- 1 cup pitted Montmorency cherries, juice drained and reserved in the freezer (we will use it later)
- 2 cups sugar
- 1 tsp Sure-jell
- 1 tsp plain gelatin dissolved in ¼ cup water

Instructions
Follow the instructions for the Vanilla Peach Bourbon Filling (p. 164). Like peaches, cherries can be very juicy, especially if you are using fresh frozen cherries. Be sure to cook at the cooking temperature and proper consistency. Do the cooling test in a bowl.

Fills 12-18 kolaches

POCEPKA KOLACHE TOPPING

Ingredients
- ½ cup sugar
- ¼ cup flour
- ¼ cup melted butter

Instructions
Mix well and use to top the kolaches. Reserve any remaining pocepka for other dessert projects.

Tops 12-18 kolaches

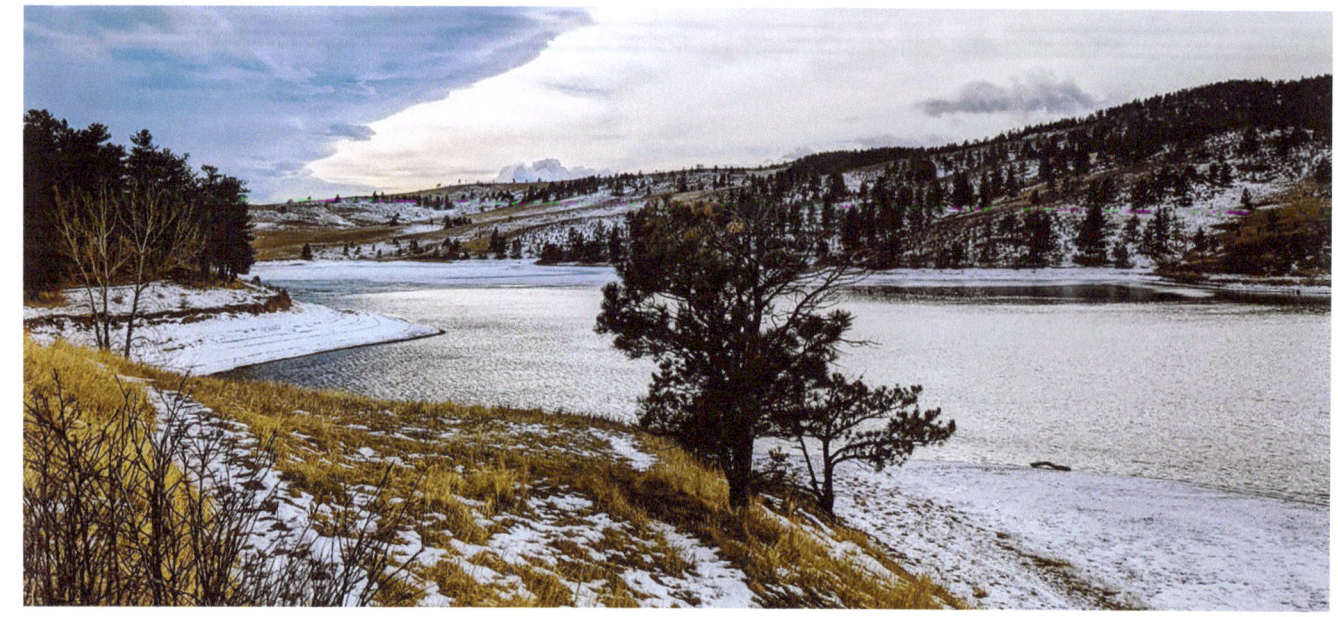
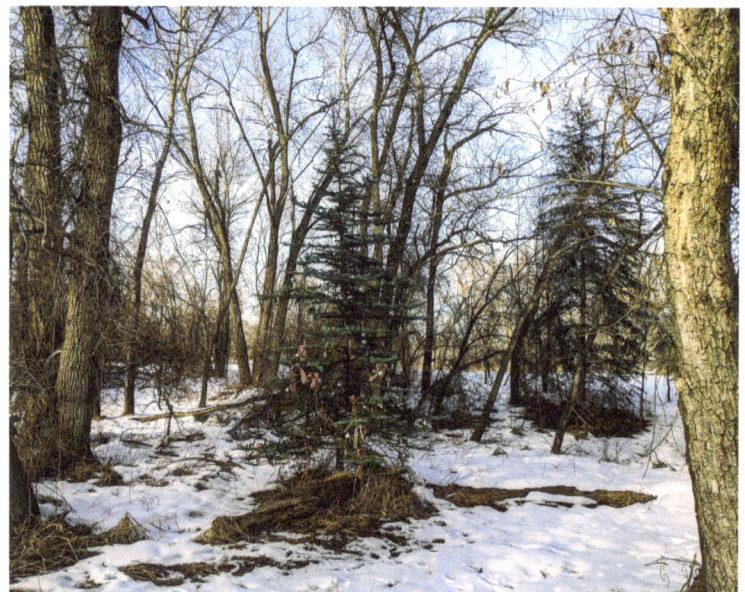
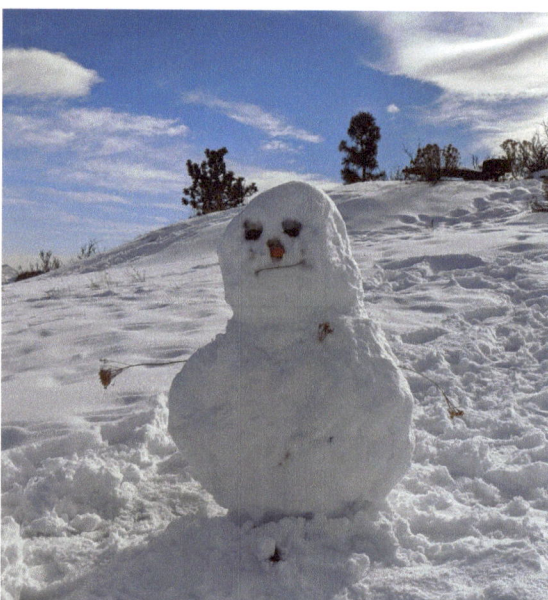
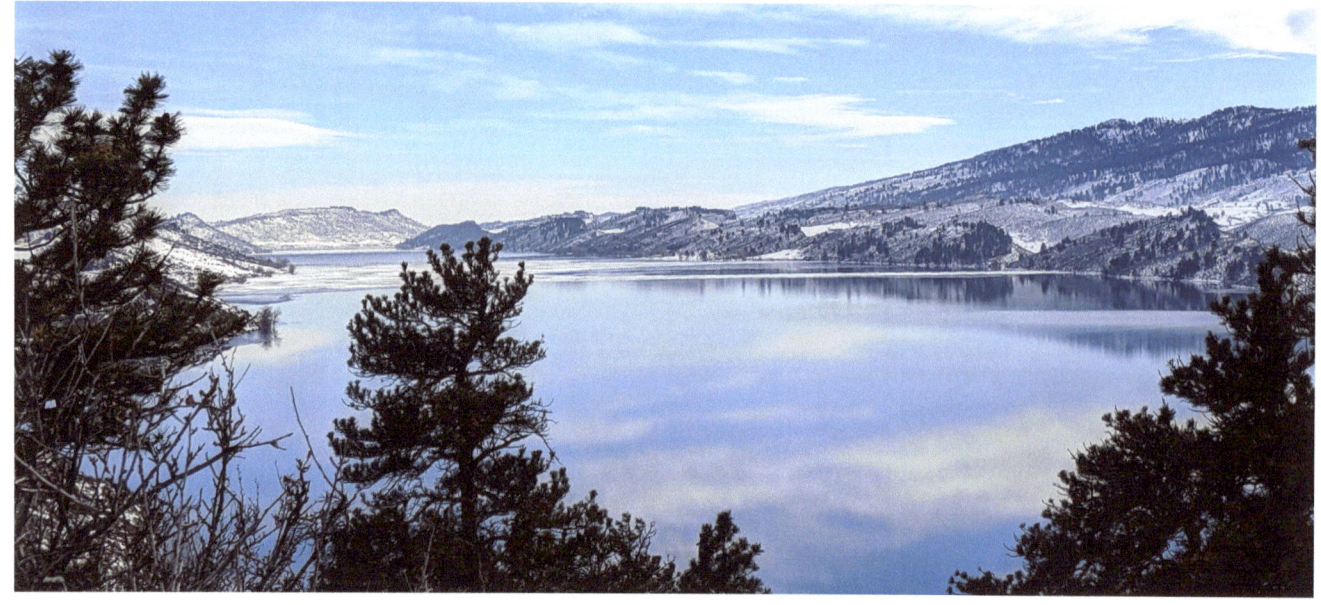

Cuisine-Related Herb, Aromatic, Spice, Nut, and Seed Pairings

Cuisine	Herbs/Aromatics	Spices	Nuts	Seeds/Other
Italian, Sicilian, Sardinian	Basil, fennel, garlic, leek, onion, marjoram, oregano, parsley, rosemary, sage, thyme	Chile, black pepper, white pepper	Almonds, hazelnuts, pine nuts	Truffle
Thai	Basil, cilantro, galangal, ginger, kaffir lime, lemongrass, mint, tamarind	Chile, coriander, cumin, turmeric, curry	Cashew, almond, peanut	Sesame
Mexican, Spanish	Cilantro, garlic, onion, parsley, saffron	Chile, cinnamon, coriander, cumin, paprika	Almonds	Sesame, pumpkin, sunflower
Moroccan, African	Chive, cilantro, garlic, ginger, mint, onion, saffron, sage, rose	Cardamom, clove, cinnamon, coriander, cumin, fenugreek	Almonds	Sesame
Japanese, Chinese	Basil, garlic, ginger, miso, scallion, vinegar, wasabi	Chile, cardamom, coriander, star anise	Peanuts, almonds, cashews	Sesame, seaweed
Turkish, Greek	Cilantro, dill, garlic, marjoram, mint, onion, oregano, parsley, saffron, thyme	Anise, cinnamon, chili, fenugreek, sesame, sumac	Almonds, pistachios, walnuts	Sesame, pine nuts, almonds, cashews
Indian	Cilantro, fennel seed, ginger, garlic, mint, onion, saffron	Anise, black pepper, cardamom, chile, cinnamon, clove, cumin, curry, garam masala, fenugreek, mustard, rose, tamarind, turmeric	Almonds, peanuts, pistachios, cashews	Sesame

ELEVATIONS: Simple Tips for Brightening Any Dish

Crispy Capers: Rinse 2 tbsp capers. Pat dry and put in a small microwaveable bowl. Add 1 tsp oil. Coat thoroughly. Microwave on high for 2-minute intervals until crispy. Let cool. Keep them in the refrigerator and use as needed.

Crispy Lentils: Mix 1 cup of cooked, French Puy lentils with 1 tbsp of your favorite spice mixture and 2 tsp olive oil. Spread on parchment-lined baking sheet. Bake in a pre-heated 400°F oven for 20-25 minutes, until crunchy but not burned.

Crispy Shallots: Thinly slice 1 shallot. Put in a small microwaveable bowl and add 1 tsp oil and a dash of sea salt. Coat thoroughly. Microwave on high for 2-minute intervals until crispy. Let cool. Refrigerate and use as needed. Shallots will continue to caramelize for a while after cooking – do not overcook.

Cuisine-Related Herb, Spice, Nut Blends: Using nutritional yeast as a base, create your own umami by adding a blend to your dish. Heat ¼ cup nutritional yeast in skillet over low heat. Add your choice of cuisine-related herb, seed, nuts, and spice ingredients to the skillet (see Cuisine-Related Pairing chart, (p. 167). Heat on low for 3-4 minutes. Do not burn. Cool and place in air-tight container. Use as a garnish on soups, salads and other vegetable medleys. You may also choose to purchase a ready-made blend from your spice store—such as Greek, French, Italian, or Mediterranean—then add the yeast, seeds, and nuts to the blend.

Furikake: This seed, seaweed, and spice mixture from Japan will elevate any stir fry, soup, or Asian rice dish. You can make your own by adding 1 tsp Nori flakes to 2 tbsp of an Everything-Bagel-type spice mix. Or you can purchase furikake online.

Grape Tomatoes: Use each of the colors now available within the varieties of grape tomatoes – green, yellow, orange, red, and dark purple. Quartered tomatoes add a bit of softness, and a bit of sweetness and tang. Depending on the dish, add a bit of olive oil and a spice mix. For example, use an adobo spice mix to elevate plain tomatoes to extraordinary.

Grated Carrot: Simple, huh? A dusting of finely grated, orange carrot sprinkled on top of a light-colored soup adds a contrast of color, and a bit of sweetness.

Gremolata: This 3-ingredient topping will add a bit of zest (literally) and color to your dish. In a mortar and pestle, grind 1 cup of roughly chopped parsley and 2 garlic cloves to a coarse mixture. Add the grated peel of 1 lemon. Combine well.

Herbs: Add freshly chopped or minced parsley, cilantro, or mint – depending on the dish. Leave a few herbs whole, or partially whole to accent the beauty of a dish.

Honey-Glazed Pecans: Combine 1 cup pecan halves, ¼ cup honey, and 1 tablespoon of sugar in a bowl. Spread on a parchment covered or silpat baking sheet, and bake at 350°F for 10-5 minutes, stirring at 5-minute intervals until caramelized, but not burnt. Cool and store in an airtight container.

Microgreens: Purchase or grow your own Daikon radish, pea, sunflower or other microgreens. Not only will you get a flavor boost and increased visual appeal, you will get added nutrition as well.

Olives: It doesn't take much of the salty, brininess of olives to add umami and flavor to a dish. I am giving a plug to Healthy Harvest Olives in Boulder, as these are some of the best olives on the market. Single estate varietals, certified organic, and non-pasteurized – preserving the live probiotics and lactobacillus bacteria on the olive and in the brine. Simple elegance.

Paprika: Paprika comes in many forms – sweet, hot, bittersweet, and smoked. Play around for your dish. Sprinkle ½ teaspoon paprika via a small sieve or strainer onto your dish for a perk of color.

Pistou: Follow the recipe for Microgreen Pistou (p. 129), but substitute basil for the microgreens.

Pomegranate Seeds: These may not be available year-round, but take advantage of them when they are – these are fruit powerhouses for nutrition, adding beauty and taste to a salad, soup, or grain dish.

Saffron, Almond, and Parsley Pesto: Place a few strands of saffron between wax paper and crush. In a mortar and pestle, grind ½ cup toasted almonds, 3 garlic cloves, and ½ cup parsley. Add the crushed saffron. Excellent on any French or Middle Eastern style bean, soup, or rice dish.

Smoked Crunchy Mushrooms: Remove the stems from one 8-ounce carton of baby bella mushrooms and chop into ½-inch pieces. Coat with 2 tbsp oil, 1 tsp soy sauce and 1 tsp liquid smoke, and 2 tsp ground black pepper. Bake at 400°F until crispy. Let cool and store in plastic container.

Smoked Soy Sauce: Smoke your own soy sauce or purchase online. A drop or a little drizzle goes a long way.

Store-bought Spice/Herb/Seed Blends: You can certainly make your own blends. I recommend purchasing quality blends from your local spice shop for the following: dukkah, berbere, and za'atar.

Toasted Chopped Nuts: Keep roasted, sliced or slivered almonds, whole or chopped pistachios, cashews, and honey-roasted pecans in your freezer. With these you can add a touch of crunch and nutrition to your dish.

Toasted Panko or Bread Crumbs: Heat 1 tbsp oil in a skillet. Add 1 cup of panko or white bread crumbs. Stir over medium heat until golden and crunchy. Salt, pepper, and herb to your taste.

6 oz Restaurant Squeeze Bottle Cuisine Sauces: To quickly finish a dish, I keep sriracha, harissa, Indian mint chutney, Indian tamarind dipping sauce, my favorite TexMex green sauce, and other sauces in these bottles to quickly and elegantly add a flavor boost to a dish.

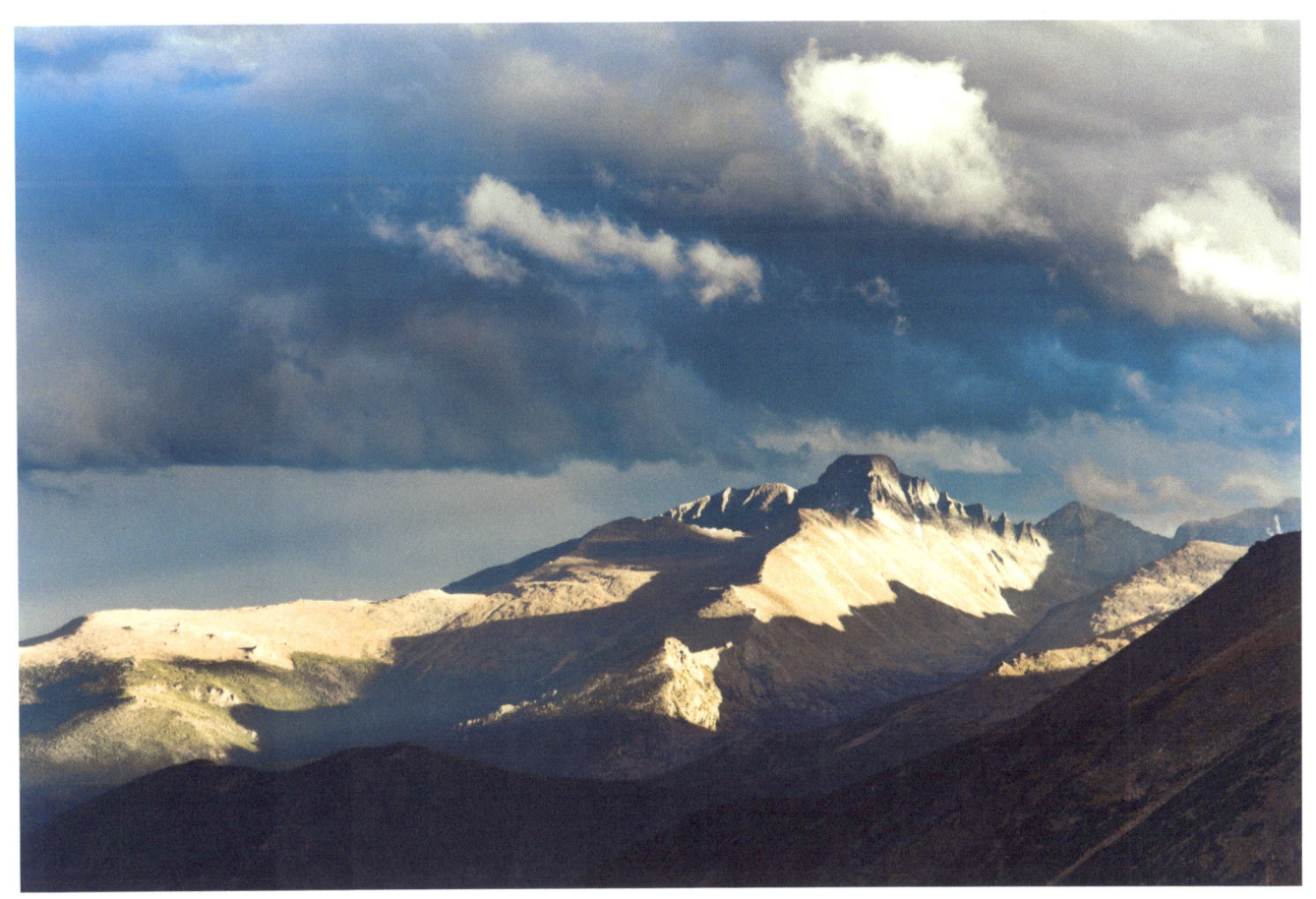

Beer Pairings by Justin Kruger

Beer and food – for the longest time I never thought of the two as a harmonious pairing. I would drink beer, and eat food. Rinse and repeat. As a chef, wine was always the obvious partner for food enjoyment – coursing, whites to start, reds to finish. Moving to Colorado and discovering a lush craft beer scene opened my eyes to so many possibilities. Beer is the perfect foil for food. The broad spectrum of flavors and aromas that beer provides allows for so many adventures for pairing beer with food.

In these pages is an amazing array of wonderful food and food opportunities for beer. The best part of exploring the many, many styles of beers is seeing how they work with food. Let's start with quick notes for pairing and eating: First, take in the aroma of the beer, then take your first bite of food. Follow with the beer, and hold the beer in your mouth for a brief second to allow the flavors to mix before swallowing. A proper pairing will bring a smile to your face. Prost!

Colorado Smoked Green Chili (p. 154): I wanted to start with a challenge. Big, bold flavors of smoke and the warming heat of green chiles. When matching beers for food, the first and most important rule is: Enjoy drinking the beer on its own. With that out of the way, there are two beer styles that I feel would be perfect with the chili. For a lighter pairing, Helles would be a wonderful counterpoint. Light in color, with malt sweetness to balance the spice, and a clean finish to highlight the smoke. The second beer is a bit more of a challenge – a smoked porter. Malty and roasty, with a firm smoke to really enhance the robust flavors of the chili. A standard porter would also pair nicely. The roast in the porter will enhance the earthiness of the chiles and temper their heat.

Fresh Fava Beans with Mint, Garlic, and Cumin (p. 34): For a chef, fava beans represent spring. I never believe spring has sprung until I am using favas in my food. They are wonderful, fresh beans with an amazing flavor. For this dish, saison screams, "Drink me." Saison, with its hints of pepper and citrus, will bring out the sweetness of the fava. The dry finish to the saison will refresh the palate for another bite. Try to avoid a dry hopped or heavy brettanomyces saison for this dish. The hop aroma of the dry hopped variant could possibly overpower the delicate flavors, and the funkiness of the brett variant should be enjoyed on its own.

Rustic Peach Crumble (p. 85): Summer in Colorado is a peach lover's paradise. We are blessed with an amazing supply of Western Colorado peaches. Bright sweetness, with a tannic balance from the skin. For a dessert like this, a proper dessert beer is needed – Belgian Tripel. An effervescent beer with hints of honey and citrus will elevate and highlight the peach. Firm bitterness to balance the sweetness, with perceived sweetness to cut the tannins.

Pasta with Pumpkin Cream Sauce (p. 119): Hard-skinned squash is a hallmark of fall. Pumpkin, butternut, and acorn – all these squashes exude sweetness and complex depth. I look for a proper brown ale for this dish. Heaps of malt sweetness and subtle bitterness to warm the soul. Easy to drink, and even easier to enjoy with this dish.

Let's finish with some general guidelines to know when pairing beer with food:

1. **IPAs, Hazy, Dry Hopped Beers:** These are best enjoyed on their own. More often than not, their bitterness will overpower the dish.
2. **Barrel Aged Beers:** For the price, use them as a nightcap. The bold flavors and high alcohol will drive everything on the palette.
3. **Sour Beer:** Some sours would pair great with certain foods, and the best part of beer pairing is the ability to experiment – but more often than not, the high levels of acid makes pairing difficult.

Wine Pairings by Ann Rawlinson, Sommelier, CMS

What's a nice, single, sommelier doing living in the "Napa Valley of Craft Beer"? Having one hell of a time, tasting and learning a lot about beer. A Cicerone in the making? Maybe. That being said, I still remember my wine pairing guidelines, like with like, or exactly the opposite – i.e. pairing a sweet dessert wine with blue cheese. Wine pairing also has to do with a balance of acid in the wine and the dish. I hope you find these pairings pleasing!

Kohlrabi Bean Barley Soup (p. 103): Born and raised in Wisconsin, I am very familiar with kohlrabi. Cooked kohlrabi is rather mellow, comparatively to raw. A Gruner Veltliner would go down a treat, as would a Fino Sherry. Don't be afraid of Sherry – it is very food-friendly!

Lentils with Celeriac Truffle Purée (p. 114): Splurge on the biggest, oakiest Napa Chardonnay you can find! The big Napa Chards have layers of flavors, hazelnut, citrus, melon, and a hint of nutmeg. Or a really nice bottle of bubbles (Brut or Extra Dry), truffles & Champagne = MAGIC!

Grilled Squash with Miso and Sesame Glaze (p. 58): California Sauvignon Blanc – with less grassy and more stone fruit flavors, it will pair nicely with the lean, green flavors of this dish. Or a really nice bottle of Rosé Sparkling wine, round enough to take the edge off.

Sardinian Saffron Fregola with Potatoes and Peas (p. 60): A big, burly Rosé. Yes, Rosé! They can be big and robust. Look for one with a deeper color. Many times, this signals a longer time that the wine spent on the skins, so more flavor and more tannins. A half-dry Chenin Blanc (Vouvray) would also pair really well with the saffron in this dish.

Three Herbs and Sumac Potatoes (p. 65): California Pinot Noir – a little more fruit, less earthy and mushroomy than other Pinot Noirs. Or try a light, bright Torrontés from Argentina. It will pair well with the lemon flavors in the Sumac.

Basil Pesto with your Choice of Pasta (p. 72): Cortese di Gavi, an Italian white wine. There's a saying in the wine biz: "What grows together, goes together." Perfect example, Pesto and Cortese. Or "lean in" with a New Zealand Sauvignon Blanc – herbaceous complements herbaceous.

Eggplant Parmesan (p. 78): An Italian or Californian Barbera. Barbera is a soft red wine from Italy – high in acid, low in tannins, it's sufficiently lush for this rich dish. Or go with a hearty Italian Rosé – this drink also has the "oomph."

Roasted Tomatoes and Mushrooms in Brandy Cream Sauce (p. 81): A brilliant, bright Oregon Pinot Noir will pair well with the sweet tomatoes and mushrooms. Or a rich, but not tannic, GSM (Grenache, Syrah, Mourvèdre) blend from the US or Australia.

Pasta with Pumpkin Cream Sauce (p. 119): I am going to suggest an Amontillado Sherry – rich and nutty, it will be lovely with the pumpkin cream. Please note that Sherry has more alcohol than regular wine. This helps cut the richness of this dish, and the flavors are complementary. Or pair with a US Viognier, which has a gorgeous, perfumed aroma and a big mouthfeel that pairs well with turmeric.

French Apple Pie (p. 120): Pair with Tokaji – a Hungarian dessert wine. Look for one that has four "Puttonyos" (or better) for this dish. Or Sauternes – a French dessert wine. Both wines go well with sweet fruit afters.

"I have found a dream of beauty
at which one might look
all one's life and sigh."

Isabella L. Bird

www.ingramcontent.com/pod-product-compliance
Lightning Source LLC
Chambersburg PA
CBHW041412160426
42811CB00107B/1787